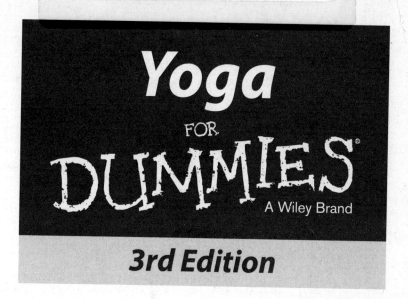

# Yoga
## FOR
# DUMMIES®
A Wiley Brand

## 3rd Edition

**by Larry Payne, PhD,
and Georg Feuerstein, PhD**

**Foreword by Felicia Tomasko, RN**
Editor in Chief,
*LA YOGA Ayurveda and Health Magazine*

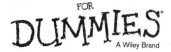

FOR
DUMMIES®
A Wiley Brand

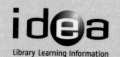

**Yoga For Dummies,® 3rd Edition**

Published by: **John Wiley & Sons, Inc.,** 111 River Street, Hoboken, NJ 07030-5774, www.wiley.com

Copyright © 2014 by John Wiley & Sons, Inc., Hoboken, New Jersey

Media and software compilation copyright © 2014 by John Wiley & Sons, Inc. All rights reserved.

Published simultaneously in Canada

For general information on our other products and services, please contact our Customer Care Department within the U.S. at 877-762-2974, outside the U.S. at 317-572-3993, or fax 317-572-4002. For technical support, please visit www.wiley.com/techsupport.

Wiley publishes in a variety of print and electronic formats and by print-on-demand. Some material included with standard print versions of this book may not be included in e-books or in print-on-demand. If this book refers to media such as a CD or DVD that is not included in the version you purchased, you may download this material at http://booksupport.wiley.com. For more information about Wiley products, visit www.wiley.com.

Library of Congress Control Number: 2013958401

ISBN 978-1-118-83956-0 (pbk); ISBN 978-1-118-83949-2 (ebk); ISBN 978-1-118-83954-6

Manufactured in the United States of America

10 9 8 7 6 5 4 3 2 1

# Contents at a Glance

# Table of Contents

# Foreword

*W*hen I first met Larry Payne, it was 1995. At the time, I was a 24-year-old Yoga student living in Boulder, Colorado, studying to be a Yoga teacher. I was also anticipating attending my first Yoga conference: Unity in Yoga, held in the stunning mountain town of Aspen.

I don't expect Larry remembered meeting me, but I remember him. I remember his confident delivery, his enthusiasm, his experience, and his three-ring binder filled with information on the business of Yoga. I remember him offering suggestions to a rapt group of students on how to grow their presence as a teacher and find new places to offer classes: churches, community centers, schools. The experience increased my love affair with Yoga; I became enamored with the possibilities of incorporating it more into my own life and sharing it with others. Larry was one of the teachers leading the movement to make Yoga more accessible and as widely practiced as it is today.

That year was before the first edition of *Yoga For Dummies* was published, before the first Yoga Journal conference took place, and before the founding of *LA YOGA Ayurveda and Health Magazine*, where I am now the editor-in-chief. It was also before interested students were able to do a Google search for Yoga centers or online videos, and before my small New England hometown sported any variety of Yoga classes.

Back when I was a high school student beginning my Yoga practice, scouring libraries and bookstores for resources, I would have loved nothing more than to have found a copy of *Yoga For Dummies*. Even 25 years into my personal practice and with 15 years of teaching, I frequently rifle through my own copy of this book. I might be searching for inspiration; suggestions on practice, teaching, or sequencing; a clear explanation of a point of practice; or other gems of grounded, practical information. With gratitude, I always find it in these pages.

Over the past two decades, since Larry and I met on that spring day on the snowy mountaintop in Aspen, not only has he written *Yoga For Dummies* (with late scholar Georg Feuerstein, PhD), but he also has founded and built the notable Yoga Therapy RX program at Loyola Marymount University, where I am honored to be among the faculty. Larry has been responsible for training thousands of students as they seek to become respected members of the growing professional community of Yoga therapists. As part of that same active Yoga community, I am honored to call Larry both a colleague and a friend.

The book you're currently holding reflects years of study and practice by the authors, all put together in an easy-to-understand format. It's a friendly guide that demystifies traditions and brand names, helping you make sense of how to prepare for your first practice or your five thousandth. Within these pages, you discover how to design your own practice (suggestions I love), as well as how to incorporate concentration, steadiness, mindfulness, and more in every part of your life. Pick up this book for your parents, your children, your favorite teacher, or yourself. Keep it nearby for when you need a reminder of something essential (even in your desk drawer or bookshelf at work). Fold over pages, write notes to yourself, travel with it.

When I began my own Yoga practice, I had no idea where it would take me, but on a daily basis, I feel grateful for what it has added to everything I do. Yoga has allowed me to find balance amid all the chapters of my life, including nursing school and the state boards, the everyday challenges of work and life in L.A., a cross-country move, time spent living overseas, health challenges, family dynamics, relationships, and more. In all the chapters of any life, Yoga offers tools for practice, helping us build resilience so that we may thrive. For this aim, *Yoga For Dummies* is a trusted companion, a steady support, a lifetime tool for practicing Yoga at any age and for any body. Use it well, and return to these pages often.

**Felicia Marie Tomasko, RN, E-RYT-500**
Editor in Chief, *LA YOGA Ayurveda and Health Magazine*
and *Find Bliss Magazine*
President, Bliss Network
Member, Board of Directors, National Ayurvedic Medical Association
and The Academic Consortium for Complementary and Alternative
Health Care

# Introduction

**M**ore than 20 million Americans practice Yoga of some kind, and many more millions of Yoga practitioners live in other parts of the world. Yoga isn't a fad. It has a history of approximately 5 millennia and has been around in the West for much more than a hundred years. Though ancient, it's especially relevant to today's hectic and stressful way of life.

By its very nature, Yoga leads you toward greater balance and relaxation. It's the ultimate mind-body practice. A Yoga practice brings a balanced mixture of alertness and relaxation with each pose. The physical movements coordinated with the breath bring bodily and mental relaxation, and the serene mind brings further relaxation to stressed and tight muscles. What results is a welcome dose of enhanced well-being. These benefits draw millions to the practice of this ancient tradition. And indeed, Yoga has never been more important. In our hectic 24/7 way of life, loaded with opportunities for constant stimulation and accumulation of stress, Yoga brings balance to all who take the time to welcome it into their lives.

Yoga has brought health and peace of mind to millions of people, and it can do the same for you. We invite you to explore Yoga in depth with *Yoga For Dummies,* 3rd Edition, as your guide. The yogic postures are an excellent starting point, but they're merely the outermost shell of a multilayered tradition. At its core, Yoga is a timeless answer for anyone seeking deeper meaning in life and that elusive treasure called abiding peacefulness.

## About This Book

Perhaps *Yoga For Dummies,* 3rd Edition, is the first book on Yoga you've ever held in your hands. In this case, we can definitely say that you're starting at the right place. More likely, however, you've leafed through quite a few other books, including some that are neither sound nor helpful. How, then, is this book different? We have a two-part answer for you.

First, the information you find in *Yoga For Dummies,* 3rd Edition, is based on our extensive study and practice of Yoga. Between us, we have more than 75 years of experience with Yoga. One author (Larry) directs a university-based Yoga therapy training program for Yoga teachers at Loyola Marymount

University; has a thriving practice as a Yoga therapist and Yoga teacher in Los Angeles, where he adapts Yoga to his clients' specific needs and health challenges (especially back problems); and has produced a popular series of Yoga DVDs. The other author (Georg) is internationally recognized as a leading expert on the Yoga tradition, has authored many seminal works on it, and has created a teacher training manual on Yoga philosophy that Yoga teachers in seven countries refer to. In this book, we merge our respective areas of expertise to create a reliable and user-friendly introductory book that can also serve you as a reference work on an ongoing basis.

Second, we're both dedicated to motivating you to practice Yoga, a system that we've seen work both minor and major miracles. We've committed our lives to making Yoga available to anyone who cares about the health and wholeness of the body and mind. In short, we can say, with all modesty, that you're in the best of hands.

This book guides you slowly, step by step, into the treasure house of Yoga. And what a treasure house it is! You find out how to strengthen your mind and enlist it to unlock your body's extraordinary potential. A sound body requires a sound mind, and we show you how to improve or regain the health and wholeness of both.

We know you're busy, so we've organized this book in the easy-access way the Dummies series is known for. You may choose to read the book from cover to cover, or you may read any section or chapter as it calls to you. Feel free to skip over the Technical Stuff, which we indicate with an icon, and the sidebars (although we think you'll find these interesting). But please, when you see a Warning icon, take note — we want your practice to be a safe one.

Whether you're interested in becoming more flexible, more fit, less stressed, or more peaceful and joyful, this book contains all the good counsel and practical exercises you need to get started.

Above all, we've endeavored to make this book relevant to busy people like you. And if, after reading this guide, you become more serious about studying and practicing Yoga, consider taking a Yoga class with a qualified instructor. This book is a great guide, but nothing compares to hands-on instruction and guidance.

## Foolish Assumptions

We know you're no dummy! But if you're a newbie to Yoga, we know you appreciate starting with the basics. No prior exposure to the many aspects of Yoga is necessary for you to benefit from this book. In fact, this book is the perfect first step in your exploration, and we invite you to continue to explore further when you have this under your belt. The Additional Yoga Resources section online at www.dummies.com/extras/yoga can help you with that, but you get more on that later in this introduction.

We also know that some of our readers may already have some experience with Yoga and want to understand the fundamentals more deeply. For you, we provide detail and a fair amount of depth across the Yoga spectrum, but always in a clear and direct manner. We assume that you're looking for sound information with a no-nonsense presentation. Let other books speak to you in an esoteric manner. For us, let's just talk Yoga!

# Icons Used in This Book

Throughout the book, you'll notice little pictures in the margins. These icons point you to information that you may not want to forget or, in some cases, you may decide to skip over.

Our tips point you toward helpful information that can make your yogic journey a little smoother.

When we point to information for you to remember, we think it's worthwhile for you to pause and make a mental note of the information; it can help you down the road in your understanding and practice.

Please take note of all warnings. Yoga is safe, but Yoga injuries can and do happen, and we don't want that to be your experience.

Consider this material "nice to know" information. We think it's interesting and can add to your experience. But feel free to skip it if you want to breeze through.

# Beyond the Book

In addition to the book content, you can find valuable free material online. We provide you with a Cheat Sheet that addresses questions that may be first and foremost in your mind: We separate Yoga facts from myths, help you find the right Yoga teacher for you, and offer tips for a successful Yoga practice. You can access this material at www.dummies.com/cheatsheet/yoga.

We've also included additional articles at `www.dummies.com/extras/yoga`. There you can read about avoiding common Yoga injuries, taking Yoga on the road with you, finding lucidity in sleep as well as wakefulness, and eating like a yogi. Plus, we've included a bonus chapter on Yoga therapy for the upper back and neck, two common areas of stress and strain, and we've detailed a Yoga therapy routine for the lower back. You can also make use of our list of additional resources when you've mastered the basics and want to learn more about Yoga.

But wait, there's more! We have 10 short videos that introduce you to great ideas for improving your Yoga practice, regardless of your age or physical abilities. Check out these tried-and-true poses and routines at `www.dummies.com/go/yoga`.

# *Where to Go from Here*

We've designed *Yoga For Dummies*, 3rd Edition, to be both an introduction and a beginner's reference work. You can read the chapters one after the other and practice along with us, or you can dip into the book here and there, reading up on the subjects that currently interest you, such as relaxation techniques or helpful props for your practice.

If you're a newcomer to Yoga, we recommend that you spend some time with the table of contents and leaf through the book to get a general sense of how we've structured and approached the material. You probably want to begin your reading with the first two chapters, which give you a picture of the Yoga landscape.

If you aren't new to Yoga and you want a refresher course, you can also use this book as a reliable guide in answering your questions. Perusing the table of contents is a good starting point for you as well. You may find yourself gravitating to later chapters that zero in on specific categories of postures, or postures and routines for specific age groups or needs, or ways to custom-design a personal practice. And of course, the index is always useful to locate specific information on any topic of interest.

Okay, then, are you ready to Yoga?

# Part I
# Getting Started with Yoga

getting started with yoga

# In this part . . .

- ✔ Familiarize yourself with the vast roadmap of Yoga
- ✔ Understand the basics, to make your practice of Yoga both enjoyable and safe
- ✔ Find a Yoga class and instructor that meet your individual needs
- ✔ Start putting the fundamentals to use: guidelines for safe practice, conscious breathing, relaxation techniques, and coordination of breath and movement

# Chapter 1

# Yoga 101: Building a Foundation

Although *Yoga* is now a household word, many people don't know exactly what it is. Far more than just physical exercise, Yoga can transform you, even if it's not your intention when you first step onto the mat. In this chapter, we clear up the confusion and explain what Yoga really is and how it relates to your health and happiness. We also help you see the richness of Yoga, with its many different branches and approaches. Yoga really does offer something for everyone.

Whatever your age, weight, flexibility, or beliefs may be, you can practice and benefit from some version of Yoga. Yoga may have originated in India, but it's for all of humanity.

## Understanding the True Character of Yoga

Whenever you hear that Yoga is *just* this or *just* that, your nonsense alert should kick into action. Yoga is too comprehensive to reduce to any one aspect — it's like a skyscraper with many floors and numerous rooms at each level. Yoga isn't *just* gymnastics, fitness training, a way to control your weight, stress reduction, meditation, or a spiritual path — it's *all* these tools and a great deal more.

The Yoga we enjoy today comes from a 5,000-year-old Indian tradition. Some of the exercises look like gymnastics and so, not surprisingly, have made their way into Western gymnastics. These exercises, or postures, help you become (and stay) fit and trim, control your weight, and reduce your stress level. Yoga also offers a whole range of meditation practices, including breathing techniques that exercise your lungs and calm your nervous system, or that charge your brain and the rest of your body with delicious energy.

You can also use Yoga as an efficient system of healthcare that has proven its usefulness in both restoring and maintaining health. Yoga continues to gain acceptance within the medical establishment; more physicians are recommending Yoga to their patients not only for stress reduction, but also as a safe and sane method of exercise and physical therapy (notably, for the back, neck, knees, and hips).

Still, Yoga is far more than a system of preventative or restorative healthcare. Yoga looks at health from a broad, holistic perspective that integrative medicine is only now rediscovering. This perspective appreciates the enormous influence of the mind — your psychological attitudes — on physical health.

## Finding unity

The word *Yoga* comes from the ancient Sanskrit language spoken by the traditional religious elite of India, the *Brahmins*. *Yoga* means "union" or "integration" and also "discipline." The system of Yoga, then, is a *unitive* or *integrating discipline*. Yoga seeks unity at various levels. First, it seeks to unite body and mind, which people all too often separate. Some people are chronically "out of the body." They can't feel their feet or the ground beneath them, as if they hover like ghosts just above their bodies. They're unable to cope with the ordinary pressures of daily life, so they collapse under stress. They don't understand their own emotions. Afraid of life, they're easily hurt emotionally.

Yoga also seeks to unite the rational mind and the emotions. People frequently bottle up their emotions and don't express their real feelings. Instead, they choose to rationalize away these feelings. Chronic avoidance can become a serious health hazard; if people aren't aware that they're suppressing feelings such as anger, the anger consumes them from the inside out.

Here's how Yoga can help you with your personal growth:

- ✔ It can put you in touch with your real feelings and balance your emotional life.

- ✔ It can help you understand and accept yourself so that you feel comfortable with who you are. You don't have to "fake it" or reduce your life to constant role playing.

- ✔ It helps you become more able to empathize and communicate with others.

Yoga is a powerful means of psychological integration. It makes you aware that you're part of a larger whole, not merely an island unto yourself. People can't thrive in isolation. Even the most independent individual is greatly indebted to others. When your mind and body are happily reunited, this union with others comes about naturally. The moral principles of Yoga are all-embracing, encouraging you to seek kinship with everyone and everything. We say more about this topic in Chapter 22.

## Finding yourself: Are you a yogi (or a yogini)?

Someone who's practicing the discipline of balancing mind and body through Yoga is traditionally called a *yogi* (if male) or a *yogini* (if female). In this book, we use both terms at random. Alternatively, we also use the English term *Yoga practitioner*. Becoming a *yogi* or *yogini* means you do more than practice Yoga postures. Yoginis embrace Yoga as a self-transforming spiritual discipline. A yogi who has really mastered Yoga is called an *adept*. If such an adept also teaches (and not all of them do), this person is traditionally called a *guru*. The Sanskrit word *guru* literally means "weighty one." According to traditional esoteric sources, the syllable *gu* signifies spiritual darkness, and *ru* signifies the act of removing. Thus, a guru is a teacher who leads the student from darkness to light.

Very few Westerners have achieved complete mastery of Yoga, mainly because Yoga is still a relatively young movement in the West. So please be careful about anyone who claims to be enlightened or to have been given the title of guru! However, at the level at which Yoga is generally taught outside its Indian homeland, many competent Yoga teachers or instructors can lend a helping hand to beginners. In this book, we hope to do just that for you.

## Considering Your Options: The Eight Main Branches of Yoga

When you take a bird's-eye view of the Yoga tradition, you see a dozen major strands of development, each with its own subdivisions. Picture Yoga as a giant tree with eight branches; each branch has its own unique character, but each is also part of the same tree. With so many different paths, you're sure to find one that's right for your personality, lifestyle, and goals. In this book, we focus on Hatha Yoga, the most popular branch of Yoga, but we avoid the common mistake of reducing it to mere physical fitness training. Thus, we also talk about meditation and the spiritual aspects of Yoga.

Here are the seven principal branches of Yoga, with an eighth branch we added at the end:

- **Bhakti *(bhuk-tee)* Yoga, the Yoga of devotion:** Bhakti Yoga practitioners believe that a supreme being (the Divine) transcends their lives, and they feel moved to connect or even completely merge with that supreme being through acts of devotion. Bhakti Yoga includes such practices as making flower offerings, singing hymns of praise, and thinking about the Divine.

- **Hatha *(haht-ha)* Yoga, the Yoga of physical discipline:** All branches of Yoga seek to achieve the same final goal, enlightenment (see Chapter 23), but Hatha Yoga approaches this goal through the body instead of through the mind or the emotions. Hatha Yoga practitioners believe that unless they properly purify and prepare their bodies, the higher stages of meditation and beyond are virtually impossible to achieve — such an attempt is like trying to climb Mt. Everest without the necessary gear. We focus on this particular branch of Yoga in this book.

  Hatha Yoga is much more than posture practice, which is so popular today. Like every form of authentic Yoga, it's a *spiritual* path.

- **Jnana *(gyah-nah)* Yoga, the Yoga of wisdom:** Jnana Yoga teaches the ideal of *nondualism* — that reality is singular and your perception of countless distinct phenomena is a basic misconception. What about the chair or sofa you're sitting on? Isn't that real? What about the light that strikes your retina? Isn't that real? Jnana Yoga masters answer these questions by saying that all these things are real at your present level of consciousness, but they aren't ultimately real as separate or distinct things. Upon enlightenment, everything melts into one, and you become one with the immortal spirit.

- **Karma *(kahr-mah)* Yoga, the Yoga of self-transcending action:** Karma Yoga's most important principle is to act unselfishly, without attachment, and with integrity. Karma Yoga practitioners believe that all actions, whether bodily, vocal, or mental, have far-reaching consequences for which they must assume full responsibility.

- **Mantra *(mahn-trah)* Yoga, the Yoga of potent sound:** Mantra Yoga makes use of sound to harmonize the body and focus the mind. It works with *mantras*, which can be a syllable, word, or phrase. Traditionally, practitioners receive a mantra from their teacher in the context of a formal initiation. They're asked to repeat it as often as possible and to keep it secret. Many Western teachers feel that initiation isn't necessary and that any sound works. You can even pick a word from the dictionary, such as *love, peace,* or *happiness.* From a traditional perspective, such words aren't really mantras, but they can be helpful nonetheless.

# The Eight Limbs of Yoga

In traditional Raja Yoga, students move toward enlightenment, or liberation, through an eight-limb approach:

✔ *Yama (yah-mah):* Moral discipline, consisting of the practices of nonharming, truthfulness, nonstealing, chastity, and greedlessness. (For an explanation of these five virtues, head to Chapter 22.)

✔ *Niyama (nee-yah-mah):* Self-restraint, consisting of the five practices of purity, contentment, austerity, self-study, and devotion to a higher principle.

✔ *Asana (ah-sah-nah):* Posture, which serves two basic purposes: meditation and health.

✔ *Pranayama (prah-nah-yah-mah):* Breath control, which raises and balances your mental energy, thus boosting your health and mental concentration.

✔ *Pratyahara (prah-tyah-hah-rah):* Sensory inhibition, which internalizes your consciousness to prepare your mind for the various stages of meditation.

✔ *Dharana (dhah-rah-nah):* Concentration, or extended mental focusing, which is fundamental to yogic meditation.

✔ *Dhyana (dhee-yah-nah):* Meditation, the principal practice of higher Yoga. (Chapter 23 explains this practice and the next.)

✔ *Samadhi (sah-mah-dhee):* Ecstasy, or the experience in which you become inwardly one with the object of your contemplation. This state is surpassed by actual enlightenment, or spiritual liberation.

✔ **Raja *(rah-jah)* Yoga, the Royal Yoga:** Raja Yoga means literally "Royal Yoga" and is also known as classical Yoga. When you mingle with Yoga students long enough, you can expect to hear them refer to the eight-fold path laid down in the Yoga-Sutra of Patanjali, the standard work of Raja Yoga. Another name for this yogic tradition is Ashtanga Yoga (pronounced *ahsh-tahng-gah*), the "eight-limbed Yoga" — from *ashta* (eight) and *anga* (limb). (Don't confuse this tradition with the Yoga style known as Ashtanga Yoga, which we discuss in "Taking a Closer Look at Hatha Yoga," later in this chapter.)

✔ **Tantra *(tahn-trah)* Yoga (including Laya Yoga and Kundalini Yoga), the Yoga of continuity:** Tantra Yoga is the most complex and most widely misunderstood branch of Yoga. In the West and India, Tantra Yoga is often confused with "spiritualized" sex; although some (so-called left-hand) schools of Tantra Yoga use sexual rituals, they aren't a regular practice in the majority of (so-called right-hand) schools. Tantra Yoga is actually a strict spiritual discipline involving fairly complex rituals and detailed visualizations of deities. These deities are either visions of the divine or the equivalent of Christianity's angels and are invoked to aid the yogic process of contemplation.

## Good karma, bad karma, no karma

The Sanskrit term *karma* literally means "action." It stands for activity in general, but also for the "invisible action" of destiny. According to Yoga, every action of body, speech, and mind produces visible and also hidden consequences. Sometimes the hidden consequences — destiny — are far more significant than the obvious repercussions. Don't

think of karma as blind destiny. You're always free to make choices. The purpose of Karma Yoga is to regulate how you act in the world so that you cease to be bound by karma. The practitioners of all types of Yoga seek to not only prevent bad karma, but also go beyond good karma, to no karma at all.

Another common name for Tantra Yoga is Kundalini Yoga (pronounced *koon-dah-lee-nee*). The latter name, which means "she who is coiled," hints at the secret "serpent power" that Tantra Yoga seeks to activate: the latent spiritual energy stored in the human body. If you're curious about this aspect of Yoga, you may want to read the autobiographical account by Gopi Krishna or my (Georg's) *Tantra: The Path of Ecstasy* (Shambhala). ***Note:*** Kundalini Yoga is also the name of a Hatha Yoga style; we discuss it in "Taking a Closer Look at Hatha Yoga," later in the chapter.

✔ ***Guru (goo-roo) Yoga,* the Yoga of dedication to a Yoga master.** This branch is one we added to the great Yoga tree. In Guru Yoga, your teacher is the main focus of spiritual practice. Such a teacher is expected to be enlightened, or at least close to being enlightened (see Chapter 23 for more about enlightenment). In Guru Yoga, you honor and meditate on your guru until you merge with him. Because the guru is thought to already be one with the ultimate reality, this merger duplicates his spiritual realization in you.

But please don't merge with your guru too readily! Guru Yoga is relatively rare in the West, so approach it with great caution to avoid possible exploitation.

# *Taking a Closer Look at Hatha Yoga*

In its voyage to modernity, Yoga has undergone many transformations. One of them was Hatha Yoga, which emerged around 1100 AD. (We focus on this branch of Yoga throughout this book.) The most significant adaptations, however, occurred during the past several decades, particularly to serve the needs or wants of Western students. Of the many styles of Hatha Yoga available today, the following are the best known:

✔ **Iyengar Yoga** is the most widely recognized approach to Hatha Yoga. Characteristics of this style include precision performance and the aid of numerous props. B.K.S. Iyengar, the brother in-law of the famous T.S. Krishnamacharya (1888–1989) and uncle of T.K.V. Desikachar, developed this approach. Iyengar has trained thousands of teachers, including many in the United States. His Ramamani Iyengar Memorial Yoga Institute, founded in 1974 and dedicated to his late wife, Ramamani, is located in Pune, India.

✔ **Viniyoga** (pronounced *vee-nee yoh-gah*) focuses on the breath and emphasizes practicing Yoga according to your individual needs and capacities. Shri Krishnamacharya first developed this approach, and his son T.K.V. Desikachar continued it. In the United States, Viniyoga is now associated with Gary Kraftsow and the American Viniyoga Institute (AVI); Desikachar has expanded his approach in conjunction with his son Kausthub under the new umbrella of The Krishnamacharya Healing and Yoga Foundation (KHYF) and Sannidhi of Krishnamacharya Yoga (SKY), headquartered in Chennai (formerly Madras), India. As the teacher of well-known Yoga masters B.K.S. Iyengar, K. Pattabhi Jois, and Indra Devi, Professor T.S. Krishnamacharya can be said to have launched a veritable Hatha Yoga renaissance in modern times that's still sweeping the world.

✔ **Ashtanga Yoga** is by far the most athletic of the three versions of Hatha Yoga. This version combines postures with breathing. Ashtanga Yoga differs from Patanjali's eightfold path (also called Ashtanga Yoga), although it's theoretically grounded in it. (We discuss the Ashtanga Yoga tradition in "Considering Your Options: The Eight Main Branches of Yoga," earlier in this chapter.) This approach originated with Shri Krishnamacharya but grew in popularity thanks to K. Pattabhi Jois. Jois was born in 1915 but had such a modern outlook that he draw eager Western students to his Ashtanga Yoga Institute in Mysore, India, until his death in 2009. He was a principal disciple of T.S. Krishnamacharya, who apparently instructed him to teach the sequences known as Ashtanga Yoga or Power Yoga.

*Power Yoga* is a generic term for any style that closely follows Ashtanga Yoga but doesn't have a set series of postures. It emphasizes flexibility and strength and was mainly responsible for introducing Yoga postures into gyms. Beryl Bender Birch, Bryan Kest, Baron Baptiste, and Sherri Baptiste Freeman are all closely associated with Power Yoga. In a similar manner, *Vinyasa Yoga* and *Flow Yoga,* developed by Ganga White and Tracey Rich, are variations of Ashtanga Yoga.

✔ **Kripalu Yoga** is a three-stage Yoga approach tailored to the needs of Western students. The first stage emphasizes postural alignment and coordination of breath and movement; you hold the postures for a short time only. The second stage adds meditation and prolongs the postures. In the final stage, practicing the postures becomes a spontaneous meditation in motion. Swami Kripalvananda (1913–1981) created Kripalu Yoga, and his disciple Yogi Amrit Desai further developed it.

# The sacred syllable *om*

The best-known traditional mantra, used by Hindus and Buddhists alike, is the sacred syllable *om* (pronounced *ommm*, with a long *o* sound). It's the symbol of the absolute reality — the Self or spirit. It consists of the letters *a, u,* and *m,* joined by the nasal humming of the letter *m.* The *a* corresponds to the waking state, *u* to the dream state, and *m* to the state of deep sleep; the nasal humming sound represents the ultimate reality. We introduce several other traditional mantras in Chapter 23 in our coverage of meditation.

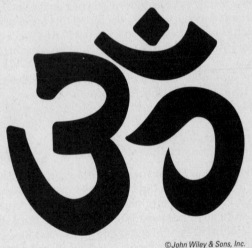

©John Wiley & Sons, Inc.

✔ **Integral Yoga** aims to integrate the various aspects of the body-mind using a combination of postures, breathing techniques, deep relaxation, and meditation. Swami Satchidananda (1914–2002), a student of the famous Swami Sivananda of Rishikesh, India, introduced this type of Yoga at the Woodstock festival in 1969, where he taught the baby boomers to chant *om.* Over the years, Integral Yoga has attracted thousands of students.

✔ **Sivananda Yoga** includes a series of 12 postures, the Sun Salutation sequence, breathing exercises, relaxation, and *mantra* chanting. It's the creation of the late Swami Vishnudevananda (1927–1993), also a disciple of Swami Sivananda of Rishikesh, India, who established his Sivananda Yoga Vedanta Center in Montreal in 1959. He trained more than 6,000 teachers, and you can find numerous Sivananda centers around the world.

✔ **Ananda Yoga** is a gentle style that prepares students for meditation. Its distinguishing features are the silent affirmations associated with holding the postures. Ananda Yoga is anchored in the teachings of Paramahansa Yogananda (1893–1952) and Swami Kriyananda (Donald Walters; 1926–2013), one of his disciples. This Yoga style includes Yogananda's unique energization exercises, first developed in 1917, which involve consciously directing the body's energy (life force) to different organs and limbs. You can find more information about the Ananda Institute of Alternative Living in Nevada City, California, in Chapter 24.

✔ **Kundalini Yoga** isn't only an independent approach of Yoga; it's also the name of a style of Hatha Yoga. Its purpose is to awaken the serpent power *(kundalini)* by means of postures, breath control, chanting, and meditation. Sikh master Yogi Bhajan (1929–2004), who came to the United States in 1969, developed the approach; he is the founder and spiritual head of the Healthy, Happy, Holy Organization (3HO), which has headquarters in Los Angeles and numerous branches around the world. (We cover the Kundalini Yoga approach in the earlier section "Considering Your Options: The Eight Main Branches of Yoga.")

✔ **Prime of Life Yoga** is my own (Larry's) creation. This style follows the principle of modifying postures to match the needs and abilities of the student. It offers a safe, user-friendly approach targeted to men and women ages 45 to 75, which represents the largest segment of the U.S. population. Hallmarks of this approach are its focus on the breath, function over form, a mix of dynamic and static movement, and Forgiving Limbs. Prime of Life Yoga has roots in the contemporary teachings of the late Sri T. Krishnamacharya and his son T.K.V. Desikachar. Sri T. Krishnamacharya altered his approach to teaching after his experience working with his first Western male student, Dr. Albert Franklin, who was the U.S. ambassador to India at that time. Not surprisingly, we cover aspects of Prime of Life Yoga in more detail throughout this book: We talk about Forgiving Limbs in Chapter 3 and explore the basics of the breath in Chapter 5. The principle of function over form shows up throughout the book in the instructions for the postures.

✔ **Somatic Yoga** is an integrated approach to the harmonious development of body and mind, based on both traditional yogic principles and modern psychophysiological research. It's the creation of Eleanor Criswell, EdD, emeritus professor of psychology at Sonoma State University in California, founding director of the Humanistic Psychology Institute (now Saybrook University, San Francisco), and emeritus professor of The International Association of Yoga therapists; she has taught Yoga since the early 1960s. This gentle approach emphasizes visualization, very slow movement into and out of postures, conscious breathing, mindfulness, and frequent relaxation between postures.

✔ **Moksha Yoga** champions a green philosophy. It uses traditional postures in a heated room and includes relaxation periods. This approach is based on the style of Bikram Yoga (listed next) and is popular in Canada.

✔ **Bikram Yoga** has a set routine of 26 postures. This very vigorous style requires a certain fitness level for participation, especially because it calls for a high room temperature. Founder Bikram Choudhury, who achieved fame as the teacher of Hollywood stars, teaches at the Yoga College of India in Bombay and other locations around the world, including San Francisco and Tokyo.

You also may hear or see mention of other Yoga styles, including Tri Yoga (developed by Kali Ray), White Lotus Yoga (developed by Ganga White and Tracey Rich), Jivamukti (developed by Sharon Gannon and David Life), Ishta Yoga (an acronym for the Integrated Science of Hatha, Tantra, and Ayurveda, developed by Mani Finger), Forrest Yoga (a mixture of Hatha Yoga and Native American ideas created by Ana Forrest), and Yin Yoga (developed by Paul Grilley).

*Hot Yoga* isn't really a style itself; it just means that the practice occurs in a high-temperature room (90°F to 100°F). It usually refers to either Ashtanga Yoga or Bikram Yoga.

# Finding Your Niche: Four Basic Approaches to Yoga

Since Yoga came to the West from its Indian homeland in the late 19th century, it has undergone various adaptations. Broadly, you can look at yoga in four overlapping approaches.

- ✔ As a method for physical fitness and health maintenance
- ✔ As a body-oriented therapy
- ✔ As a comprehensive lifestyle
- ✔ As a spiritual discipline

The first two approaches are often categorized as Postural Yoga; it contrasts with Traditional Yoga, which generally encompasses the last two approaches. As its name suggests, Postural Yoga focuses (sometimes exclusively) on Yoga postures. Traditional Yoga seeks to adhere to the traditional teachings taught anciently in India. We take a look at the four basic approaches in the upcoming sections.

## Yoga as fitness training

The first approach, Yoga as fitness training, is the most popular way Westerners practice Yoga. It's also the most radical revamping of Traditional Yoga. More precisely, it's a modification of traditional Hatha Yoga. Yoga as fitness training is concerned primarily with the physical body's flexibility, resilience, and strength.

Fitness is how most newcomers to Yoga encounter this great tradition. Fitness training is certainly a useful gateway into Yoga, but later, some people discover that Hatha Yoga is a profound *spiritual* tradition. From the earliest times, Yoga masters have emphasized the need for a healthy body — but they've also always pointed beyond the body to the mind and other vital aspects of the being.

If what motivates you is the prospect of having tighter buns or improving your golf game, you can certainly find that through Yoga. As you progress with a dedicated practice, your body will become stronger and more agile, and your buns will tighten, too. As a "meditation in motion," though, Yoga also can impact your performance on the green. The focus and coordination you develop on your Yoga mat will spill over to your swing — and to the rest of your life.

## Yoga as therapy

The second approach, Yoga as therapy, applies yogic techniques to restore health or full physical and mental function. While the idea behind as a therapy is quite old, it's growing into a whole new professional discipline. Different from even a highly experienced Yoga teacher, Yoga therapists have specialized training to apply the tools of Yoga to promote and support healing. Commonly, Yoga is intended for people who don't suffer from disabilities or ailments that require remedial action and special attention. Yoga therapy, on the other hand, addresses these special needs and enables people who cannot participate in a typical group setting to enjoy Yoga's many fruits. Chapter 24 delves deeper into this facet of Yoga.

## Yoga as a lifestyle

Yoga as a lifestyle enters the proper domain of Traditional Yoga. Although practicing Yoga only once or twice a week for an hour or so and focusing on its fitness training aspect is beneficial, you unlock the real potency of Yoga when you adopt it as a lifestyle — *living* Yoga and practicing it every day through physical exercises or meditation. Above all, when you adopt Yoga as a lifestyle, you apply the wisdom of Yoga to your everyday life and live with awareness. Yoga has much sage advice about everyday living, including diet and sleep habits, how you relate to others, and where you focus your attention and energy. It offers a total system of conscious and skillful living.

In modern times, a Yoga lifestyle includes caring for the ailing environment, an idea especially captured in Green Yoga. (Check out the sidebar "Healing the planet through Green Yoga" in this chapter for more information.) Lifestyle Yoga, which emphasizes being kind to others and the planet, is a fundamental concept in Yoga. It's where you begin. Just make a few simple adjustments in your daily schedule and keep your goals vividly in front of you. Whenever you're ready, make further positive changes one step at a time. See Chapter 22 for more on working Yoga into your whole day.

## *Yoga as a spiritual discipline*

Lifestyle Yoga (see the preceding section) is concerned with healthy, wholesome, functional, and benevolent living. Yoga as a spiritual discipline, the fourth approach, is concerned with all that *plus* the traditional ideal of *enlightenment* — that is, discovering your spiritual nature. This approach is often equated with Traditional Yoga. (We discuss the journey to enlightenment in Chapter 22.)

Different people understand the word *spiritual* differently, so we need to explain how we use it here. *Spiritual* relates to *spirit*, your ultimate nature. In Yoga, it's called the *atman* (pronounced *aht-mahn*) or *purusha (poo-roo-shah)*.

According to nondualistic (based in one reality) Yoga philosophy, the *spirit* is one and the same in all beings and things. It's formless, immortal, superconscious, and unimaginably blissful. It's transcendental because it exists beyond the limited body and mind. You discover the spirit fully in the moment of your enlightenment.

---

### Feeling enlightened

To get a sense of the nature of enlightenment, sit in a warm room, as still as possible, with your hands in your lap. Now sense your skin all over; it's your body's boundary separating you from the air surrounding you. As you become more aware of your body's sensations, pay special attention to the connection between your skin and the air. After a while, you realize that no sharp boundary really exists between your skin and the outside air. In your imagination, you can extend yourself further and further beyond your skin into the surrounding space. Where do you end, and where does the space begin? This experience can give you a sense of the all-comprising expansiveness of enlightenment, which knows no boundaries.

---

## What most approaches to Yoga have in common

Most traditional or tradition-oriented approaches to Yoga share two fundamental practices, the cultivation of awareness and relaxation.

- ✔ *Awareness* is the peculiarly human ability to pay close attention to something, to be consciously present, and to be mindful. Yoga is attention training. To see what we mean, try this exercise: Pay attention to your right hand for the next 60 seconds. Feel your right hand, and do nothing else. Chances are, your mind drifts off after only a few seconds. Yoga asks you to rein in your attention whenever it strays.

- ✔ *Relaxation* is the conscious release of unnecessary tension in the body.

Both awareness and relaxation go hand in hand in Yoga. Without bringing awareness and relaxation to Yoga, the movements are merely exercises — not *Yoga*.

*Conscious breathing* often joins awareness and relaxation as a third foundational practice. Normally, breathing happens automatically. In Yoga, you bring awareness to this act, which then makes it a powerful tool for training your body and your mind. We say much more about these aspects of Yoga in Chapter 5.

# Pointing the Way to Happiness: Health, Healing, and Yoga

The source of your health and happiness lies within you. Outside agents such as physicians, therapists, or remedies can help you through major crises, but you yourself are primarily responsible for your own health and happiness.

What is health? Most people answer this question by saying that health is the opposite of illness, but *health* is more than the absence of disease — it's a positive state of being. Health is wholeness. To be healthy means not only to possess a well-functioning body and a sane mind, but also to vibrate with life, to be vitally connected with your social and physical environment. To be healthy also means to be happy.

## No such thing as a free lunch

You get out of Yoga what you put into it. You're probably familiar with the adage of our data-crunching age: "Garbage in, garbage out." It captures a simple truth: The quality of a cause determines the quality of the effect — what you get out of any endeavor is only as good as what you put in. In other words . . .

✔ Don't expect health from junk food.

✔ Don't expect happiness from miserable attitudes.

✔ Don't expect good results from shoddy Yoga practice.

✔ Don't expect something from nothing.

Yoga is a powerful tool, but you must learn to use it properly. You can buy the latest-generation computer with a dizzying array of functions, but if you only know how to use it as a typewriter, that's all it is.

Life is constant movement, and health is, too. In today's world, your body must handle an onslaught of toxins that's unique to our times. During the course of your life, you can expect inevitable fluctuations in your state of health; even cutting your finger with a knife temporarily upsets the balance. Your body reacts to the cut by mobilizing all the necessary biochemical forces to heal itself. Regular Yoga practice can create optimal conditions for self-healing. You achieve a better baseline of health, with an improved immune system that enables you to stay healthy longer and heal faster.

Yoga is about healing, not curing. Like a really good physician, Yoga takes deeper causes into account; it doesn't just slap a bandage on surface symptoms. Often these causes are rooted in the mind — in the way you live and how you think. For this reason, Yoga masters recommend self-understanding. Instead of waiting until something goes wrong and then relying on a pill or a physician to fix the problem, Yoga encourages you to take the initiative in preventing illness and restoring or maintaining your health. We're not talking about self-doctoring (which can be dangerous); instead, you need to take responsibility for your health. A good physician knows that a patient's active participation in the process greatly facilitates healing.

Yoga points the way to happiness, health, and life-embracing meaning by suggesting that the best possible meaning you can find for yourself springs from the well of joy deep within you. That joy or bliss is the very nature of the spirit, or the transcendental Self (refer to "Yoga as a spiritual discipline," earlier in this chapter). Joy is like a 3D lens that captures life's bright colors and motivates you to embrace life in all its countless forms.

# Balancing Your Life with Yoga

The Hindu tradition explains Yoga as the discipline of balance, another way of expressing the ideal of unity through Yoga. Everything in you must harmonize to function optimally. A disharmonious mind is disturbing in itself, but sooner or later, it also causes physical problems. An imbalanced body can easily warp your emotions and thought processes. If you have strained relationships with others, you cause distress not only for them, but also for yourself. And when your relationship with your physical environment is disharmonious, well, you trigger serious repercussions for everyone.

A beautiful and simple Yoga exercise called the tree (see Chapter 8) improves your sense of balance and promotes your inner stillness. Even when conditions force a tree to grow askew, it always balances itself out by growing a branch in the opposite direction. In this posture, you stand still like a tree, perfectly balanced.

Yoga helps you apply this principle to your life. Whenever life's demands and challenges force you to bend to one side, your inner strength and peace of mind serve as counterweights. Rising above all adversity, you can never be uprooted.

---

## Healing the planet through Green Yoga

Climate change and other aspects of environmental degradation are on everyone's mind. Contemporary Yoga philosophy encourages applying Yoga's ethical standards to the health of the ailing planet. Georg and Brenda Feuerstein explain this Green Yoga approach in their book *Green Yoga* (Traditional Yoga Studies).

Green Yoga is Yoga that incorporates environmental mindfulness and activism in its spiritual orientation. It centers on a deep reverence for all life and a lifestyle of voluntary simplicity; it believes the time has come to make Yoga count in more than personal terms.

Carpooling or biking to your next class and using an environmentally friendly Yoga mat are just a couple ways to get started.

# Locating Your Starting Place in the World of Yoga

Now that you know the lay of the land, consider what motivates you to practice Yoga, as well as your lifestyle, physical style, and any limitations. Then find the style of Yoga and practice environment that's a good fit for you.

- ✔ Are you primarily looking for a method of stress management?
- ✔ Do you need to get your body moving after spending long hours in front of your computer?
- ✔ Do you seek quiet time and decompression after running after the kids all day?
- ✔ Are you drawn to a mental image of yourself with six-pack abs and tight buns?
- ✔ Do you aspire to reach transcendence?
- ✔ Are you a spiritual person in search of an outlet?
- ✔ Are you a secular person who yearns for moments of focus and balance?
- ✔ Do you have health concerns, such as lower back problems, that might limit your movement?
- ✔ Are you an athletic person looking for variety?
- ✔ Have you been a couch potato until now?

If your goals are entirely spiritual, choose a branch of Yoga that can best help you achieve those goals. You may resonate with Bhakti Yoga, Jnana Yoga, Raja Yoga, Karma Yoga, or Tantra Yoga. If your main interest is in improving your health or overall physical well-being, or if you primarily want to become fit and flexible, select a style of Hatha Yoga that fits you best. To help you wind down, go with one of the more restorative styles. To get the juices flowing and blood pumping, try one of the flow styles. And Viniyoga and Prime of Life styles of Yoga are especially well suited for people with physical concerns such as achy backs and shoulders.

All forms of Yoga, when done with intention, can help you relax and give you a feeling of oneness. That oneness is Yoga.

# Chapter 2

# Ready, Set, Yoga!

This chapter gives you everything you need to prepare for your Yoga practice, whether you opt to take part in a class or practice solo. We discuss rounding up the gear you want to have, finding enough time to practice, cultivating an attitude that helps you get the most out of your practice, and more.

Make sure you're physically ready before you begin this new venture with Yoga — or any fitness activity, for that matter. If you have an existing health challenge, consult your doctor before embarking on your new activity. Keep in mind that one of the bounties of Yoga is that, even if your medical history includes hypertension, heart problems, arthritis, or chronic back pain, you can benefit from it. You just need to approach it with respect for your body's needs and limits, as well as its possibilities. Chapter 26 gives pointers on how to practice safely.

If you have any serious physical limitations or concerns, you may want to work closely with a competent Yoga therapist to create just the right routines and to monitor your progress. You can find out more about Yoga therapy and Yoga therapists in Chapter 24.

## Make a promise to yourself

Most people are aware of how fast time flies in the 24 hours they're given each day. If you've picked up this book and are reading these words, chances are, you want to practice Yoga. To have the time to practice Yoga, decide to *make* the time. Do you have an idle 15 minutes somewhere in your busy day? If so, why not roll out the mat? Can you find a place either before or after the things you must do, to fit in something you will grow to love? If so, you can fit in a class here and there. If improving your health and well-being is important, and you've chosen Yoga as the way to do it, make a commitment to yourself as you would to another person, and follow through.

If you think practicing Hatha Yoga is beyond you because it requires too much flexibility or is otherwise too physically demanding, know that you can be as stiff as a board and still benefit from Yoga. Surprising? The yogic postures help you become more flexible, whatever your starting point. Don't gauge yourself by the photos you see in some Yoga books; they usually show advanced practitioners at their best. This book focuses on the needs of beginners. After you take the first few steps, you may be quite surprised at where you find yourself.

# Finding Suitable Yoga Instruction

Okay, you've decided to try Yoga. What's the next step? Safest is to set your sights on a suitable Yoga class or teacher instead of plowing forward as a strict do-it-yourselfer. Although you can explore some basic practices by reading about them (this book makes sure of that!), a full-fledged, safe Yoga routine really requires proper instruction from a qualified teacher. The following sections help you determine what kind of class to seek out.

Most people go for group instruction, but if you can afford private lessons, even a few sessions can be extremely beneficial. Importantly, if you have a serious health challenge, you need to work privately with a Yoga therapist.

## Checking out classes and teachers

These days, it seems you can find a Yoga class on every corner in large cities, so urbanites have lots of choices. But even country folk should be able to find an option that works. Here are some suggestions for finding the Yoga class that's right for you, wherever you live:

- Put out the word that you're looking. You may get lots of referrals and suggestions.

- Search online for studios and classes in your area. If you find a site that rates the offerings, check out the comments and see what others say.

- ✔ Stop in at your local YMCA/YWCA or adult education center to check class offerings.

- ✔ Look into the possibilities at your local health club. However, before you join a Yoga session there, make sure the teacher is really qualified. How much training has he had? Has she been certified by a recognized or registered Yoga teacher training school or instructor?

- ✔ Explore online Yoga sites that offer taped or streamed Yoga classes. Many sites offer classes in a range of styles for a variety of abilities and preferences.

We think that visiting a few places and teachers is important before you commit to a course or a series of classes. When you visit a Yoga center or classroom, pay attention to your intuitive feelings about the place. Consider how the staff treats you and how you respond to the people attending class. Stroll around the facility and feel its overall energy. First impressions are often (although not always) accurate. Some teachers even let you quietly look in on a class, although others find this practice too distracting for their students.

Bring a written checklist to your class visit. Don't feel embarrassed about being thorough. If you don't want to be so obvious, memorize the points you want to check out. Here are some ideas for your list:

- ✔ How do I feel about the building or classroom atmosphere?

- ✔ What's my gut response to the teacher? Does he create a safe environment that inspires trust?

- ✔ Do I prefer a male or female teacher?

- ✔ Does the teacher or school have a good reputation?

- ✔ How large are the classes? Will I be able to receive individual attention from the teacher as I practice in the class?

When checking out a Yoga center, don't hesitate to ask questions of the instructor or other staff members about any concerns you have. In particular, find out what style of Hatha Yoga the center offers. Some styles — notably Ashtanga, or Power Yoga — demand athletic fitness. Others embody a more relaxed and adaptable approach. In this book, we favor the latter. However, we can readily appreciate that some vigorous people may feel attracted to and benefit from yogic routines that are the equivalent of a workout and that call for strength, endurance, high flexibility, and a drench of perspiration.

If you're not familiar with the style of a particular school, don't hesitate to ask for an explanation (check out our explanation of styles in Chapter 1). Yoga practitioners are usually pretty friendly folk, eager to answer your questions and put your mind at ease. If they aren't, make a mental note. Everyone has an occasional off day, including Yoga teachers, but if you don't feel welcome and comfortable on your first visit, you probably won't receive any better treatment later.

## What makes a good teacher?

A good Yoga teacher is an example of what Yoga is all about: a balanced person who's not only skillful in the postures, but also courteous of and thoughtful toward others, as well as adaptive and attentive to everyone's individual needs in class. Check out the teacher's credentials to be sure she has been properly trained or is certified in one of the established traditions.

We caution you to steer clear of teachers who have taken only a few workshops on Yoga or received their diplomas after a 3-day course. They may be excellent aerobics instructors who know nothing about Yoga. Also avoid the drill sergeant type or anyone who makes you feel intimidated about your level of skill in performing the postures. By the way, under no circumstances must you allow your instructor to push or coerce you into a posture that doesn't feel right or that causes you pain.

## *Making sure the course fits your experience level*

Many Yoga studios and community centers that teach Yoga offer introductory courses (4 to 6 weeks), so you don't have to jump into the deep end. If you're a beginner, look for a beginner's course. You're likely to feel more comfortable in a group that's starting at the same skill level instead of being surrounded by advanced practitioners who can perform difficult postures easily and elegantly. Whatever the skill level of a class, don't feel self-conscious. None of the advanced students will stare at you to see whether the new kid in class is any good. You may get a few encouraging smiles, though.

Beginner's classes are sometimes advertised as *Easy Does It Yoga* or *Gentle Yoga*.

As a beginner, stay away from overly large classes (more than 20 students) or mixed-level classes that lump together Yoga freshmen with postgraduates. While some highly skilled and experienced teachers can manage such classes well, chances are, the teacher can't give you the attention you need to ensure your safety. The dilemma is that many of the more experienced teachers are quite popular, and their classes tend to be large. If you find yourself as a newbie in a large class, let the teacher know you're a beginner, and bring up any physical limitations you may have. Then stake out a spot where the instructor can observe you throughout the class, or at least from time to time.

After a few classes and with the benefit of an instructor's step-by-step guidance, you can certainly continue practicing and exploring Yoga on your own (see the section "Going for It on Your Own," later in this chapter). Indeed, practicing on your own in between classes is a great way to solidify Yoga as an integral part of your life. However, if your solo practice is in lieu of class attendance, consider checking in with a teacher every so often, just to make sure you haven't acquired any bad habits in your practice style along the way.

## Backyard studios and home classes

Throughout the world, many Yoga teachers hold sessions in their homes or in backyard studios. Don't let this practice turn you off — you may find a great opportunity. Some of the most dedicated Yoga teachers work this way because they want to avoid commercialism and the details of administering a full-scale center. Backyard studios often offer a great sense of community, and you can also expect lots of valuable personal attention from the teacher because the groups tend to be smaller than in larger centers.

# *Taking other important considerations into account*

Just as not all Yoga classes and Yoga teachers are alike, the length of the class and the cost per class both vary, depending on the mode of instruction you choose. Your level of commitment plays a role in how much your individual sessions cost.

- ✓ **Time commitment:** The length of a group Yoga class varies from 50 to 90 minutes. Health clubs, fitness spas, and corporate classes are normally 50 to 60 minutes long, but beginning classes at Yoga centers usually last for 75 to 90 minutes. A private Yoga lesson customarily lasts 1 hour.

- ✓ **Cost:** In general, group Yoga classes are pretty affordable. The cheapest classes are usually available at adult education centers and at community and senior centers. YWCA classes also tend to be reasonably priced. If you have a health club membership, check to see if your gym includes free Yoga classes as part of the package. Most regular Yoga centers in metropolitan areas charge an average of $15 to $20 per class. A one-time drop-in fee (for anyone who hasn't committed to taking more than one class) is usually a few dollars higher. Some schools offer the first class free, and others may charge as much as $25. On the other end, many Yoga studios now offer community classes at a reduced fee or on a donation basis.

When you're considering a commitment to a Yoga center, check into the larger packages — they're often a good investment. Obviously, private lessons are quite a bit more expensive than group classes and range from $50 to $250. Whenever you smell commercialism, you can be fairly sure your nose isn't deceiving you. If you're uncomfortable with the price you're quoted for Yoga classes, continue to seek out a more reasonable offer. Remember, though, Yoga teachers need to pay the rent, too.

# Preparing for Group Practice

When you choose a class you think can work for you, you may be nervous about actually taking the plunge and heading to your first session. The following sections answer your questions about what to wear and take, as well as how to stay safe (and in the good graces of your classmates) as you begin your group Yoga journey.

## Deciding what to wear

Yoga practitioners wear a wide variety of exercise clothing. When selecting your own Yoga wardrobe, your most important consideration needs to be whether the clothing allows you to move and breathe freely. Another practical matter is dressing for the temperature of the room. It's wise to have an extra layer that you can wear in the beginning until you warm up and that you can put back on toward the end as you cool down.

## Packing your Yoga class kit

If you're serious about your Yoga practice (and if you're concerned about hygiene), we recommend that you invest in your own personal mat and possibly other practice items. Although many Yoga centers furnish mats, as well as blocks, straps, blankets, and bolsters, consider bringing your own. If you ever have to pick from the bottom of the bin after yet another sweaty class, you'll know what we mean. Note, however, that not every teacher uses props to the same extent, and the need for these various Yoga helpers varies with the style of the class (as we discuss in Chapter 1) and the teacher's lineage and preferences.

Before attending a class, find out what kind of floor it practices on. If the floor is carpeted, a towel or a sticky mat works (we describe sticky mats and similar useful items in Chapter 20). A hardwood floor may require more padding, especially if your knees are sensitive. In that case, bring along a thick Yoga mat or a rug remnant that's a little longer than your height and a little wider than your shoulders. A folded blanket is also helpful if you need a pad under your head when you're lying down. If you tend to get cold, bring along a blanket to cover yourself during final relaxation. You want to make this item your own because you use it not just for support, but also to cover your body.

As your teacher becomes familiar with your unique needs, she may suggest some other personalized props for you to bring to class:

- Your own Yoga mat or rug.
- A towel.
- A blanket.

- Extra clothing to layer on if the room is too cool or to take off if you're too warm.

- A bottle of water to satisfy your thirst and keep you well hydrated. We recommend a Green Yoga (discussed in Chapter 1) approach: Use a steel flask or a glass bottle to bring your own water instead of toting commercial water in a plastic bottle.

- Enthusiasm, motivation, and good humor.

## Putting safety first

The most important factor for determining the safety of a Yoga class is your personal attitude. If you participate with the understanding that you aren't competing against the other students or trying to impress the teacher, and that you also must not inflict pain upon yourself, you can enjoy a safe Yoga practice. The popular maxim "No pain, no gain" doesn't apply to Yoga. "No gain with negative pain" is a better mindset. Consider the difference between pain and the feeling of your body at work.

By *negative pain,* we mean discomfort that causes you distress or increases the likelihood of injury. Of course, if you haven't exercised for a while, you can expect to encounter your body's resistance at the beginning. You may even feel a little working soreness the next day, which just reflects your body's efforts and its adjustment to the new adventure. The key to avoiding injury is to proceed gently — better to err on the side of gentleness than to face torn ligaments. A good teacher always reminds you to ease into the postures and work creatively with your body's physical resistance. Nonharming is an important moral virtue in Yoga — and observing this foremost Yoga principle applies not just to how you treat others, but also to how you treat yourself!

If you have any physical limitations (recent surgeries; knee, neck, or back problems; and so on), be sure to inform the center and the teacher beforehand. In a classroom setting, instructors have to split their attention among many students; your upfront communication can help prevent personal injury.

If a teacher insists that you do an exercise or a routine that feels very uncomfortable or that you think may hurt you, take a break on your mat or, if that isn't possible, just walk out of the class. Try to stay cool, and register your complaint with the school afterward. Fortunately, this situation rarely happens.

## Paging Miss Manners

In all social settings, common courtesy calls for sensitivity to others; those same rules of responsible conduct apply to your participation in Yoga group sessions. So sift through all the good manners you've acquired from a lifetime of human interaction, and pack them as required equipment for your next trip to class. Before you go, check your bags for these etiquette essentials:

- Arrive on time. Wandering into class "fashionably" late is rude and disturbs others.

- If you arrive early and students from the previous class are still relaxing or meditating, respect their quiet time until your own session formally begins.

- Leave your shoes, gum, and cellphone outside the classroom.

- If you're smelling kind of ripe from a hard day's work, find some time to bathe or freshen up first.

- Keep classroom conversation to a minimum — some people arrive early to meditate or to just sit quietly.

- Remove your socks for better traction, but don't leave them near your neighbor's face.

- Avoid noisy and clanky jewelry.

- Be sure that your, ahem, private parts remain private and appropriately covered if you choose to wear loose-fitting shorts, or, against our advice, super-tight outfits.

- Don't wear perfume or cologne. Some people have allergies or sensitivities.

- Take a space near the door or a window if you require a lot of air.

- Park yourself near the instructor if you have hearing difficulties; many teachers speak softly to generate a meditative mood.

- If you've borrowed any of the studio's props, put them away neatly after class.

## Eating before Yoga practice

Whether you're taking a Yoga class or practicing on your own, the guidelines for eating before Yoga practice are similar to the advice for most physical activities. With even the lightest meal, such as fruit or juice, allow at least 1 hour before class. For larger meals with vegetables and grains, allow 2 hours, and for heavy meals with meat, wait 3 to 4 hours. Eating right after class is okay — you may even have worked up a good appetite.

# Going for It on Your Own

Traditionally, Yoga is passed down from teacher to student. However, a few accomplished yogis and yoginis are self-taught. These independent spirits set a precedent for students who enjoy exploring new territory on their own. If you live in an isolated area and don't have easy access to a Yoga instructor or class, don't be disheartened. You still have several choices that can help you begin your yogic journey.

- ✔ Taped or streamed classes on the Internet
- ✔ DVDs
- ✔ Books
- ✔ Newsletters (hard copy or online)
- ✔ Magazines
- ✔ Newspapers
- ✔ Television

Because Yoga is a motor skill, most people who practice without access to a teacher rely on a DVD or video for instruction. If you opt for this particular approach, we recommend that you learn a routine and then begin listening only to the instructor's voice instead of focusing on the screen. Yoga emphasizes more inner work than outer activity, and watching the screen interferes with this process. Listening to a disembodied voice works better. According to Yoga, the eye is an active and even aggressive sense, whereas the ear is a more passive receptor. CDs can also work well for this reason, as long as they're accompanied by informative illustrations.

We prefer a good Yoga book to magazine or newspaper articles, simply because creating a book usually requires more in-depth, detailed consideration of subject matter and presentation. Plus, books have fewer advertisements taking up valuable space than periodicals do. But don't discount the value of a newsletter from a backyard Yoga studio. The publication can be a real find if it comes from a legitimate source.

The difficulty with self-tutoring at the beginning is that you may have trouble judging good form from bad — and by *good*, we mean "safe." We also mean form that helps you build your foundation for more advanced practice, not one that aims to appear beautiful and fits the common stereotype of what Yoga is "supposed to" look like. You need time to understand how your body responds to the challenge of a posture and determine the proper adjustments for your body's own optimal form. Some people use a mirror to check the postures, but that tells only one side of the story. More importantly, it externalizes the whole process too much.

Become comfortable with checking from the inside, through inwardly *feeling* your body. Until you're proficient at doing so, seek out a competent instructor, if at all possible. Another person sees you objectively — from all sides — and can thus give you valuable feedback about your body's specific resistances and requirements.

# Fulfilling Your Promise to Yourself: Making Time for Yoga Practice

For centuries, the traditional time for Yoga practice has been sunrise and sunset, which are thought to be especially auspicious. Today's busy lifestyles, however, can undermine your best intentions, so be pragmatic and arrange your Yoga practice at your convenience. Just keep in mind that, statistically, you have a 30 percent greater chance of accomplishing a fitness goal if you practice in the morning. More important than holding tight to a preset time is just making sure that you work Yoga into your schedule *somewhere* — and stick with it.

Practicing at roughly the same time during the day can help you create a positive habit, which may make it easier to maintain your routine. Experiment to see what works in your life, and stick to it. Mix and match from these suggestions:

✔ A short daily practice of 10 to 15 minutes

✔ A Yoga class two or three times per week

✔ Short breathing and meditation breaks throughout the day

The amount of time you dedicate to Yoga is a personal choice — no need to feel guilty about your decision. Guilt is counterproductive and has no place in Yoga practice.

# Chapter 3

# Preparing for a Fruitful Yoga Practice

*I*n Yoga, what you do and how you do it are equally important, and both mind and body contribute to your actions. Yoga respects the fact that you're a thinking, feeling body as well as a physical one. Full mental participation in even the simplest of physical exercise enables you to tap into your deeper potential as a human being.

This chapter is about cultivating the right attitude toward your Yoga practice, which is the best preparation for success in Yoga. We encourage you to find your own pace without pushing yourself and risking injury, and to leave your competitive spirit to other endeavors. We also emphasize function over form, proposing that a modified version of the "ideal form" of a posture that suits your needs is the right form for you. Yoga is a creative endeavor that asks you to call upon the powers of your own mind as you explore and enjoy the possibilities.

## Cultivating the Right Attitude

*Attitudes* are enduring tendencies in your mind that show themselves in your behavior as well as your speech. Yoga encourages you to examine all your basic attitudes toward life to discover which ones are dysfunctional so that you can replace them with more appropriate ones.

## What's in a number?

Traditional Sanskrit texts of Hatha Yoga utilize numerology (as do many other contemplative and mystical traditions) and draw upon the number 84 as having significance. For instance, it's stated that 8.4 million postures exist, which corresponds to the suspected number of species of living creatures. However, of these, it was said that only 84 are useful to humans. No worries — we moderns can comfortably rely on the 20 or so easily accessible poses and their variations for a full and fruitful Yoga practice.

One attitude worth cultivating is balance in everything, which is a top yogic virtue. A balanced attitude in this context means that you're willing to build up your Yoga practice step by step instead of expecting instant perfection. It also means not basing your practice on incorrect assumptions, including the notion that Yoga is about tying yourself in knots. On the contrary, Yoga loosens all your bodily, emotional, and intellectual knots. The following sections give you some guidelines for getting in the right Yoga mindset.

## Leave pretzels for snack time

Many people are turned off by magazine covers showing photographs of experts in advanced postures with their limbs tied in knots. What these publications may fail to disclose is that most of these yogis and yoginis have practiced Yoga several hours a day for many years to achieve their level of skill. Trust us, you don't have to be a pretzel to experience the undeniable benefits of Yoga. The benefit you derive from Yoga comes from practicing at a level appropriate for you, not from striking an advanced or "ideal" form.

## Practice at your own pace

Some people are natural pretzels. If you (like most) aren't inherently noodle-like, regular practice can increase your flexibility and muscular strength. We advocate a graduated approach. In Chapters 6 through 13, you can find all the preparatory and intermediary steps that lead up to the final forms for the various postures. The late Yoga master T. S. Krishnamacharya of Chennai (Madras), India, the source of most of the best-known orientations of modern Hatha Yoga, emphasized tailoring Yoga instruction to the needs of each individual and advised Yoga teachers to take into account a student's age, physical ability, emotional state, and occupation. We agree and offer this sound advice: Proceed gently but steadfastly.

*Note:* If you like to learn Yoga from books, choose carefully. Do the exercise descriptions include all the stages of developing comfort with a particular posture? Asking a middle-aged newcomer to Yoga to imitate the final form of many of the postures without providing suitable transitions and adaptations is a prescription for disaster. For instance, in almost every book on Hatha Yoga — except ours — you see the headstand featured quite prominently. This posture has become something of a symbol for Yoga in the West. Headstands are powerful postures, to be sure, but they also count among the more advanced poses. Because this beginner's book emphasizes exercises that are both feasible and safe, we've chosen not to include the headstand. We say more about this decision in Chapter 10, which introduces safe inversion practices. Instead, we give you several adaptations that are easier to perform and have no risk attached.

## Send the scorekeeper home

American children often grow up in a highly competitive environment. From childhood on, they're pressured to do more, push harder, and win. Young athletes grow up with the spirit of competition. Although competition has its place in society, this type of competitive behavior has no place in the practice of Yoga.

Yoga is about peace, compassion, and harmony — the exact opposite of the competitive mindset. Yoga doesn't require you to fight against anyone, least of all yourself, or to achieve some goal by force. On the contrary, you're invited to be kind to yourself and others and, above all, to collaborate with your body rather than coerce it or do battle with your mind.

---

### No pain, no gain — not!

The idea of *no pain, no gain* — a completely mistaken notion — often reinforces competitiveness. Although pain and discomfort are part of life, you don't have to invite them. Yoga doesn't ask you to be a masochist. On the contrary, the goal of Yoga is to still the mind and experience freedom and liberation from suffering. Therefore, never flog your body; only coax it gently. Our motto is, "No gain from pain."

---

Heed our cautionary tale: Many years ago, a middle-aged man came to one of our classes. He was a friendly enough fellow but was extremely competitive and hard on himself. He announced right away that he was intent on mastering the lotus posture within a few weeks and pushed himself to do so during our classes. We urged him repeatedly to proceed more slowly. After only a few visits, he failed to show up and never returned. Later we learned from a mutual friend that, in his competitive zeal, he had asked his wife to sit on his legs to force them into the lotus posture. Her weight had seriously injured both his knees!

## Picture yourself in the posture

We encourage you to use visualization in executing postures. For example, before you do the cobra, shoulder stand, or triangle — or any pose, for that matter — take 10 seconds or so to visualize yourself moving into the final posture. Make your visualization as vivid as possible. Enlist the powers of your mind!

# Enjoying a Peaceful Yoga Practice

As you travel through yogic postures, you begin to build awareness of the communications taking place between your body and mind. Do you feel peacefully removed from the raging storm of life around you, comfortable and confident with your strength, range of motion, flexibility, and steadiness? Or are you painfully noting the slow passage of time, sensing a physical awkwardness or strain in your movements? Listen to your own feelings and sensations, and acknowledge their importance, to help make your Yoga experience an expression of peace, calm, and security. That positive message is what Yoga practice is all about.

## Busting the perfect posture myth

Some modern schools of Hatha Yoga claim that they teach "perfect" postures that you can slip into as easily as a tailor-made suit. But how can the same posture be perfect for both a 15-year-old athlete and a 60-year-old retiree? Besides, these schools disagree among themselves about what constitutes a perfect posture. To spell it out, the perfect posture is a perfect myth.

As the great Yoga master Patanjali explained nearly 2,000 years ago, posture has only two requirements: A posture should be steady and easeful:

- ✔ **Steady posture:** A *steady* posture is a posture that you hold stable for a certain period of time. The key isn't freezing all movement, though. Your posture becomes steady when your mind is steady. As long as your thoughts run wild, including your negative emotions, your body also remains unsteady. As you become more skilled in self-observation, you begin to notice the ever-revolving carousel of your mind and become sensitive to the tension in your body. That tension is what Yoga means by *unsteadiness*.

- ✔ **Easeful posture:** A posture is *easeful* when it's enjoyable and enlivening rather than boring and burdensome. An easeful posture increases the principle of clarity — *sattva* — in you. But easefulness isn't slouching. *Sattva* and joy are intimately connected. The more *sattva* is present in your body-mind, the more relaxed and happy you are.

Although Patanjali was thinking primarily, perhaps even exclusively, in terms of meditation postures, his formula applies to all postures equally.

## Listening to your body

No one knows your body like you do. The more you practice Yoga, the better you become at determining your limitations, as well as your strengths, within each posture. Each posture presents its own unique challenges. You want to feel encouraged to explore and expand your physical and emotional boundaries without risking strain or injury to yourself.

Some teachers speak of practicing at the *edge,* the point at which the intensity of a posture challenges you but doesn't cause you pain or unusual discomfort. The idea is to slowly and carefully push that edge further back and open up new territory. Cultivate self-observation and pay attention to the feedback from your body to be able to practice at the edge.

Each Yoga session is an exercise in self-observation without being judgmental. Listen to what your body is telling you. Train yourself to become aware of the signals that continually travel from your muscles, tendons, ligaments, bones, and skin to your brain. Be in dialogue with your body instead of indulging in a mental monologue that excludes bodily awareness. Pay particular attention to signals coming from your neck, lower back, jaw muscles, abdomen, and any known problem or tension areas of your body.

To gauge the intensity of a difficult Yoga posture, use a scale from 1 to 10, with 10 being your threshold for tolerable pain. Imagine a flashing red light and an alarm bell going off after you pass level 8. Notice the signals and heed them, particularly your breath. If your breathing becomes labored, it usually indicates that, figuratively, you're going over the edge and you might want to back off. You're the world's foremost expert on what your body is trying to tell you.

Beginners commonly experience trembling when holding certain Yoga postures. Normally, the involuntary motion is noticeable in the legs or arms and is nothing to worry about, as long as you aren't straining. The tremors are simply a sign that your muscles are working in response to a new demand. Instead of focusing on the feeling that you've become a wobbly bowl of jelly, lengthen your breath a little, if you can, and allow your attention to go deeper within. If the trembling starts to go off the Richter scale, either ease up a little or end the posture altogether.

## Moving slowly but surely

All postural movements are intended to be executed slowly. Unfortunately, most people are usually on automatic with movements that tend to be unconscious, too fast, and not particularly graceful. Most people are generally unaware of their bodies, but yogic postures lead you to adopt a different attitude. Consider the advantages of slow motion:

- ✔ Enhanced awareness, which enables you to listen to what your body is telling you and to practice at the edge.
- ✔ Safer practice. Slowing down lowers the risk of straining or spraining muscles, tearing ligaments, and overtaxing your heart.
- ✔ Arrival at a deep stage of relaxation more quickly.
- ✔ Improved breathing and breathing stamina.
- ✔ Shared workload among more muscle groups.

For the best results, practice your postures at a slow, steady pace while calmly focusing on your breath and the postural movement (flip to Chapter 5 for more info on breathing and movement). Resist the temptation to speed up; instead, savor each posture. Relax and be present here and now. If your breathing becomes labored or you begin to feel fatigued, rest until you're ready to go on.

If you find yourself rushing through your program, pause and ask yourself, "Why the hurry?" If you're truly short on time, shorten your program and focus on fewer postures. But if you just can't shake the feeling of being pressured by time, consider postponing your Yoga session altogether and practice conscious breathing (which we discuss in Chapter 5) while you go about your other business.

If you're rushing through your program because you're feeling bored or generally distracted, pause and remind yourself why you're practicing Yoga in the first place. Renew your motivation by telling yourself that you have plenty of time to complete your session. Boredom is a sign that you're detached from your own bodily experience and aren't living in the present moment. Participate fully in the process. If you need more than a mental reminder, use one of the relaxation techniques in Chapter 4 to slow yourself down. As we explain in Chapter 5, full yogic breathing in one of the resting postures also has a wonderful calming effect.

## Practicing function over form with Forgiving Limbs

In Yoga, as in life, function is more important than form. The function, not the form, of the posture gives you its benefits. Beginners, in particular, need to adapt postures to enjoy their function and benefits right from the start.

We call one useful adaptive device *Forgiving Limbs.* With Forgiving Limbs, you give yourself permission to slightly bend your legs and arms instead of keeping them fully extended. Bent arms and legs enable you to move your spine more easily, which is the focus of many postures and the key to a healthy spine.

For example, the primary mechanical function of a standing forward bend is to stretch your lower back. If you have a good back, take a moment to see what we mean in this adapted posture that's safe for beginners:

1. **Stand up straight and,** *without forcing anything,* **bend forward and try to place your head on your knees, with the palms of your hands on the floor (see Figure 3-1a), or hold the backs of your ankles.**

   Few men or women can actually do this, especially beginners.

2. **Now stand up again, separate your feet to hip width, and bend forward, allowing your legs to bend until you can place your hands on the floor and almost touch your head to your knees (see Figure 3-1b).**

   When bending forward, be sure not to bounce up and down, as most people are inclined to do. You're not a bungee cord!

As you become more flexible — and you will! — gradually straighten your legs until you can come closer to the ideal posture. Note, however, that standing forward bends are quite different from seated ones. A common lower back injury occurs when weekend warriors inspired by young, nubile instructors, as well as their own progress, try to do the seated version of the straight-legged forward bend and push too far.

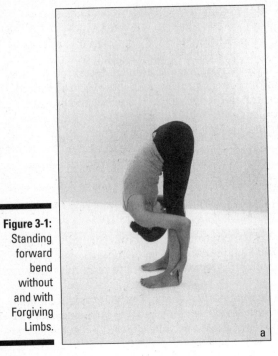 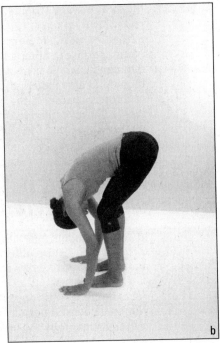

**Figure 3-1:**
Standing
forward
bend
without
and with
Forgiving
Limbs.

a

b

*Photograph by Adam Latham*

# Chapter 4

# Relaxed Like a Noodle: The Fine Art of Letting Go of Stress

• • • • • • • • • • • • • • • • • • • • • • • • • • • • • • • • • • • • • • • • • • • • • • • • • • • • •

## In This Chapter
▶ Understanding and dealing with stress
▶ Relaxing the body through mental and physical exercises

• • • • • • • • • • • • • • • • • • • • • • • • • • • • • • • • • • • • • • • • • • • • • • • • • • • • •

*L*ife in general — not merely modern life — is inherently stressful. Even an inanimate object such as a rock can experience an element of stress. Not all stress is bad for you, however. The question is whether that stress is helping you or hurting you.

Psychologists distinguish between *distress* and *eustress* (good stress). Yoga can help you minimize distress and maximize good, life-enhancing stress. For example, a creative challenge that stimulates your imagination and fires your enthusiasm but doesn't cause you anxiety or lost sleep is a positive event. Even a joyous celebration is, strictly speaking, stressful, but the celebration isn't the kind of stress that harms you — at least not in modest doses. On the other hand, doing nothing and feeling bored to tears is a form of negative stress.

In this chapter, we talk about how you can control negative stress not only through various yogic relaxation techniques, but also by cultivating appropriate attitudes and habits.

## The Nature of Stress

Stress is a fact of life. Some estimates indicate that 80 percent of all illnesses result from the stress we experience from what we perceive to be negative events or situations. Endocrinologist Hans Selye, who pioneered stress research in the mid–20th century, distinguished three phases of the stress syndrome: alarm, resistance, and exhaustion. *Alarm* can be a harmless activity, like stepping from a warm house into the cold air or receiving an upsetting phone call. Both situations require the body to make an adjustment, which is a kind of *resistance*.

When the demand on the body goes on for too long, the stage of *exhaustion* sets in, which can lead to a complete breakdown of the body and the mind — be it heart disease, hypertension, failure of the immune system, or mental illness.

Your body has evolved to handle episodes of physical stress that arise and then subside. The fight-or-flight response you experience when you're in stressful situations helps you react to real threats in your physical environment. The alertness and physical energy you feel when your physical safety is threatened are truly life saving. These circumstances were the ones for which this capacity evolved.

Contrast this with the constant stress experienced in the course of modern life. The relentless demands — work, money woes, noise, pollution, a packed schedule, and so on — can put you in a chronic state of alertness that's extremely draining to your body's energies and resources. Instead of getting you to safety, the chronic stress that's part of today's lifestyles creates an imbalance in the body and the mind, causing you to tense your muscles and breathe in a rapid and shallow manner, perhaps with little relief. Under such chronic stress, your adrenal glands work overtime and your blood may become depleted of oxygen, thus starving your cells.

How can you deal with your stress response efficiently? Yoga suggests a three-pronged solution:

- ✔ Correct stress-producing attitudes.
- ✔ Change habits that invite stress into your life.
- ✔ Release existing tension in the body on an ongoing basis.

Stress can occur without any obvious unpleasant stimulus. Even a birthday celebration can cause you stress, usually because of some hidden anxiety (like another year to mark off). Stress can be cumulative and can creep up on you so gradually that it's imperceptible — until its acute and adverse symptoms manifest.

## Correcting wrong attitudes

Yoga's integrated approach works with both the body and the mind, offering potent antidotes to just the sort of attitudes that make you prone to stress, especially egotism, extreme competitiveness, perfectionism, and the sense of having to accomplish everything right now and by yourself. In all matters, Yoga seeks to replace negative thoughts and attitudes with positive mental dispositions; it asks you to be kind to yourself. Yogic practice helps you understand that everything has its proper place and time.

## Wherever ego, I go

The ultimate source of stress is the ego, or what the Yoga masters call the "I-maker" *(ahamkara)*, from *aham* ("I") and *kara* ("maker"). From the perspective of Yoga, the ego is a mistaken notion in which people identify with their particular bodies instead of with the universe as a whole. Consequently, they experience fear of change and attachment to the body and the mind. This attachment, which is the survival instinct, gives rise to all those many emotions and intentions that make up the game of life. Keeping this artificial center — the ego — going is inherently stressful. Yoga masters all agree that relaxing the grip of the ego allows you to experience greater peace and happiness. Happy letting go!

If you, like so many stress sufferers, have a hard time asking for help, Yoga can give you a real appreciation that everyone is interdependent. If it's your nature to distrust of others, Yoga puts you in touch with the part of your psyche that naturally trusts life itself. It shows you that you don't need to feel as if you're under attack, because your real life — your spiritual identity — can never be harmed or destroyed.

## *Changing poor habits*

Everything in the universe follows an ebb-and-flow pattern that you can count on. Seasons change, and newborn babies grow and eventually become elderly adults. Yogic wisdom recommends that you adopt the same natural patterns in your personal life. Notice and appreciate the cyclical change of the seasons, the myriad ways that you and your environment change and evolve. You may spend much of your time being serious, but you need to play, too. In fact, you need to make time to *just be*, with no expectations and no guilt. Taking time to just be is good for your physical and mental health. Work and rest, tension and relaxation belong together as balanced pairs.

Often people desperately maintain a hectic schedule because they can't envision an alternative that includes time out. They fear what may happen if they slow down. But money and standard of living aren't everything; the *quality* of your life is far more important. Besides, if stress undercuts your health, you have to go into low gear anyway, and your climb back to health may prove costly. Yoga gives you a baseline of tranquility to deal with your fears and anxieties effectively — as long as you engage it at the mental level and not just the physical level.

# Detach yourself

Yoga shows you how to cultivate the *relaxation response* throughout the day by letting go of your hold on things. Herbert Benson, MD, coined this phrase and was among the first to point out the hidden epidemic of hypertension (high blood pressure) as a result of stress. In his national bestseller *The Relaxation Response* (Harper Paperbacks), he calls the relaxation response "a universal human capacity" and "a remarkable innate, neglected asset."

Yoga teaches you how to tap into that underused capacity of your own body-mind. The yogic equivalent of the relaxation response is *vairagya*, which means, literally, "dispassion" or "nonattachment." We call it "letting go." Feeling passionate about what you do (as opposed to having a lukewarm attitude) is good, but at the same time, you merely invite suffering when you become too attached to people,

situations, expectations, and the outcome of your actions. For most people, this lesson is difficult to learn; it's pretty much a lifelong lesson. You can start any time, but the best time to begin is now.

Yoga recommends an attitude of inner detachment in all matters. This detachment doesn't spring from boredom, failure, fear, or apathy — it comes from inner wisdom. Unfortunately, you can't turn on some tap to pour forth wisdom whenever you want it. You must acquire wisdom, either bit by bit as life presents opportunities or deliberately through an intelligent study of the yogic tradition. The latter approach can involve listening directly to the teachings of bona fide masters or studying the same teachings in book form. Yoga's traditional teachings fill many books — all translated from the Sanskrit language for the benefit of contemporary students.

Your inner wisdom tells you that your body and mind are subject to change and that nothing in your environment permanently stays the same. Therefore, there's no point in anxiously clinging to anything. Yoga recommends that you constantly remember your spiritual nature, which is beyond the realm of change and ever blissful and at peace. However, it also asks you to care for others and the world you live in, all while appreciating that you can't step into the same river twice.

For example, if you're a mother, you love and take tender care of your children. But if you're also a yogini, you don't succumb to the stress-producing illusion that you *own* your children. Instead, you always remain aware of the fact that your sons and daughters have their own lives to live, which may turn out to be quite different from yours. You know that all you can do is guide them as best you can.

Of course, you can take many practical steps, described in books on stress management, to reduce stressful situations. These suggestions include not waiting until the last minute to start or finish projects, improving your communication with others, avoiding unnecessary confrontations, and accepting that we live in an imperfect world.

Your daily Hatha Yoga routine, especially the relaxation exercises, can help you extend the feeling of peacefulness or calmness beyond the Yoga session to the rest of the day. Pick some activities or situations that you repeat several times a day as reminders to consciously relax, such as when you go to the bathroom, wait at a traffic light, sit down, open or close a door, or look at your watch. Whenever you encounter these activities, exhale deeply and consciously relax, remembering the peaceful feeling evoked in your daily session.

## Releasing bodily tension

Yoga pursues tension release through all its many different techniques, including breathing exercises and postures, but especially relaxation techniques. The former are a form of *active* or *dynamic relaxation*; the latter are a form of *passive* or *receptive relaxation*.

# Relaxation Techniques That Work

The Sanskrit word for relaxation is *shaithilya*, which is pronounced *shy-theel-yah* and means "loosening." It refers to the loosening of physical and mental tension and effort — all the knots that you tie when you don't go with the flow of life. These knots are like kinks in a hose that prevent the water from flowing freely. Keeping muscles in a constant alert state expends a great amount of your energy, which then is unavailable when you call upon your muscles to really function. Conscious relaxation trains your muscles to release their grip when you don't use them. This relaxation keeps the muscles responsive to the signals from your brain telling them to contract so that you can perform the countless tasks of a busy day.

Relaxation isn't quite the same as doing nothing. Often when you believe you're doing nothing, you're actually busy contracting muscles quite unconsciously. Relaxation is a conscious endeavor that lies somewhere between effort and noneffort. To truly relax, you have to understand and practice the skill.

Relaxation doesn't require any gadgets, but you may want to try the following:

- ✔ Practice in a quiet environment where you're unlikely to be disturbed by others or the telephone.

- ✔ Try placing a small pillow under your head and a large one under your knees, for support and comfort in the *supine*, or lying, positions. Alternatively, use a folded blanket.

- ✔ Ensure that your body stays warm. If necessary, heat the room first or cover yourself with a blanket.

- ✔ Don't practice relaxation techniques on a full stomach; it can cause reflux.

# Deep relaxation: The corpse posture

The simplest, yet most difficult, of all Yoga postures is the corpse posture (*savasana,* from *shava* and *asana,* pronounced *shah-vah sah-nah*).This posture is the simplest because you don't have to use any part of your body at all, and it's the most difficult precisely because you're asked to do nothing whatsoever with your limbs. The corpse posture is an exercise in mind over matter. The only props you need are your body and mind.

If you're high-strung, *asana* practice helps make the corpse posture more easily accessible.

Here's how you do the corpse posture:

1. **Lie flat on your back, with your arms stretched out and relaxed by your sides, palms up (or whatever feels most comfortable).**

   Place a small pillow or folded blanket under your head, if you need one, and another large one under your knees for added comfort.

2. **Close your eyes.**

   Check out Figure 4-1 for a look at the corpse posture.

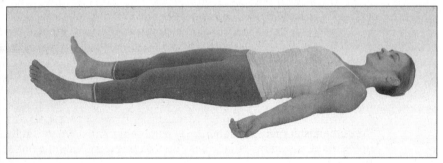

**Figure 4-1:** The corpse is the most popular of all Yoga postures.

*Photograph by Adam Latham*

3. **Form a clear intention to relax.**

   Some people picture themselves lying in white sand on a sunny beach.

4. **Take a couple deep breaths, lengthening exhalation.**

5. **Contract the muscles in your feet for a couple seconds and then consciously relax them; do the same with the muscles in your calves, thighs, buttocks, abdomen, chest, back, hands, forearms, upper arms, shoulders, neck, and face.**

6. **Periodically scan all your muscles, from your feet to your face, to check that they're relaxed.**

   You can often detect subtle tension around the eyes and the scalp muscles. Also relax your mouth, jaw, and tongue.

7. **Focus on the growing bodily sensation of no tension, and let your breath be free.**

8. **At the end of the session, before opening your eyes, form the intention to keep the relaxed feeling for as long as possible.**

9. **Open your eyes, stretch, roll to one side, and get up slowly.**

Practice 10 to 30 minutes; the longer the duration, the better. But watch out — relaxing for too long can make you drowsy.

### Ending relaxation peacefully

Allowing relaxation to end on its own is best — your body knows when it has benefited sufficiently and naturally brings you out of relaxation. However, if you have only a limited time for the exercise, set your mental clock to 15, 20, or however many minutes after closing your eyes, as part of your intention.

If you need to have a sound to remind you to return to ordinary waking consciousness, you can find any number of free or low-cost apps for your smartphone. You can set the timer for the length you like and be awakened by a pleasant sound of your choosing, like a bell or gong.

### Staying awake during relaxation

If it looks like you're going to fall asleep while doing the corpse posture, try bringing your feet closer together. Also, periodically pay attention to your breathing, making sure it's even and unforced. Catnaps are generally excellent; if you're experiencing insomnia, however, we recommend saving your sleep until you go to bed at night. (For good anti-insomnia exercises, check out "Relaxation before sleep" and "Insomnia buster," later in this section.) In any case, the benefits of conscious relaxation are more profound than any catnap. The beautiful part of relaxation is that you're conscious throughout the experience and can control it to some extent. Through relaxation, you get more in touch with your own body, which benefits you throughout the day: You detect stress and tension in your body more readily and then take appropriate action. Also, you avoid the risk of feeling drowsy afterward because you inadvertently entered into a deeper sleep. Remember that sleep isn't necessarily relaxing — people sometimes wake up feeling like they've done heavy work in their sleep.

# Afternoon delight

When your energies flag in the afternoon, try the following exercise as a great stress buster. You can practice it at home or in a quiet place at the office. Just make sure that you aren't interrupted. For this exercise, you need a sturdy chair, one or two blankets, and a towel or an eye pillow (see Chapter 20 for more on this additional yoga resource). Allow 5 to 10 minutes.

1. **Lie on your back and put your feet on the chair, which faces you (see Figure 4-2).**

   Make sure your legs and back are comfortable. Keep your legs 15 to 18 inches apart. You can also put your legs and feet up on the edge of a bed. If none of the feet-up positions feels good, just lie on your back with your legs bent and feet placed on the floor. If the back of your head isn't flat on the floor, and if your neck and throat feel tense or your chin is pushed up toward the ceiling, raise your head slightly on a folded blanket or a firm, flat cushion so that you feel more comfortable.

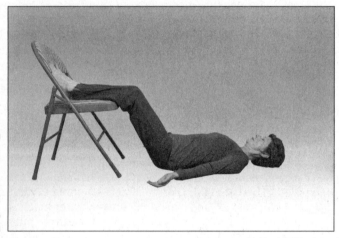

**Figure 4-2:**
Lie on your back and put your feet on a chair.

*Photograph by Adam Latham*

2. **Cover your body from the neck down with one of the blankets.**

   Don't let your body cool down too quickly; it not only feels uncomfortable and interferes with your relaxation, but it also can cramp your muscles.

3. **Place the eye pillow or towel folded lengthwise over your eyes.**

4. **Rest for a few moments, and get used to the position.**

5. **Visualize a large balloon in your stomach: As you inhale through your nose, expand the imaginary balloon in all directions; as you exhale through your nose, release the air from the balloon.**

   Repeat this step several times until it becomes easy for you.

6. **Inhale freely, and begin to make your exhalation longer and longer.**

   Inhale freely, exhale forever.

7. **Repeat Step 6 at least 30 times.**

8. **When you finish the exercise, allow your breath to return to normal and rest for a minute or so, enjoying the relaxed feeling.**

   Don't rush getting up.

## Magic triangles: Relaxing through visualization

The following relaxation technique utilizes your power of imagination. If you can picture images easily in your mind, you may find the exercise enjoyable and refreshing. For this exercise, you need a chair and a blanket (if necessary). Allow 5 minutes.

1. **Sit up tall in a chair, with your feet on the floor and comfortably apart, and your hands resting on top of your knees, as in Figure 4-3.**

   If your feet aren't comfortably touching the floor, fold the blanket and place it under your feet for support.

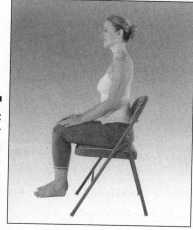

**Figure 4-3:** Sit with your feet on the floor and your hands on your knees.

*Photograph by Adam Latham*

2. **Breathe through your nose, but allow your breath to move freely.**

3. **Close your eyes and focus your attention on the middle of your forehead, just above the level of your eyebrows.**

   Make sure you don't crinkle your forehead or squint your eyes.

4. **Visualize as vividly as possible a triangle connecting the forehead point and the palms of both hands.**

   Register (but don't think about) any sensations or colors that appear on your mental screen while you hold the triangle in your mind. Do this visualization for 8 to 10 breaths, and then dissolve the triangle.

5. **Visualize a triangle formed by your navel and the big toes of your feet; retain this image for 10 to 12 breaths.**

   If any part of the mental triangle is difficult to connect, keep focusing on that part until the triangle fully forms.

6. **Keeping your eyes closed, visualize again the first triangle formed between your forehead and your two palms, and then simultaneously visualize the second triangle (navel to toes).**

   This final step is more challenging. Picture both triangles together for 12 to 15 breaths, and then dissolve them.

## Relaxation before sleep

If you want to enjoy deep sleep or you're experiencing insomnia (but you don't want to count sheep), the following exercise can help you. Many people don't make it to the end of this relaxation technique without falling asleep. For this exercise, you need the following props: a bed or other comfortable place to sleep, two pillows, and one or two blankets. Allow 5 to 10 minutes.

1. **Prepare yourself for sleep and get into bed, lying on your back under the blankets.**

   Your legs can be straight or bent at the knees, with your feet flat on the mattress.

2. **Place one pillow or a folded blanket under your head, and have the other one nearby.**

3. **With your eyes closed, begin to breathe through your nose, making your exhalation twice as long as your inhalation.**

   Keep your breathing smooth and effortless. Also, don't try to direct your breath to any part of your body. Let the breathing pattern be effortless, something you can keep up.

4. **Remain on your back for 8 breaths. Then roll onto your right side and place the second pillow between your knees.**

   Now use the same breathing ratio from Step 3 for 16 breaths.

5. **Finally, roll onto your left side, with the second pillow still between your knees, and use the breathing ratio for 32 breaths.**

## Insomnia buster

This exercise is for people who suffer from insomnia but have an active imagination. Instead of watching your mind weave tale after tale when you can't sleep at night, why not recruit your imagination for the purpose of falling soundly asleep? Here's how.

If you're claustrophobic, this exercise may not necessarily work for you. But before giving up, you may first want to try evoking feelings of security and comfort, as when in a mother's womb or a favorite place in nature.

1. **Prepare yourself for sleep, and lie down comfortably in bed in any position.**

2. **With closed eyes, breathe evenly through your nose for a while.**

3. **Now visualize yourself snugly enfolded in a protective cocoon of purple.**

4. **While feeling safe in your purple environment, visualize a thin line of white light extending from the crown of your head to your solar plexus, just below your navel.**

This technique works even while traveling on a plane, with the jets roaring next to your ears. Just tell the flight attendant not to disturb you while you're sleeping.

# Yoga Nidra: Catch Up on Your Sleep Quotient with Yogic Sleep

If your body-mind is slow to wind down to get its well-deserved rest, here's a potent technique to entice Mr. Sandman to visit you regularly. Yogic Sleep is a powerful relaxation technique that you can do when you gain some control over the relaxation response (which we discuss in the earlier "Detach yourself" sidebar). When practiced successfully, this technique can be as restorative as sleep — except that you remain fully aware throughout.

To induce Yoga Nidra, you must listen to a set of instructions, similar to guided meditation. You can listen to a friend reading the instructions, but listening to a recording by someone else or by you yourself is more practical.

One feature of this practice is to focus in relatively quick succession on individual parts of the body. Mentally name each part, and then sense it as distinctly as possible.

In the beginning, you may find actually feeling certain body parts difficult. Don't let this setback dismay you; continue to rotate your awareness fairly swiftly. With practice, you can include in this circuit even your inner organs and all kinds of mental states.

Practicing Yoga Nidra before sleep is best because it's an excellent technique for inducing lucid dreaming and out-of-body experiences during sleep. *Lucid dreaming* refers to the kind of dream in which you're aware that you're dreaming. Great Yoga masters remain aware even during deep sleep. Only the body and brain are fast asleep, whereas awareness is continuous.

## Formulating your intention

Yoga Nidra serves as a potent tool for reprogramming your brain. If you do it correctly, it can accelerate your inner or spiritual growth. It allows you to cultivate good habits and attitudes. First, consider which specific habit or attitude you really want to replace with a more positive habit or attitude. This phase is called *formulating your intention*. Take your time to consider what you want to change about yourself.

Phrase your chosen intention in the following way: *I will become more [this or that]*. This wording affirms your life's future trajectory by enlisting the unconscious mind. Worthy intentions may be to become more patient, more tolerant, or more loving. We recommend that your chosen intention not contradict any of Yoga's high moral virtues, which we discuss in Chapter 22. Also make your intention realistic and specific. An intention like "I will become enlightened" is specific enough but perhaps not very realistic. By contrast, an intention like "I will become a better person" is too vague. A better intention is something more along the lines of "I am becoming more relaxed within myself," "I will become more tolerant toward others," or "I will become more patient." You want your intention to be something you can stick with until you realize it in your life, not one you have to abandon because it was too lofty or undefined.

When formulating your intention, try to evoke the corresponding feeling inside you so you know what it feels like to be loving, patient, forgiving, or whatever.

After you set an intention, you formally apply it during the actual Yoga Nidra exercise (described in the following section) by repeating it when prompted.

## Performing Yoga Nidra

The following steps show you how to perform Yoga Nidra.

1. **Choose a clear intention (as we describe in the preceding section), and lie flat on your back, with your arms stretched out by your sides (or however feels most comfortable).**

   Place a pillow or folded blanket behind your neck for support, and use another pillow or folded blanket under your knees for added comfort. Refer to Figure 4-1, earlier in the chapter, for an illustration.

2. **Close your eyes.**

3. **Repeat the clear intention you chose in Step 1 three times.**

4. **Take a couple deep breaths, emphasizing exhalation.**

5. **Starting with your right side, rotate your awareness through all parts on that side of your body — limb by limb — in fairly quick succession.**

   Follow this progression: each finger, palm of the hand, back of the hand, hand as a whole, forearm, elbow, upper arm, shoulder joint, shoulder, neck, each section of the face (forehead, eyes, nose, chin, and so on), ear, scalp, throat, chest, side of the rib cage, shoulder blade, waist, stomach, lower abdomen, genitals, buttocks, whole spine, thigh, top and back of knee, shin, calf, ankle, top of foot, heel, sole, each toe.

6. **Be aware of your body as a whole.**

7. **Repeat the rotation in Step 5 on the left side, ending with the whole-body awareness described in Step 6.**

8. **Repeat Steps 5 through 7 one or more times until you achieve an adequate level of relaxation.**

9. **Continue to be aware of the whole body and the space surrounding it, feeling the stillness and peace.**

10. **Reaffirm your initial intention three times.**

11. **Mentally prepare to return to ordinary consciousness.**

12. **Gently move your fingers for a few moments, take a deep breath, and then open your eyes.**

No time limit applies to your Yoga Nidra performance unless you impose one. Expect to come out of Yogic Sleep naturally, whether you return after only 15 minutes or a whole hour. Or you may just fall asleep. If you have things to do afterward, make sure you set your phone or meditation app for a gentle wake-up call. Don't rush! Take your time to reintegrate with the ordinary world.

I (Georg) swear by this practice. It's the most powerful yogic technique for personal change at the beginner level. Only the ecstatic state *(samadhi)* is more transformative. Several good recordings for practicing Yoga Nidra are available, but don't be surprised to discover that the instructions vary from recording to recording. Check out our section on additional Yoga resources at Dummies.com.

# Chapter 5

# Breath and Movement Simplified

. . . . . . . . . . . . . . . . . . . . . . . . . . . . . . . . . . . . . . . . . . . . . . . . . .

### In This Chapter

▶ Understanding breathing basics

▶ Detailing yogic breathing mechanics

▶ Linking breath and postural movement

▶ Adding sound to postural practice

▶ Introducing traditional methods of breath control

. . . . . . . . . . . . . . . . . . . . . . . . . . . . . . . . . . . . . . . . . . . . . . . . . .

*T*he masters of Yoga discovered the usefulness of the breath thousands of years ago and, in Hatha Yoga, have perfected a system for the conscious control of breathing. In this chapter, we share their secrets with you. In the ancient Sanskrit language, the word for "breath" is the same as the word for "life" — *prana* (pronounced *prah-nah*) — which gives you a good clue about how important Yoga thinks breathing is for your well-being. Yoga without *prana* is like putting an empty pot on the stove and hoping for a delicious meal. In this chapter, we show you how to use conscious breathing in conjunction with the Yoga postures. We also introduce several breathing exercises that you do seated either on a chair or in one of the Yoga sitting postures (if you're up to that).

## Breathing Your Way to Good Health

Think of your breath as your most intimate friend. Your breath is with you from the moment you're born until you die. In a given day, you take between 20,000 and 30,000 breaths. Most likely, barring any respiratory problems, you're barely aware of your breathing. This state is akin to taking your best friend so for granted that the relationship gets stale and is put at risk. Although the automatic nature of breathing is part of the body's machinery that keeps you alive, having breathing occur automatically isn't necessarily to your advantage; *automatic* doesn't always mean "optimal." In fact, most people's breathing habits are quite poor and to their great disadvantage. Stale air accumulates in their lungs and becomes as unproductive as a stale friendship. Poor breathing is known to cause and increase stress. Conversely, stress shortens your breath and increases your level of anxiety.

You can help alleviate stress through the simple practice of yogic breathing. Among other benefits, breathing loads your blood with oxygen, which, by nourishing and repairing your body's cells, maintains your health at the most desirable level. Shallow breathing, which is common, doesn't efficiently oxygenate the 10 pints of blood circulating in your arteries and veins. Consequently, toxins accumulate in the cells. Before you know it, you feel mentally sluggish and emotionally down, and eventually organs begin to malfunction. Is it any wonder that the breath is the best tool you have to profoundly affect your body and mind?

Bad breath is improved by brushing your teeth regularly and occasionally sucking on a mint. Bad breathing, however, is a bad habit that requires a bit more to change: You must retrain your body through breath awareness.

In Yoga, consciously regulated breathing has three major applications. Use it in these ways:

- ✔ In conjunction with the various postures to achieve the deepest possible effect and to prepare the mind for meditation
- ✔ As breath control (called *pranayama,* pronounced *prah-nah-yah-mah*) to invigorate your vitality and reduce your anxiety
- ✔ As a healing method in which you consciously direct the breath to a particular part or organ of the body to remove energetic blockages and facilitate healing

## Taking high-quality breaths

Before you jump right in and make drastic changes to your method of breathing, take a few minutes to assess your current breathing style. You may find it helpful to keep a log of your breathing habits over the course of a couple days, noting how your breathing changes in accordance with the situations around you and your states of mind. Check your breathing by asking yourself the following questions:

- ✔ Is my breathing shallow (my abdomen and chest barely move when I fill my lungs with air)?
- ✔ Do I often breathe erratically (my breathing rhythm isn't harmonious)?

✔ Do I easily get out of breath?

✔ Is my breathing labored at times?

✔ Do I hold my breath in stressful situations?

✔ Do I generally breathe too fast?

If your answer to any of these questions is yes, you're an ideal candidate for yogic breathing. Even if you didn't answer yes, practicing conscious breathing still benefits your mind and body.

Men take an average of 12 to 14 breaths per minute, and women take 14 to 15. Breathing at a markedly faster pace — usually associated with *chest breathing* — qualifies as hyperventilation, which leads to carbon dioxide depletion (your body needs some of this gas to maintain the right acid–alkaline balance of the blood).

## *Relaxing with a couple of deep breaths*

Think about the many times you've heard someone say, "Now, just take a couple of deep breaths and relax." This recommendation is so popular because it really works! Pain clinics across the country use breathing exercises for pain control. Childbirth preparation courses teach Yoga-related breathing techniques to both parents to aid in the birthing process. Moreover, since the 1970s, wellness experts have taught yogic breathing to corporate America with great success.

### The cosmic side of breathing

The Yoga scriptures state that humans take an average of 21,600 breaths per day. This number, which falls within the range accepted by modern research, is profoundly symbolic. Here's why: 21,600 is one-fifth of 108,000. The number 108, or multiples of it, is charged with special significance in India. The importance relates to the astronomical fact that the distance between the sun and Earth is 108 times greater than the sun's diameter. The symbolism is represented in the 108 beads of the mala (similar to a rosary) many Yoga practitioners in India use. A full round on the mala is a symbolic journey from Earth to heaven — that is, from ordinary consciousness to higher consciousness. Even the one-fifth is significant; 5 is the number associated with the air element. This correlation is one of many that Yoga masters profess between the human body–mind and the universe at large.

Yogic breathing is like texting your nervous system with the message to relax. One easy way to experience the effect of simple breathing is to try the following exercise:

1. **Sit comfortably in your chair.**

2. **Close your eyes and visualize a swan gliding peacefully across a crystal-clear lake.**

3. **Now, like the swan, let your breath flow along in a long, smooth, and peaceful movement, ideally through your nose.**

   If your nose is plugged up, try to breathe through your nose and mouth, or just through your mouth.

4. **Extend your breath to its comfortable maximum capacity for 20 rounds; then gradually let your breath return to normal.**

5. **Afterward, take a few moments to sit with your eyes closed, and notice the difference in how you feel overall.**

   Can you imagine how relaxed and calm you can feel after 10 to 15 minutes of conscious yogic breathing?

## Practicing safe yogic breathing

As you look forward to the calming and restorative power of yogic breathing, take time to reflect on a few safety tips that can help you enjoy your experience.

✔ If you have problems with your lungs (such as a cold or asthma), or if you have heart disease, consult your physician before embarking on breath control, even under the supervision of a Yoga therapist (unless your therapist happens to be a physician as well).

✔ Don't practice breathing exercises when the air is too cold or too hot.

✔ Avoid practicing in polluted air, including the smoke from incense. Whenever possible, practice breath control outdoors or with an open window, where you maximize exposure to *negative ions* (atoms with a negative electronic charge). Negative ions in moderation are considered beneficial for health. On the other hand, positive ions, which your TV and computer produce, have been connected with fatigue, headaches, and respiratory problems.

✔ Don't strain your breathing — remain relaxed while doing the breathing exercises.

✔ Don't overdo the number of repetitions. Stay within our guidelines for each exercise.

✔ Don't wear constricting clothing.

## Real-life story on the benefits of yogic breathing

The late T. Krishnamacharya of Chennai (Madras), India — one of the great Yoga masters of the 20th century — is a classic illustration of the benefits of yogic breathing. On his 100th birthday celebration, he initiated the ceremony by chanting a 30-second-long continuous *om* sound. He also sat up perfectly straight on the floor for many hours every day during the festivities, which lasted several days. Not bad for a centenarian!

## *Reaping the benefits of yogic breathing*

In addition to relaxing the body and calming the mind, yogic breathing offers an entire spectrum of other benefits that work like insurance, protecting your investment in a longer and healthier life. Consider these six important advantages of controlled breathing:

- ✔ It steps up your metabolism (which helps with weight control).
- ✔ It uses muscles that automatically improve your posture, preventing the stiff, slumped carriage characteristic of many older people.
- ✔ It keeps the lung tissue elastic, which allows you to take in more oxygen to nourish the 50 trillion cells in your body.
- ✔ It tones your abdominal area, a common site for health problems because many illnesses begin in the intestines.
- ✔ It strengthens your immune system.
- ✔ It reduces your levels of tension and anxiety.

## *Breathing through your nose (most of the time)*

No matter what anybody else tells you, yogic breathing typically occurs through the nose, during both inhalation and exhalation. For traditional yogis and yoginis, the mouth is meant for eating and the nose for breathing. We know at least three good reasons for breathing through the nose:

- ✔ It slows the breath because you're breathing through two small openings instead of the one big opening in your mouth, and slow is good in Yoga.
- ✔ The air is hygienically filtered and warmed by the nasal passages. Even the purest air contains, at the least, dust particles and, at the worst, all the toxic pollutants of a metropolis.

✔ According to traditional Yoga, nasal breathing stimulates the subtle energy center — the so-called *ajna-cakra* (pronounced *ah-gyah-chuk-rah*) located near sinuses in the spot between the eyebrows. This very important location is the meeting place of the left (cooling) and the right (heating) currents of vital energy *(prana)* that act directly on the nervous and endocrine systems. (For the two currents, see the "Alternate nostril breathing" section later in this chapter.)

Folk wisdom teaches that every rule has its exception, which is definitely the case with the yogic rule of breathing through the nose. A few classical yogic techniques for breath control require you to breathe through the mouth. When we present a mouth-breathing technique, we alert you to that fact.

### What if I can't breathe through my nose?

Some folks suffer from various physiological conditions that prevent them from breathing through their noses. Of course, Yoga is flexible. If you have difficulty breathing when lying down, try sitting up. The time of day can also make a difference in your ability to breathe. For example, you may be more congested or exposed to more allergens in the morning than in the afternoon. Of course, you can detect the differences.

If you're still not sure how to settle on a comfortable breathing method, first try inhaling through your nose and exhaling through your mouth. Failing this, just breathe through your mouth and don't worry for now; worry is always counterproductive.

### What about breathing through my nose all the time?

Many Americans participate in more than one kind of physical activity or exercise discipline. Each has its own guidelines and rules for breathing, which we recommend you follow. For example, the majority of aerobic activities — running, walking, weight lifting, and so on — recommend that you inhale through the nose and exhale through the mouth. The reason: You need to move a lot of air quickly in and out of your lungs. And breathing only through the nose while swimming can be very dangerous. In fact, we don't recommend underwater *pranayama* unless you enjoy a snootful of water making its way to your lungs.

In the beginning, save yogic breathing for your Yoga exercises. Later, when you become more skillful at it, you may want to adopt nasal breathing during all normal activities. You can then benefit from its calming and hygienic effects throughout the day.

## Notice your breath

When you pay close attention to the rhythm of your breath, you may be surprised to notice that it has several parts. According to Yoga, the four aspects of controlled breathing are as follows:

✔ Inhalation (*puraka*, pronounced *poo-rah-kah*)

✔ Retention, or holding, after inhalation (*antar-kumbhaka*, pronounced *ahn-tahr-koom-bhah-kah*)

✔ Exhalation (*recaka*, pronounced *reh-chah-kah*)

✔ Retention, or holding, after exhalation (*bahya-kumbhaka*, pronounced *bah-yah-koom-bhah-kah*)

In this book, we emphasize exhalation. Some classical Yoga authorities also refer to a type of retention that occurs spontaneously and effortlessly in some higher states of consciousness. This retention is known as *kevala-kumbhaka* (pronounced *keh-vah-lah-koom-bhah-kah*), or absolute retention.

# Mastering the Mechanics of Yogic Breathing

Most people are either shallow chest breathers or shallow belly breathers. Yogic breathing incorporates a complete breath that expands both the chest and the abdomen on inhalation either from the chest down or from the abdomen up. Both are valid techniques. (Figures 5-2 and 5-3, later in the chapter, show you each of these techniques.)

Yogic breathing involves breathing much more deeply than usual, which, in turn, brings more oxygen into your system. Don't be surprised if you feel a little lightheaded or even dizzy in the beginning. If this situation happens during your Yoga practice, just rest for a few minutes or lie down until you feel like proceeding. Remind yourself that you don't need to rush.

Some Yoga practitioners think that you can breathe into parts of the body other than the lungs. Not so. You inhale the breath through either your nose or your mouth, and it then expands into the lungs. You may perceive that the breath is moving up and down throughout the body, but you're actually feeling muscle contraction. Any suggestion of an up or down movement of the breath is due entirely to the sequence of your muscular control and the flow of your attention.

In both chest and abdominal breathing, the abdomen draws in on exhalation. From a mechanical standpoint, Yogic breathing moves the spine and works the muscles and organs of respiration, which primarily include the diaphragm, *intercostal* (between the ribs) and abdominal muscles, and the lungs and heart. The diaphragm pulls down when it contracts, which creates more space for the lungs during inhalation. The chest noticeably widens. When the diaphragm relaxes, it moves back into its upward curve, forcing the air out of the lungs.

The *diaphragm* is a vaulted muscle sheath that separates the lungs and heart from the stomach, liver, kidneys, and other abdominal organs. It's attached all around the lower border of the ribcage and, by a pair of powerful muscles, to the first through fourth lumbar vertebrae. The diaphragm and the chest muscles activate the lungs, which don't have muscles.

## Understanding how your emotions affect your diaphragm

Psychologically, people tend to use the diaphragm as a lid to bottle up their undigested or unwanted emotions of anger and fear. Chronic contraction of the diaphragm makes it inflexible and blocks the free flow of energy between the abdomen (the nether region of the bowels) and the chest (the feelings associated with the heart). Yogic breathing helps restore flexibility and function to the diaphragm and removes obstructions to the flow of physical and emotional energy. You can then experience liberation of your emotions, which can lead you to integrate them with the rest of your life.

Deep breathing not only affects the organs in your chest and abdomen, but also reaches down into your gut emotions. Don't be surprised if sighs and perhaps even a few tears accompany the tension release your breath work achieves. These are welcome signs that you're peeling off the muscular armor you have placed around your abdomen and heart. Instead of feeling concerned or embarrassed, rejoice in your newly gained inner freedom! Yoga practitioners know that real men (and women) do cry.

## Appreciating the complete yogic breath

If shallow or erratic breathing puts your well-being at risk, the complete yogic breath is your ticket to excellent physical and mental health. If you do no other Yoga exercise, the complete Yoga breath — integrally combined with relaxation — can still be of invaluable benefit to you. It's your secret weapon, except that Yoga doesn't advocate the use of force.

## Belly breathing

Before you jump into practicing the complete yogic breath, try out this exercise:

1. **Lie flat on your back, and place one hand on your chest and the other on your abdomen, as in Figure 5-1.**

   Place a small pillow or folded blanket under your head if you have tension in your neck or if your chin tilts upward. Place a large pillow under your knees if your back is uncomfortable.

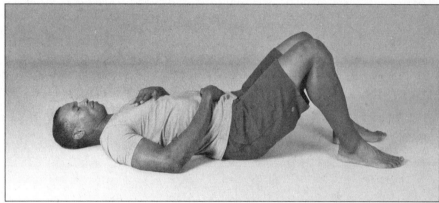

**Figure 5-1:**
Your hand position helps you detect motion during belly breathing.

*Photograph by Adam Latham*

2. **Take 15 to 20 slow, deep breaths. During inhalation, expand your abdomen; during exhalation, contract your abdomen but keep your chest as motionless as possible.**

   Your hands act as motion detectors.

3. **Pause for a couple seconds between inhalation and exhalation, keeping the throat soft.**

## Belly-to-chest breathing

In belly-to-chest breathing, you really exercise your chest and diaphragm muscles as well as your lungs, and you treat your body with oodles of oxygen and life force *(prana)*. When you're done, your cells are humming with energy and your brain is grateful to you for the extra boost. You can use this form of breathing before you begin your relaxation practice, before and where indicated during your practice of the Yoga postures, and whenever you feel so inclined throughout the day. You don't necessarily have to lie down as we describe in the following exercise; you can be seated or even walking. After practicing this technique for a while, you may find that it becomes second nature to you.

1. **Lie flat on your back, with your knees bent and your feet on the floor at hip width, and relax.**

   Place a small pillow or folded blanket under your head if you have tension in your neck or if your chin tilts upward. Place a large pillow under your knees if your back is uncomfortable.

2. **Inhale while expanding your abdomen, your ribs, and then your chest; pause for a couple seconds.**

3. **Exhale while releasing your chest and shoulder muscles, gently and continuously contracting or drawing in your abdomen (see Figure 5-2); pause again for a couple seconds.**

4. **Repeat Steps 2 and 3 from 6 to 12 times.**

**Figure 5-2:**
The classic
Yoga breath.

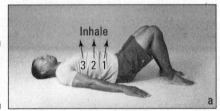
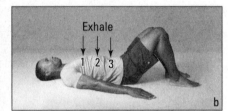

*Photograph by Adam Latham*

You can greatly enhance the value of this exercise and others by fully participating with your mind. Feel the air fill your lungs. Feel your muscles work. Feel your body as a whole. Visualize precious life energy entering your lungs and every cell of your body, rejuvenating and energizing you. To help you experience this exercise more profoundly, keep your eyes closed. Place your hands on your abdomen and feel it expand upon inhalation.

### Chest-to-belly breathing

Classically, yoga teachers taught yogic breathing from the abdomen up on inhalation (see the preceding section), which you can see in numerous publications on Yoga. This method works well for many people. However, in the 1960s, Yoga master T.K.V. Desikachar, with the guidance of his father, the late T. Krishnamacharya, began to adapt the traditional yogic breathing to the needs of Western students. Think about it: Folks in the West sit in chairs and bend forward too much. The daily sitting routine begins in the early morning when they go to the bathroom and then lean over the sink to brush their teeth and do whatever else they do to their faces. They sit at the breakfast table and then again while they commute to their workplaces, where they clock a lot more time sitting and slouching in front of a computer or typewriter or bending over a machine. Finally, in the evening, they go home and sit down for dinner; afterward, perhaps, they sit in front of the television or their computer until their eyes get blurry.

The chest-to-belly breathing emphasizes arching the spine and the upper back to compensate for all this bending forward throughout the day, and it also works well for moving into and out of Yoga postures. Chest-to-belly breathing is also an excellent energizer in the morning; you can do it even before you hop out of bed. We don't recommend this exercise late at night, though, because it's likely to keep you awake.

The following exercise complements the belly-to-chest breathing we cover in the preceding section. As with that technique, you can practice the following exercise lying down, seated, or even while walking.

1. **Lie flat on your back, with your knees bent and your feet on the floor at hip width, and relax.**

   Place a small pillow or folded blanket under your head if you have tension in your neck or if your chin tilts upward. Place a large pillow under your knees if your back is uncomfortable.

2. **Inhale while expanding the chest from the top down and continuing this movement downward into the belly, as in Figure 5-3a; pause for a couple seconds.**

**Figure 5-3:**
The new
Yoga breath.

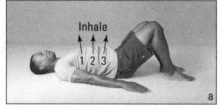
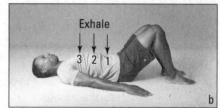

*Photograph by Adam Latham*

3. **Exhale while gently contracting and drawing the belly inward, starting just below the navel (see Figure 5-3b); pause for a couple seconds.**

4. **Repeat Steps 2 and 3 from 6 to 12 times.**

## Starting out with focus breathing

If you have a little difficulty synchronizing yourself with the rhythm of the complete Yoga breathing techniques, you may first want to try a simpler method we call *focus breathing*. Focus breathing is a great stepping stone to all the other techniques. The following list walks you through the phases of focus breathing:

✔ **Phase 1:** During your Yoga practice, simply follow the directions we give you about when to inhale and exhale for each posture, breathe only through the nose, and make the breath a little longer than normal. That's all you have to do! Don't worry about where the breath is starting or ending — just breathe slowly and evenly. (We present the postures in Part II.)

> ✔ **Phase 2:** When you're used to the Phase 1 practice, just add a short pause of 1 or 2 seconds after inhalation and another one after exhalation.
>
> ✔ **Phase 3:** When you're comfortable with the practices of Phases 1 and 2, add drawing in the belly during exhalation without force or exaggeration.

## Realizing the power of a pause

During your normal shallow breathing, you notice a slight natural pause between inhalation and exhalation. This pause becomes important in yogic breathing; even though it lasts only 1 or 2 seconds, the pause is a natural moment of stillness and meditation. If you pay attention to this pause, it can help you become more aware of the unity among body, breath, and mind — all are key elements in your Yoga practice. With the help of a teacher, you also can discover how to lengthen the pause during various Yoga postures to heighten its positive effects.

# Seeing How Breath and Postural Movement Work Together

In Hatha Yoga, breathing is just as important as the postures, which we describe in Part II. How you breathe when you're moving into, holding, or moving out of any given posture can greatly increase the efficiency and benefits of your practice. Think of the breath as mileage plus. The more you use breathing consciously, the more mileage you gain for your health and longevity. Consider some basic guidelines:

> ✔ **Let the breath surround the movement.** The breath leads the movement by a couple of moments — that is, you initiate breathing (both inhalation and exhalation) and then you make the movement. When you inhale, the body opens or expands, and when you exhale, the body folds or contracts.
>
> ✔ **Both the inhalation and the exhalation end with a natural pause.**
>
> ✔ **In the beginning, let the breath dictate the length of the postural movement.** For example, if you're raising your arms as you inhale and you run out of breath before you reach your goal, just pause your breathing for a moment and bring your arms back down as you exhale. With practice, your breath will gradually get longer.
>
> ✔ **Let the breath itself be your teacher.** When your breath sounds labored, you need to back off or come out of a posture.
>
> ✔ **Try to visualize the breath flowing into the area you're working with in any given posture.**

## Breathing in four directions

You can move your body in four natural directions:

- ✔ **Flexion:** Bending forward
- ✔ **Extension:** Bending backward
- ✔ **Lateral flexion:** Bending sideways
- ✔ **Rotation:** Twisting your body

Normally, when people move, they tend to hold or strain their breath. In Yoga, you simply follow the natural flow of the breath. As a rule, adopt this pattern:

- ✔ Inhale when moving into back bends (see Figure 5-4a).
- ✔ Exhale when moving into forward bends (see Figure 5-4b).
- ✔ Exhale when moving into side bends (see Figure 5-4c).
- ✔ Exhale when moving into twists (as shown in Figure 5-4d).

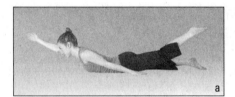 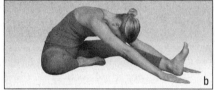

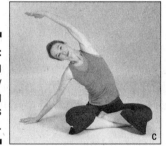 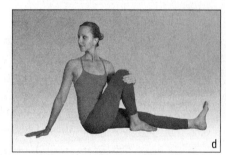

**Figure 5-4:**
Breathing
properly
during
postures is
important.

Photograph by Adam Latham

## Recognizing the distinct roles of movement and holding in Yoga postures

Most Yoga books talk about *stationary* or *held* Yoga postures *(asanas)*. We recommend that, before you try to hold a posture, you first become acquainted with moving in and out of most of the postures we recommend in this book, following the rules of breath and movement in the preceding section. When you can move in and out of a given posture easily and confidently, try holding the posture for a short period *without* holding or straining your breath. You know you're straining when your face turns into a grimace or you feel it going red like a tomato. Getting a handle on moving into and out of the postures before adding the element of holding is important for three reasons:

✔ It helps prepare your muscles and joints by bringing circulation to the area. It's like juicing up your joints, which adds a safety factor.

✔ It helps you experience the intimate connection among body, breath, and mind.

✔ In the case of stretching postures, moving into and out of a given posture before holding the posture supports the concept of *proprioceptive neuromuscular facilitation* (PNF). If you tighten a muscle before stretching it, either by gentle resistance *(isotonic)* or by pushing against a fixed force *(isometric)*, the subsequent stretch is deeper than just using a static pose. Scientific research supports this phenomenon; numerous physical therapy texts refer to it as PNF.

## Achieving a deeper stretch with The Yoga Miracle

To see and experience firsthand the power of PNF (we introduced PNF in the preceding section) in the context of Yoga, grab yourself a partner and follow these instructions for what we call The Yoga Miracle. You can achieve a deeper stretch than normal with this exercise.

1. **Lie on your back, with your left leg bent and your left foot on the floor; your right leg is up in the air and slightly bent.**

   Ask your partner to kneel in the lunge position near your feet.

2. **Have your partner test the flexibility of your hamstrings by holding the back of your right heel and pushing it gently toward you until you reach the first resistance point.**

   The partner on the floor must be relaxed, without resisting. (See Figure 5-5a.) Be sure not to force anything.

3. **Bring your right leg back to the starting point, and then begin to push against the kneeling partner's hand, as in Figure 5-5b.**

   The kneeling partner now either gently resists your right foot completely (isometrically) or allows your foot to move a little with resistance (isotonically).

   Both tests produce the same effect. As you push against your partner's hand, your right hamstring muscles tighten. You want these muscles to tighten for about 10 seconds.

4. **After approximately 10 seconds, the partner on the ground relaxes the right leg and then allows the standing partner to repeat Step 2 (see Figure 5-5c).**

    Compare the results to the ones from the original Step 2 stretch, and behold The Yoga Miracle!

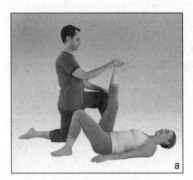 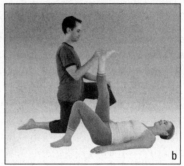

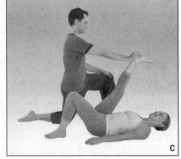

**Figure 5-5:** Test your new flexibility and behold The Yoga Miracle.

*Photograph by Adam Latham*

 Don't try to push your partner over — just push until you feel your leg muscles tighten. Next, after about 10 seconds, release your leg and allow your partner to stretch you again by gently pushing against your heel, causing your leg to move toward you in a stretch that's not forced, as in Figure 5-5c. See how far you can extend this time. You may be pleasantly surprised!

## *Answering common breath and movement questions*

Getting the hang of breath and movement takes a bit of work when you tackle them separately, and combining them successfully can be even trickier. The following sections give you some tips on handling both.

### How much should I move and how long should I hold?

We note the number of repetitions and how long to hold them in all our recommended programs. With practice, you develop an idea of what's right for you; a lot depends on how you feel at any given moment. In general, we recommend at least three but no more than eight repetitions for a *dynamic*, or moving, posture. You can put together a program that has only moving postures, but normally we recommend a combination of both *static* (still) and dynamic postures.

We often ask you to hold a posture for 6 to 8 breaths, which translates to roughly 30 seconds. Keep breathing when you hold a posture — don't hold your breath.

### What about bouncing when I hold a stretching posture?

Now and then, we still see eager Yoga practitioners seeking to achieve better flexibility by bouncing during the holding phase of a stretching posture. This practice is part of old-school training, which really isn't such a good habit after all. Bouncing not only tends to disconnect you from the breath, but it also can be risky, especially if your muscles are stiff or not adequately warmed up. Be kind to yourself!

### How do I start combining breath with movement?

The arrows in the following exercise and wherever they appear in this book tell you the direction of postural movement and the part of the breath that goes with the movement. *Inhale* means inhalation, *exhale* means exhalation, and *breaths* means the number of breaths defining the length of a postural hold.

1. **Lie on your back comfortably, with your legs straight or bent; place your arms at your sides near your hips, with your palms turned down (see Figure 5-6a).**

2. **Inhale through your nose and, after 1 or 2 seconds, begin to slowly raise your arms over your head — in sync with inhalation — until they touch the ground behind you (see Figure 5-6b).**

    Leave your arms slightly bent.

3. **When you reach the end of inhalation, pause for 1 or 2 seconds, even if your arms don't make it to the floor; then exhale slowly through your nose and bring your arms back to your sides along the same path.**

4. **Repeat Steps 2 and 3 with a nice, slow rhythm.**

    Remember, open or expand as you inhale; fold or contract as you exhale.

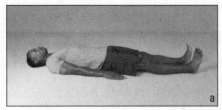 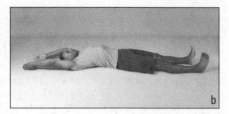

**Figure 5-6:**
The breath
surrounds
the
movement.

*Photograph by Adam Latham*

When you become comfortable with this exercise, combine it with our recommended breathing techniques from earlier in this chapter: focus breathing (which we cover in "Starting out with Focus Breathing") or any of the techniques in "Appreciating the complete yogic breath" (belly breathing, belly-to-chest breathing, or chest-to-belly breathing). You can decide which technique you prefer as you begin combining breathing with movement.

# Infusing Sound into Yogic Breathing

Sound, which is a form of vibration, is one of the means by which Yoga harmonizes the vibration of your body and mind. In fact, the repetition of special sounds is one of the oldest and most potent techniques of Yoga. Here we show you how to try this technique in conjunction with conscious breathing. A good way to start is to use the soft-sounding syllables *ah*, *ma*, and *sa*. (We're not asking you to chant, although chanting can be a great and useful experience as well.) Sound makes your exhalation longer and also tightens your abdominal muscles.

Try the following exercise while sitting in a chair or on the floor:

1. **Take a deep breath and then, as you exhale, make a long *ah* sound in a way that you find pleasing and comfortable.**

   Continue the same sound for as long as your exhalation lasts. Then take a resting breath in between and repeat the exercise five times.

2. **Relax for a few moments, and then do five repetitions with the sound *ma*.**

3. **Relax again, and conclude by making the sound *sa* five times.**

   After you complete the full cycle, sit quietly for a few minutes and notice how relaxed you feel.

## Good vibes

Yoga masters have long known that the universe is an ocean of vibrations. Some practitioners have maintained that even the ultimate reality is a state of continuous vibration — but a vibration that exceeds the three dimensions of space. Some quantum physicists call this entity a *holomovement*. The Sanskrit word for "vibration" is *spanda* (pronounced *spun-dah*). According to Yoga, the human body and mind are constantly vibrating. However, this vibration is more or less disharmonious and out of sync with the super-vibration of the *ultimate reality*. This disharmony creates unhappiness, alienation, and a sense of being separate from the physical world. The purpose of Yoga is to remove this disharmony and synchronize the body and mind with the ultimate reality, restoring joy and the sense of being connected with everyone and everything.

True yogic breathing also includes the *throat sound*, which forms part of the traditional practice of *ujjayi* (pronounced *ooh-jah-yee*), or "victorious" breath control. This more advanced technique is often mistakenly identified as sound breathing. The *ujjayi* sound is produced with the mouth closed and by breathing through the nose. By slightly constricting the throat during inhalation and exhalation, you produce a soft hissing sound similar to a distant ocean wave. This technique is easiest to pick up during exhalation; you can then gradually apply it to the inhalation phase. If you're making the sound properly, you notice a slight contraction of your abdomen. You want your exhale to be audible to you, but not to someone standing 4 feet away from you. Certainly, don't strain to the point that you make a grimace! If the throat sound doesn't happen for you right away, just leave it until later — no need to rush.

This kind of breathing stimulates the energetic center at the throat and is quite relaxing. Some evidence states that it slows the heart rate, lowers blood pressure, and induces a deeper and more restful sleep.

## *Breath Control the Traditional Way*

Hatha Yoga includes various methods of breath control, all of which belong to the more advanced practices and traditionally follow extensive purification of body and mind. Some Western teachers have incorporated these methods into their beginner classes, but our experience shows us that they're best at the intermediary to advanced levels. We believe three methods are suitable for beginners if you practice them with the necessary modifications and precautions.

Traditional Hatha Yoga emphasizes holding the breath — not a good idea for beginners. In this section, we focus on techniques that are safe for any healthy person to practice.

## Expanding the life force through Yoga

According to Yoga, the breath is just the material aspect of an energy that's far more subtle and universal. Called *prana* (pronounced *prah-nah*), which means both "breath" and "life," this energy corresponds to the Chinese concept *chi,* known to a growing number of Westerners from acupuncture and Far Eastern martial arts.

This life force underlies everything that exists and, ultimately, is the power *(shakti,* pronounced *shuk-tee)* aspect of the spirit itself. When *prana* leaves the body, a person dies. Thus, the practitioners of Hatha Yoga seek to carefully preserve the life force and enhance or expand it as much as possible. The most significant practice for doing so is *pranayama* (pronounced *prah-nah-yah-mah),* a Sanskrit term that is often incorrectly explained as consisting of *prana* and

*yama* ("control"). In fact, it drives from *prana* and *ayama* (pronounced *ah-yah-mah)* — the expansion or extension of the life force. So although the term is conveniently translated as "breath control," it's actually much more.

Science has solved many mysteries but is still puzzled about life itself. Some scientists now believe that a subtle, vital energy that can't be reduced to biochemistry does indeed operate in the body. They have named it *bioenergy* or *bioplasma.* Through Yoga, especially yogic breathing, you can come to control that energy, whatever you want to call it, in your own body. Some Yoga masters can even influence the life force in someone else's body, helping them to heal or speeding up their spiritual awakening.

The cooling methods in this section are best done in warm weather, to avoid overcooling.

## Alternate nostril breathing

Lab researchers have demonstrated what Yoga masters have known for hundreds, if not thousands, of years: Humans don't breathe evenly through both nostrils. In a 2-to-3-hour cycle, the nostrils become alternately dominant. It appears that left-nostril breathing is particularly connected with functions of the left cerebral hemisphere (notably verbal skills), and right-nostril breathing seems to connect more with the right hemisphere (notably spatial performance).

The technique called *alternate nostril breathing* goes by various others names, including *nadi-shodhana* ("channel cleansing," pronounced *nah-dee-shod-hah-nah).* The following steps help you tackle it at the beginning level:

1. **Sit comfortably on a chair or in one of the yogic sitting postures, with your back straight (see Chapter 7).**

2. **Check which nostril has the most air flowing through it, and begin alternative breathing with the open nostril.**

   If both are equally open, all the better. In that case, begin with the left nostril.

You can check which nostril is dominant simply by breathing through one nostril and then the other, and comparing the two flows.

3. **Place your right hand so that your thumb is on the right nostril and the little finger and ring finger are on the left nostril, with the index and middle fingers tucked against the ball of the thumb.**

   *Note:* According to some authorities, you place the index and middle fingers on the spot between the eyebrows (known as the *third eye*). We recommend the other method if it feels comfortable to you.

4. **Close the blocked nostril and, mentally counting to 5, inhale gently but fully through the open nostril — don't strain (see Figure 5-7).**

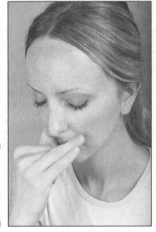

**Figure 5-7:**
Alternate
nostril
breathing.

*Photograph by Adam Latham*

5. **Open the blocked nostril and close the other nostril, and exhale, again mentally counting to 5.**

6. **Inhale through the same nostril to the count of 5, and exhale through the opposite nostril, repeating 10 to 15 times.**

As your lung capacity improves, you can make your inhalations and exhalations longer, but *never* force the breath. Gradually increase the overall duration of the exercise from, say, 3 minutes to 15 minutes.

## The cooling breath

This technique, which in Sanskrit is called *shitali* (pronounced *sheet-ah-lee*), gets its name from the cooling effect that it has on the body and the mind. Traditionally, the cooling breath is believed to remove fever, still hunger, quench thirst, and alleviate diseases of the spleen. Here's how you practice it:

1. **Sit in a comfortable Yoga posture or on a chair, and relax your body.**

2. **Curl your tongue lengthwise, and let its tip protrude from your mouth, as in Figure 5-8.**

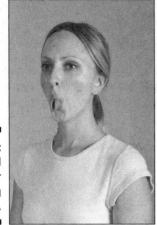

Photograph by Adam Latham

**Figure 5-8:**
Curled
tongue for
cooling
breath.

3. **Slowly suck in air through the tube your tongue forms, and exhale gently through the nose; repeat this breath 10 to 15 times.**

If you can't curl your tongue — which is a genetic ability — you can practice the Crow's Beak instead. This technique is technically known as *kaki-mudra* ("crow's gesture," pronounced *kah-kee-moo-drah*). Here you pucker your mouth, leaving just a small space for the air to pass through. Inhale through the mouth and exhale through the nose, as with *shitali*.

## *Shitkari: Inhalation through the mouth*

*Shitkari* (pronounced *sheet-kah-ree*) is another technique that calls for inhalation through the mouth, and its effects are similar to the cooling breath we discuss in the preceding section. The term means "that which makes a sucking sound." Sitting upright and relaxed, move through the following routine:

1. **Open your mouth, but keep your teeth closed, as if you're going to brush your front teeth.**

2. **Place the tip of the tongue against the palate behind the upper teeth; keep your eyes closed, and make sure you don't squint your face.**

3. **Inhale through your teeth and breathe out through your nose; repeat the inhalation and exhalation 10 to 15 times.**

If your gums are sensitive or a visit to the dentist is long overdue, avoid this practice when the air is cool.

## Kapala-bhati: Frontal sinus cleansing

*Kapala-bhati* (pronounced *kah-pah-la-bhah-tee*) literally means "skull luster" and is also known as *frontal sinus* (or *brain*) *cleansing*. The curious Sanskrit name is explained by the fact that the technique causes a sense of luminosity in the head, as well as lightheadedness, especially when you're overdoing it. Sometimes this breathing method is wrongly equated with *bhastrika* ("bellows"), which is a more advanced technique of rapid breathing, but *kapala-bhati* belongs to the preparatory practices of traditional Hatha Yoga. The technique requires rapid inhalation and exhalation through the nose with short, staccato breaths, with emphasis on exhalation.

*Kapala-bhati* is an energizing technique that you can use to combat physical or mental fatigue, so if you value your sleep, don't practice it at night. It can also warm your body (but avoid practicing this technique in cold air). Before attempting the following exercise, get the hang of relaxing your abdomen during inhalation and pulling it in during exhalation. Gradually shorten the exhalations.

1. **Sit, if you can, in a comfortable cross-legged posture, holding your spine straight and resting your hands in your lap.**

2. **Take a few deep breaths and, after your last inhalation, do 15 to 20 fast exhalations, each followed by a short inhalation, using the nose to inhale and exhale; repeat this step twice.**

   With each exhalation, which lasts only for half a second, pull in your abdomen.

If you're contracting your facial or shoulder muscles during *kapala-bhati,* you're not practicing correctly. Remember to stay relaxed and let the abdominal muscles do most of the work.

---

## I've got the whole world in my breath

According to Yoga, everyone is interconnected and part of the same single reality. You can make this abstract fact more concrete and personal when you consider the breath. Each breath you take contains about 10 sextillion atoms, which is the number 1 followed by 22 zeroes. Multiply this by 6 billion people and roughly 21,000 exhalations per day. Every time you take a breath, you inhale an average of one atom from the exhaled atoms in the atmosphere. Upon exhalation, you contribute to the collective store of exhaled breaths. Therefore, you're literally sharing other people's breaths and life energies, and they're sharing yours.

# Part II
# Moving into Position: Basic Yoga Postures

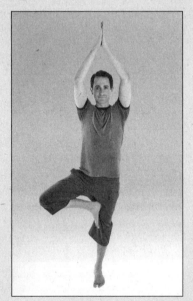
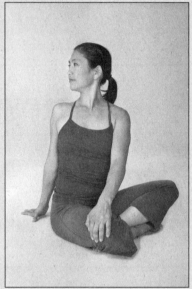
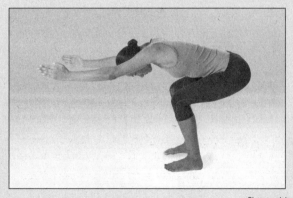

Photograph by Adam Latham

Yoga is a safe and life-enhancing practice. Yet when zeal and carelessness collide, injuries can — and do — occur from time to time. Learn how to develop safe habits from the start so you can enjoy your Yoga practice without fear of injury. Visit www.dummies.com/extras/yoga to read about avoiding common Yoga injuries.

# In this part . . .

- Ease into dozens of Hatha Yoga postures, step by step, for a safe and balanced program
- Focus on the basic categories of Yoga postures: sitting, standing, bending, twisting, balancing, inverted, and dynamic poses
- Begin your Yoga practice by following our sample beginner's routine

# Chapter 6

# Please Be Seated

Culture greatly influences the way humans sit. People in the Eastern Hemisphere favor squatting on their haunches or sitting cross-legged on the floor, but most Westerners are comfortable only sitting on chairs — as you're probably doing right now as you read this book. Actually, your everyday sitting preferences have a decided effect on your capacity to feel steady and comfortable in the Yoga postures, whether standing or sitting.

If you're new to Yoga and its sitting postures, you'll soon discover that a lifetime of chair sitting exacts a stiff price. Your work with the postures in this book can help you gradually improve your floor sitting, but until you're ready to make the transition to the floor, use a chair when you sit for formal practice. After all, two of the largest Yoga organizations in the world, The Self-Realization Fellowship (SRF) and Transcendental Meditation (TM), encourage their Western practitioners to use a chair for meditation and breathing exercises.

In this chapter, we describe the following sitting postures you can use for relaxation, meditation, breath control, and various cleansing practices — or as a starting point for other postures:

- ✔ Chair-sitting posture
- ✔ Easy posture
- ✔ Thunderbolt posture
- ✔ Auspicious posture
- ✔ Perfect posture

Yoga makes use of many other sitting postures as well; you can gradually add to your basic repertoire as your joints become more flexible and your back muscles gain strength.

# Understanding the Philosophy of Sitting

Beyond increasing strength and flexibility, Yoga postures, or *asanas* (pronounced *ah-sah-nahs*) in Sanskrit, help you get in tune with yourself, your body, and your environment. Traditional Yoga manuals tell us that the main purpose of *asana* is to prepare the body to sit quietly, easily, and steadily for breathing exercises and meditation. So when you're in the right position, you can begin to see yourself as one with your environment.

For traditional Yoga masters, *asanas* are just one part of the yogic system. Postures are the basis of the third limb of the classical eightfold path of Yoga formulated by Yoga master Patanjali. (Flip to Chapter 20 for more on the eightfold path.)

Yogic postures are more than mere bodily poses — they're also expressions of your state of mind. An *asana* is poise, composure, carriage — all words suggesting an element of balance and refinement. The postures demonstrate the profound connection between body and mind. Flopping down on a chair isn't Yoga, but when you sit with intention, awareness, and balance, it is.

Traditional Yoga experts view the body as a temple dedicated to the spirit. They believe you must keep the body pure and beautiful to honor the spiritual reality it houses. Each posture is another way of remembering the higher principle — commonly called the *spirit, divine,* or *transcendental Self* — that the body enshrines. If you prefer to practice Yoga without such ideas, you can still use posture as a way of connecting with nature because your body isn't totally isolated from its environment. Where exactly does your body

## Asana by any other name

The term *asana* simply means "sitting." It can denote both the surface you sit on and the bodily posture. An alternative term is *tirtha,* or "pilgrimage center," which suggests that practitioners should approach Yoga postures not casually, but respectfully, with great mental focus.

Some postures are called *mudras* (pronounced *moo-drahs*), or "seals," because they're especially effective in keeping the life energy *(prana)* sealed within the body. Adopting these postures leads to greater vitality and better mental focus. Life energy is everywhere, both inside and outside the body, but you must properly harness it within the body to promote health and happiness.

end, and where exactly does the surrounding space begin? How much does your body's electromagnetic field extend beyond your skin? How far away did the oxygen particles that are now part of your body originate?

The way you sit is an important foundation technique for these practices; when you perform them properly, the sitting postures act as natural "tranquilizers" for the body — and when the physical vehicle is still, the mind soon follows.

If your knees are more than a few inches higher than your hips when you sit cross-legged on the floor, it's an indication that your hip joints are tight. If you try to sit for a long time in this position for meditation or breathing exercises, you may well end up with an aching back. Don't feel bad — you're not alone. Accept your current limitations in this area, and use a prop, like a firm cushion or thickly folded blanket, to raise your buttocks off the floor high enough to drop your knees at least level with your hips.

If you attend a lecture or other special gathering at a Hatha Yoga center, remember that few, if any, chairs are usually available, so be prepared to sit on the floor. If you aren't accustomed to sitting cross-legged on the floor with an unsupported back, bring along a prop, such as a firm cushion or a blanket, to raise your buttocks (see Chapter 19). Arrive early so that you can find a wall or post to sit against to support your back. If none of these ideas sits well with you (no pun intended), just bring your own folding chair and sit near the rear of the room.

# Adding Varity to Your Sitting Postures

Some contemporary Hatha Yoga manuals feature more than 50 sitting postures, which demonstrate not only the inventiveness of Yoga practitioners, but also the body's amazing versatility. But half a dozen yogic sitting postures is plenty for your repertoire . The following sections describe some good sitting postures and show you how to execute them.

For postures that involve sitting on the floor, raising your buttocks off the floor on a firm cushion or thickly folded blanket is helpful because it allows you to sit in a comfortable and stable position without slumping.

Be sure to alternate the cross of your legs from day to day when practicing any of the sitting postures — you don't want to become lopsided.

## Chair-sitting posture

Cultural habits inspire most Westerners to sit in a chair when they meditate, so floor sitting is usually something folks have to work up to with practice. Over time, your *asana* practice can help you build comfort with sitting on the floor for exercises. As Figure 6-1 shows, your ear, shoulder, and hip are in alignment, as viewed from the side. The following steps walk you through the chair-sitting posture:

1. **Use a sturdy armless chair, and sit near the front edge of the seat without leaning against the chair back.**

   Make sure your feet are flat on the floor. If they don't quite reach, support them with a block, folded blanket, or phone book.

2. **Rest your hands on your knees with your palms down, and then close your eyes.**

3. **Rock your spine a few times, alternately slumping forward and arching back to explore its full range of motion.**

   Settle into a comfortable upright position midway between the two extremes.

4. **Lift your chest, without exaggerating the gentle inward curve in your lower back, and balance your head over your torso.**

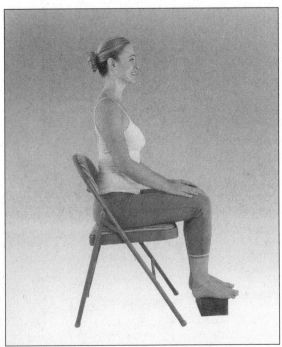

**Figure 6-1:**
The chair-sitting posture.

*Photograph by Adam Latham*

# The easy posture: Sukhasana

According to Yoga master Patanjali, a posture must be "steady" *(sthira)* and "easeful" *(sukha)*. The basic Yoga sitting position is called, appropriately, the easy/easeful posture *(sukhasana)*; Westerners sometimes call it the *tailor's seat.* We strongly recommend that beginners start their floor sitting practice with the easy posture, which Figure 6-2 illustrates.

The easy posture is a steady and comfortable sitting position for meditation and breathing exercises. The posture also helps you become more aware of and actually increase the flexibility in your hips and spine. It's good preparation for more advanced postures.

Here's how it works:

1. **Sit on the floor with your legs straight out in front of you; place your hands on the floor beside your hips, with your palms down and fingers pointing forward.**

   Shake your legs up and down a few times to get the kinks out.

2. **Cross your legs at the ankles with the left leg on top and the right leg below.**

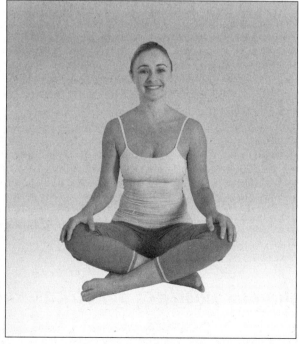

**Figure 6-2:**
Be sure you're steady and comfortable in the easy posture.

*Photograph by Adam Latham*

3. **Press your palms on the floor, and slide each foot toward the opposite knee until your right foot is underneath your left knee and your left foot is underneath your right knee.**

4. **Lengthen the spine by stretching your back in an upward motion, and balance your head over your torso.**

*Note:* In the classic (traditionally taught) posture, you drop your chin to your chest, extend your arms, and lock your elbows. We recommend, however, that you rest your hands on your knees with your palms down and elbows bent, and keep your head upright; that modification is more relaxing for beginners.

## The thunderbolt posture: Vajrasana

The thunderbolt posture is one of the safest sitting postures for students with back problems. *Vajrasana* increases the flexibility of your ankles, knees, and thighs; improves circulation to the abdomen; and aids in digestion.

Use the following steps to practice this posture:

1. **Kneel on the floor and sit back on your heels; position each heel under the buttocks on the same side, and rest your hands on the tops of your knees, with your elbows bent and your palms down.**

2. **Lengthen your spine by stretching your back in an upward motion, balance your head over your torso, and look straight ahead, as in Figure 6-3.**

*Note:* In the classic posture, which we don't recommend for beginners, the chin rests on the upper chest, and the arms extend until the elbows are locked and the hands are on the knees.

If you have trouble sitting back on your heels because of tightness in your thigh muscles or pain in your knees, put a cushion or folded blanket between your thighs and calves. Increase the thickness of your lift until you can sit comfortably. If you feel discomfort in the fronts of your ankles, put a rolled towel or blanket underneath them.

The Sanskrit word *vajra* (pronounced *vahj-rah*) means "thunderbolt" or "adamantine." So this posture is also known as the *adamantine posture*.

## The auspicious posture: Svastikasana

Before its perversion in Nazi Germany, the *svastika* served as a solar symbol for good fortune. It has the same meaning in Yoga. The term is made up of the prefix *su* ("good") and *asti* ("is") — hence, "It's good."

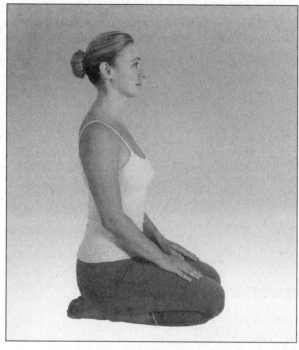

**Figure 6-3:**
A safe
sitting
posture for
lower back
problems.

*Photograph by Adam Latham*

The *svastikasana* improves the flexibility of the hips, knees, and ankles and also strengthens the back. The following instructions help you get the hang of this posture.

Use the preparation series for advanced sitting postures in Chapter 6 to improve your performance for this posture.

1. **Sit on the floor with your legs straight out in front of you; place your hands on the floor beside your hips, with your palms down and fingers pointing forward.**

   Shake your legs up and down a few times to get the kinks out.

2. **Bend your left knee, and place the sole of your left foot against the inside of your right thigh, with your left heel close to your groin.**

   If this step is difficult, don't use this pose.

3. **Bend your right knee toward you, and take hold of your right foot with both hands.**

4. **Grip the front of your ankle with your right hand and the ball of your big toe with your left hand; slide the little-toe side of your foot between your left thigh and calf until only your big toe is visible, and wiggle the big-toe side of your left foot up between the right thigh and calf, if you can.**

5. **Rest your hands on your knees, with your arms relaxed and palms down.**

6. **Lengthen your spine by stretching your back in an upward motion, balance your head over your torso, and look straight ahead, as in Figure 6-4.**

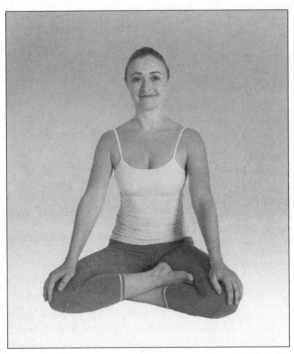

**Figure 6-4:**
The auspicious posture.

*Photograph by Adam Latham*

*Note:* In the classic posture, the chin rests on the chest with the arms straight down and palms open in *jnana mudra* at the knees. The bottom (left) foot is pulled up and wedged between the right calf and the thigh.

*Jnana mudra* (pronounced *gyah-nah moo-drah*), or "wisdom seal," is one of several hand positions used in Yoga. To do this *mudra*, bring the tip of your index finger to the tip of your thumb to form a circle; extend the three remaining fingers, keeping them close together (as in Figure 6-5). This hand gesture makes a good circuit, sealing off the life energy *(prana)* in your body. (Check out Chapter 5 for more on *prana*.)

## The perfect posture: Siddhasana

The Sanskrit word *siddha* (pronounced *sidd-hah*) means both "perfect" and "adept." In Yoga, an *adept* isn't just a skillful practitioner, but an accomplished master who has attained inner freedom.

Many Yoga masters in bygone eras preferred this posture and used it often in place of the lotus posture. We don't cover either the half lotus or the full lotus position in this book because they're suitable only for more experienced students.

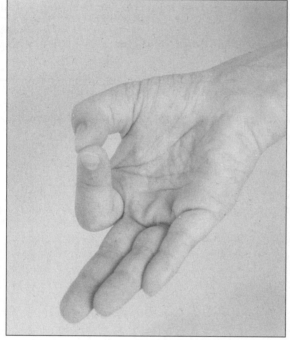

**Figure 6-5:**
This hand
position
seals in
life energy
called
*prana*.

*Photograph by Adam Latham*

The *siddhasana* improves the flexibility of your hips, knees, and ankles, and strengthens the back. It differs from svastikasana, in that you tuck your feet into your thighs between the thighs and calves on both sides. The posture is considered the perfect meditation posture for anyone practicing celibacy. Siddhasana is also beneficial for men with various prostate problems.

The preparation series for advanced sitting postures in Chapter 6 can help you with this posture.

Here's how you do it:

1. **Sitting on the floor with your legs straight out in front of you, place your hands at your sides (close to your hips), with your palms down and fingers forward.**

   Shake your legs out in front of you a few times.

2. **Bend your left knee, and bring your left heel into your groin near the *perineum* (the area between the anus and the genitals).**

   Stabilize your left ankle with your left hand.

3. Bend your right knee and slide your right heel toward the front of your left ankle.

4. Lift your right foot, position your right ankle just above your left ankle, and bring your right heel into the genital area.

5. Tuck the little-toe side of your right foot between your left thigh and your calf.

6. Place your hands, palms down, on the same-side knee, with your arms relaxed.

7. Straighten and extend your back and neck, bringing your head up nice and tall; look straight ahead, as in Figure 6-6.

You can use a cushion to raise your hips so they're level with your knees.

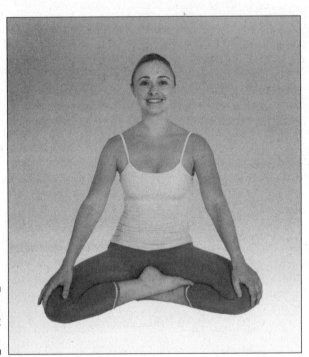

**Figure 6-6:**
The perfect
posture.

*Photograph by Adam Latham*

***Note:*** In the classic posture, which we don't recommend for beginners, the chin rests on the chest, the arms are straight down, the elbows are locked, and the palms are open in *jnana mudra* (which we discuss in the preceding section) at the knees. The big-toe side of the left foot is pulled up and wedged between the right calf and the thigh.

# Chapter 7

# Standing Tall

*In This Chapter*

▶ Standing as an art

▶ Using standing postures to enhance body and mind

▶ Practicing fundamental standing postures

Standing upright is a uniquely human trait, and Yoga is a uniquely human practice. In this chapter, we discuss standing from the Yoga perspective, with an emphasis on the difference between just standing and the more quintessential version of standing. The simple act of standing upright brings your spine, muscles, tendons, and ligaments into play. Ordinarily, these parts do their assigned tasks quite automatically. But to stand efficiently and elegantly, you also need to bring awareness to the act, and that's where Yoga enters the picture.

In this chapter, we give you ten of the most common and favored Yoga standing postures to practice. They can help you discover the art of standing consciously, efficiently, and beautifully.

## Standing Strong

We are human in large part because, hundreds of thousands of years ago, our ancestors figured out how to literally stand on their own two feet. Appropriately, the yogic standing postures make up the foundation of *asana* practice.

The way you stand says a lot about you. These days, a person who stands tall usually sucks in the belly and sticks out the chest and chin in military fashion. But you can stand tall and straight and be relaxed at the same time.

---

# You're grounded!

Calling yogic standing posture an *asana*, or "seat," may seem contradictory, but the posture helps you become firmly grounded. In Yoga, grounding is as important as reaching up. You can reach the heights of Yoga only when you're as sturdy as a mountain or a sequoia.

---

Body and mind form a unit; they're the outside and inside of the same person: you. In a way, your body is a map of your mind. Through regular Yoga practice, you can use the feedback from your body to discipline your mind, and use the feedback from your mind (particularly your emotions) to train your body.

The standing postures are a kind of microcosm of the practice of *asana* as a whole (except for inversions, or upside-down postures, which Chapter 10 explores); you may hear that you can derive everything you need to know to master your physical practice from the standing postures. The standing postures help you strengthen your legs and ankles, open your hips and groin, and improve your sense of balance. In turn, you develop the ability to "stand your ground" and "stand at ease," which are important aspects of the yogic lifestyle.

The standing postures are versatile. You can use them in the following ways:

- ✔ As a general warm-up for your practice.
- ✔ In preparation for a specific group of postures (we like to think of the standing forward bends, for example, as a kind of on-ramp to the seated forward bends).
- ✔ For compensation (or to counterbalance another posture, such as a back bend or side bend). For more information, see Chapter 15.
- ✔ For rest.
- ✔ As the main body of your practice.

You can creatively adapt many postures from other groups to a standing position, which you can then use as a learning (or teaching) tool, or for therapeutic purposes. Consider, for example, the well-known cobra posture, a back bend that many beginning students find hard on the lower back (see Chapter 11). By performing this same posture in a standing position near a wall, you can use the changed relationship to gravity, the freedom of not having your hips blocked by the floor, and the pressure of the hands on the wall to free your lower back. Then you can apply this newly won understanding about your back in your practice of the more demanding traditional form of the cobra posture — or any other posture that you choose to modify at the wall.

# *Exercising Your Standing Options*

In this section, we introduce you to ten standing postures and describe the step-by-step process for each exercise. We also discuss the benefits and the classic (traditionally taught) version of the posture. We don't recommend the classic version for beginners because, in most cases, the postures are more difficult and sometimes risky. Here are a few tips before you get started with the standing postures:

- Many of these postures start in the mountain posture, so be sure to check out the "Mountain posture: Tadasana" section.

- When you try the postures on your own, follow the instructions for each exercise carefully, including the breathing. Always move into and out of the posture slowly and pause after the inhalation and exhalation (flip to Chapter 5 for more on breathing). Complete each posture by relaxing and returning to the starting place.

- When you bend forward from all the standing postures, start with your legs straight (without locking your knees), and then soften your knees when you feel the muscles pulling in the back of your legs.

- When you come up out of a standing forward bend, choose one of three ways:

  - The easiest and safest way is to roll your body up like a rag doll, stacking your vertebrae one on top of the other, with your head coming up last.

  - The next level of difficulty is to bring your arms up from the sides like wings as you inhale and raise your back.

  - The third and most challenging way is to start with the inhalation and extend your arms forward and up alongside your ears. Then continue raising the upper, middle, and lower back until you're straight up and your arms are overhead, if possible.

## *Mountain posture: Tadasana*

The mountain posture is the foundation for all the standing postures. *Tadasana* aligns the body, improves posture and balance, and facilitates breathing.

1. **Stand tall but relaxed, with your feet at hip width (down from the sits bones, not the outer curves), and hang your arms at your sides, with your palms turned toward your legs.**

The *sits bones*, also know as the *ischial tuberosity,* are the bony parts you feel underneath you when you sit up straight on a firm surface.

2. **Visualize a vertical line connecting the opening in your ear, your shoulder joint, and the sides of your hip, knee, and ankle.**

   Look straight ahead, with your eyes open or closed, as in Figure 7-1.

3. **Remain in this posture for 6 to 8 breaths.**

*Note:* In the classic version of this posture, the feet are together and the chin rests on the chest.

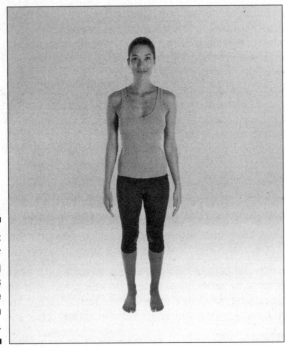

**Figure 7-1:** Start your standing postures with the mountain posture.

*Photograph by Adam Latham*

## Standing forward bend: Uttanasana

The Sanskrit word *uttana* (pronounced *oo-tah-nah*) means "extended," and this posture certainly fits that bill. The standing forward bend (see Figure 7-2) stretches the entire back of the body and decompresses the neck (makes space between the vertebrae). When a person stands in an upright posture, the cervical spine and the neck muscles work hard to balance the head. Because most people generally don't pay enough attention to this part of their anatomy, they tend to accumulate a lot of tension in their necks, which can lead to headaches. This posture frees the cervical spine and allows the neck muscles to relax. It also improves overall circulation and has a calming effect on the body and mind. The following steps walk you through the process.

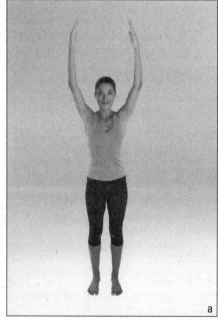 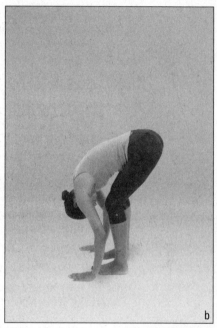

**Figure 7-2:**
The standing forward bend.

a

b

*Photograph by Adam Latham*

Be careful of all forward bends if you're having a disc problem. If you're unsure, check with your doctor or health professional.

1. **Start in mountain posture and, as you inhale, raise your arms forward and then up overhead (see Figure 7-2a).**

2. **As you exhale, bend forward from your hips.**

   When you feel a pull in the back of your legs, soften your knees (as in the Forgiving Limbs discussion in Chapter 3) and hang your arms.

3. **If your head isn't close to your knees, bend your knees more.**

   If you have the flexibility, straighten your knees but keep them soft. Relax your head and neck downward, as Figure 7-2b illustrates.

4. **As you inhale, roll up slowly, stacking the bones of your spine one at a time from bottom to top, and then raise your arms overhead.**

   Rolling is the safest way to come up. If you don't have back problems, after a few weeks, you may want to try the two more advanced techniques we discuss earlier in the section.

5. **Repeat Steps 1 through 4 three times, and then stay in the folded position (Step 3) for 6 to 8 breaths.**

*Note:* In the classic posture, the feet are together and the legs are straight. The forehead presses against the shins, and the palms are on the floor.

## Half standing forward bend: Ardha uttanasana

The Sanskrit word *ardha* (pronounced *ahrd-ha*) means "half." The half standing forward bend strengthens your legs, back, shoulders, and arms, and improves stamina.

1. **Start in the mountain posture and, as you inhale, raise your arms forward and then up overhead, as in the standing forward bend (see the preceding section).**

2. **As you exhale, bend forward from your hips; soften your knees and hang your arms.**

3. **Bend your knees and, as you inhale, raise your torso and arms up from the front so that they're parallel to the floor, as in Figure 7-3.**

   If you have any back problems, keep your arms back by your sides; then over a period of time, gradually stretch them out to the sides like a *T* and eventually in front of you so they're parallel to the floor.

4. **Bring your head to a neutral position so that your ears are between your arms; look down and a little forward.**

   To make the posture easier, move your arms back toward your hips instead of having them extend forward or out to the sides — the farther back, the easier.

5. **Repeat Steps 1 through 4 three times, and then stay in Step 4 for 6 to 8 breaths.**

*Note:* In the classic version of this posture, the feet are together and the legs and arms are straight.

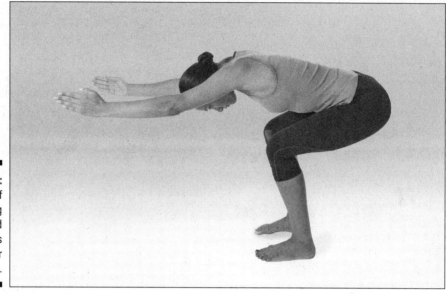

**Figure 7-3:**
The half standing forward bend is great for stamina.

*Photograph by Adam Latham*

# Asymmetrical forward bend: Parshva uttanasana

The asymmetrical forward bend stretches each side of the back and hamstrings separately. The Sanskrit word *parshva* (pronounced *pahr-shvah*) means "side" or "flank," and this posture indeed opens the hips, tones the abdomen, decompresses the neck, improves balance, and increases circulation to the upper torso and head.

1. **Stand in the mountain posture and, as you exhale, step forward about 3 to 3 ½ feet (or the length of one leg) with your right foot.**

   Your left foot turns out naturally, but if you need more stability, turn it out even more — but not past 45 degrees.

2. **Place your hands on the top of your hips, and square the front of your pelvis; release your hands and hang your arms.**

3. **As you inhale, raise your arms forward and then overhead, as in Figure 7-4a.**

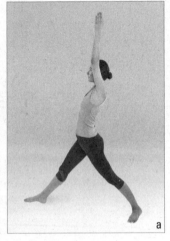
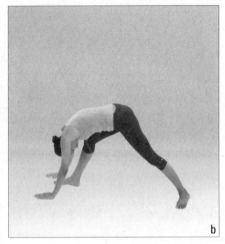

**Figure 7-4:**
This exercise stretches each side of the back and hamstrings separately.

a

b

*Photograph by Adam Latham*

4. **As you exhale, bend forward from the hips, soften your right knee and both arms, and hang down, as Figure 7-4b illustrates.**

   If your head isn't close to your right knee, bend your knee more. If you have the flexibility, straighten your right knee — but keep it soft.

5. **As you inhale, roll up slowly, stacking the bones of your spine one at a time from the bottom up, and then raise your arms overhead; relax your head and neck downward.**

   Rolling up is the safest way to come up, but if you don't have back problems, you may want to try the more advanced techniques we cover earlier in the section after a few weeks.

6. **Repeat Steps 3 and 4 three times, and then stay in Step 4 for 6 to 8 breaths.**

7. **Repeat the same sequence on the left side.**

*Note:* In the classic version of this posture, both legs are straight and the forehead presses against the forward leg.

To make the posture more challenging, square your hips forward and rotate your back foot inward.

## Triangle posture: Utthita trikonasana

The Sanskrit word *utthita* (pronounced *oot-hee-tah*) means "raised," and *trikona* (pronounced *tree-ko-nah*) means "triangle." The latter term is often mispronounced as *try-ko-nah*. The triangle posture stretches the sides of the spine, the backs of the legs, and the hips. It also stretches the muscles between the ribs (the *intercostals*), which opens the chest and improves breathing capacity.

1. **Stand in the mountain posture, exhale, and step out to the right about 3 to 3 ½ feet (or the length of one leg) with your right foot.**

2. **Turn your right foot out 90 degrees. On your left foot, have your toes turned slightly in rather than straight ahead.**

    An imaginary line drawn from the right heel (toward the left foot) should bisect the arch of the left foot.

3. **Face forward and, as you inhale, raise your arms out to the sides parallel to the line of the shoulders (and the floor) so that they form a *T* with your torso (see Figure 7-5a).**

4. **As you exhale, reach your right hand down to your right shin as close to the ankle as is comfortable for you, and then reach and lift your left arm; as much as you can, bring the sides of your torso parallel to the floor.**

    Bend your right knee slightly, as in Figure 7-5b, if the back of your leg feels tight.

5. **Soften your left arm and look up at your left hand.**

    If your neck hurts, look down or halfway down at the floor.

6. **Repeat Steps 3 through 5 three times, and then stay in Step 5 for 6 to 8 breaths.**

7. **Repeat the same sequence on the left side.**

*Note:* In the classic version of this posture, the arms and legs are straight and the trunk is parallel to the floor. The right hand is on the floor outside the right foot.

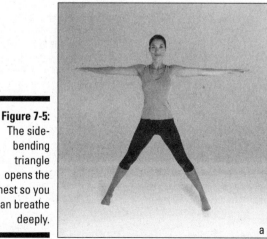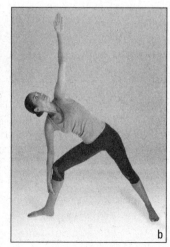

**Figure 7-5:** The side-bending triangle opens the chest so you can breathe deeply.

a

b

*Photograph by Adam Latham*

## Reverse triangle posture: Parivritta trikonasana variation

The Sanskrit word *parivritta* (pronounced *pah-ree-vree-tah*) means "revolved," which makes perfect sense with this posture. You can compare the action of twists, including the reverse triangle, on the discs between the spinal vertebrae (intervertebral discs) to the action of squeezing and then releasing a wet sponge: First you squeeze out the dirty water, and then you sponge up the clean water. The action of twisting and untwisting increases circulation of fresh blood to these discs and keeps them supple as you grow older. The reverse triangle also stretches the backs of your legs, opens your hips, and strengthens your neck, shoulders, and arms.

1. **Standing in the mountain posture, exhale and step the right foot out to the right about 3 to 3 ½ feet (or the length of one leg).**

2. **As you inhale, raise your arms out to the sides parallel to the line of your shoulders (and the floor) so that they form a *T* with your torso, as Figure 7-6a illustrates.**

3. **As you exhale, bend forward from your hips and then place your right hand on the floor near the inside of your left foot.**

4. **Raise your left arm toward the ceiling and look up at your left hand; soften your knees and your arms, and then bend your left knee, or move your right hand away from your left foot (and more directly under your torso), as in Figure 7-6b, if necessary.**

If you feel neck strain, turn your head toward the floor.

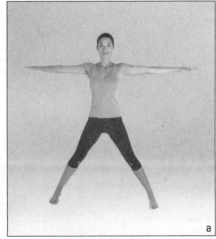 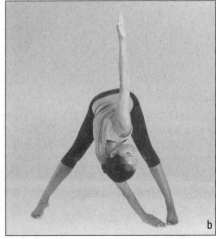

**Figure 7-6:**
The reverse triangle posture.

a

b

*Photograph by Adam Latham*

5. **Repeat Steps 2 through 4 three times, and then stay in Step 4 for 6 to 8 breaths.**

6. **Repeat the same sequence on the left side.**

*Note:* In the classic version of this posture, the feet are parallel and the legs and arms are straight. The torso is parallel to the floor, and the bottom hand rests lightly outside the opposite side foot.

# Warrior 1: Vira bhadrasana 1

The Sanskrit word *vira* (pronounced *vee-rah*) is often translated as "hero," and *bhadra* (pronounced *bhud-rah*) means "auspicious." This posture, also known as just *warrior*, strengthens your legs, back, shoulders, and arms; opens your hips, groin, and chest; increases strength and stamina; and improves balance. As its name suggests, this posture instills a feeling of fearlessness and inner strength.

1. **Stand in the mountain posture and, as you exhale, step forward approximately 3 to 3 ½ feet (or the length of one leg) with your right foot (see Figure 7-7a).**

   Your left foot turns out naturally, but if you need more stability, turn it out more (so that your toes point to the left).

2. **Place your hands on the top of your hips, and square the front of your pelvis; release your hands and hang your arms.**

3. **As you inhale, raise your arms forward and overhead, and bend your right knee to a right angle (so that your knee is directly over your ankle and your thigh is parallel to the floor), as in Figure 7-7b.**

   If your lower back is uncomfortable, lean your torso slightly over your forward leg until you feel a release of tension in your back.

4. **As you exhale, return to the starting place in Figure 7-7a; soften your arms and face your palms toward each other, and look straight ahead.**

5. **Repeat Steps 3 and 4 three times, and then stay in Step 3 for 6 to 8 breaths.**

6. **Repeat Steps 1 through 5 on the left side.**

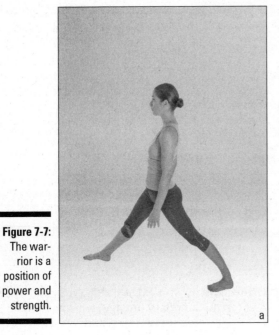
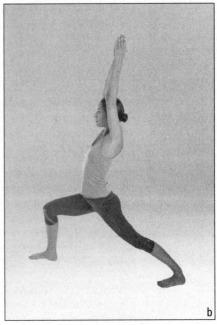

**Figure 7-7:**
The warrior is a position of power and strength.

*Photograph by Adam Latham*

# Warrior II: Vira bhadrasana II

Like the warrior I posture we cover in the preceding section, warrior II strengthens your legs, back, shoulders, and arms. It focuses more on your hips and groin, and it increases strength and stamina; it also improves balance. Use the following steps as your guide.

1. **Stand in the mountain posture; exhale and step out to the right about 3 to 3 ½ feet (or the length of one leg) with your right foot.**

2. **Turn your right foot out 90 degrees, and have the toes of your left foot turned slightly in rather than forward.**

   An imaginary line drawn from your right heel toward your left foot should bisect the arch of your left foot.

3. **Face forward and, as you inhale, raise your arms out to the sides, parallel to the line of your shoulders (and the floor), so that they form a *T* with your torso (see Figure 7-8a).**

4. As you exhale, turn your right foot out 90 degrees and bend your right knee over your right ankle so that your shin is perpendicular to the floor, as in Figure 7-8b; if possible, bring your right thigh parallel to the floor.

5. Repeat Steps 3 and 4 three times, keeping your arms in a T; then turn your head to the right, looking out over your right arm, and stay for 6 to 8 breaths.

6. Repeat Steps 1 through 5 on the left side.

Be careful not to force your hips open — it may cause problems with your knees.

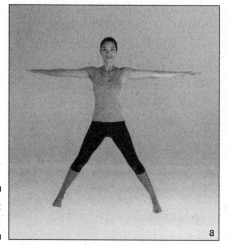
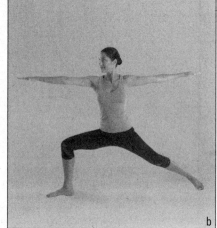

**Figure 7-8:**
Warrior II.

a

b

*Photograph by Adam Latham*

# Standing spread-legged forward bend: *Prasarita pada uttanasana*

The Sanskrit word *prasarita* (pronounced *prah-sah-ree-tah*) means "outstretched," and *pada* (pronounced *pah-dah*) means "foot." This posture, also called the wide-legged standing forward bend, stretches your hamstrings and your *adductors* (on the insides of the thighs) and opens your hips. The hanging forward bend increases circulation to your upper torso and lengthens your spine. Figure 7-9 illustrates this posture.

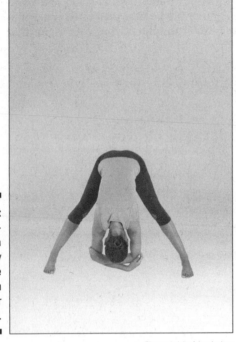

**Figure 7-9:**
This posture is a great way to release pressure in your lower back.

*Photograph by Adam Latham*

1. **Stand in the mountain posture, exhale, and step your right foot out to the right about 3 to 3½ feet (or the length of one leg).**

2. **As you inhale, raise your arms out to the sides, parallel to the line of your shoulders (and the floor), so that they form a *T* with your torso.**

3. **As you exhale, bend forward from the hips and soften your knees.**

4. **Hold your bent elbows with the opposite-side hands, and hang your torso and arms.**

5. **Stay in Step 4 for 6 to 8 breaths.**

*Note:* In the classic version of this posture, the legs are straight, the head is on the floor (and the chin presses the chest), and the arms reach back between the legs, with the palms on the floor.

## Half chair posture: Ardha utkatasana

The Sanskrit word *ardha* (pronounced *ahrd-ha*) means "half," and *utkata*, (pronounced *oot-kah-tah*) translates as "extraordinary." The half chair posture strengthens the back, legs, shoulders, and arms, and builds overall stamina. If you find this posture difficult or you have problem knees, you may want to skip this position for now and return to it after your leg muscles become a little stronger. Don't overdo this exercise (either by holding the position too long or by repeating it more than we recommend), or you'll have sore muscles the next day. But there's no harm in experiencing some muscle soreness, either, especially if you haven't exercised in a long time. Check out Figure 7-10 for guidance.

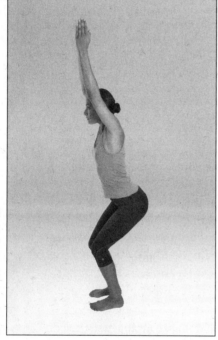

**Figure 7-10:** The half chair is a great posture for overall stamina.

*Photograph by Adam Latham*

1. **Start in the mountain posture and, as you inhale, raise your arms forward and up overhead, with your palms facing each other.**

2. **As you exhale, bend your knees and squat halfway to the floor.**

3. **Soften your arms, but keep them overhead; look straight ahead.**

4. **Repeat Steps 1 through 3 three times, and then stay in Step 3 for 6 to 8 breaths.**

*Note:* In the classic version of this posture, the feet are together and the arms are straight, with the fingers interlocked and the palms turned upward. The chin rests on the chest.

# Downward-facing dog: Adhomukha shvanasana

The Sanskrit word *adhomukha* (pronounced *ahd-ho-mook-hah*) means "downward facing," and *shvan* (pronounced *shvahn*) means "dog." Yoga masters were great observers of the world around them. They particularly noticed the behavior of animals, which is why the dog's leisurely stretching inspired them to create a similar posture for humans. The practice of downward-facing dog stretches the entire back of your body and strengthens your wrists, arms, and shoulders. This posture is a good alternative for beginning students who aren't yet ready for inversions like the handstand and headstand. Because the head is lower than the heart, this *asana* circulates fresh blood to the brain and acts as a quick pick-me-up when you're fatigued.

1. **Start on your hands and knees; straighten your arms, but don't lock your elbows (see Figure 7-11a).**

   Be sure that the heels of your hands are directly under your shoulders, with your palms on the floor, your fingers spread, and your knees directly under your hips. Emphasize pressing down with the thumbs and index fingers, or the inner web of your hand.

2. **As you exhale, lift and straighten (but don't lock) your knees; as your hips lift, bring your head to a neutral position so that your ears are between your arms.**

3. **Press your heels toward the floor and your head toward your feet, as in Figure 7-11b.**

   If your hamstrings feel tight, try putting a little bend in your knees to help you straighten your spine.

   Don't complete this step if doing so strains your neck.

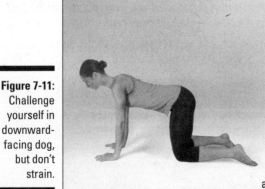
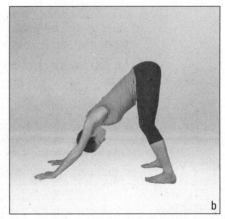

**Figure 7-11:** Challenge yourself in downward-facing dog, but don't strain.

*Photograph by Adam Latham*

4. **Repeat Steps 1 through 3 three times, and then stay in Step 3 for 6 to 8 breaths.**

*Note:* In the classic posture, the feet are together and flat on the floor, the legs and arms are straight, and the top of the head is on the floor, with the chin pressed to the chest.

Be careful not to hold this posture too long if you have problems with your neck, shoulders, wrists, or elbows.

# Chapter 8

# Steady as a Tree: Mastering Balance

. . . . . . . . . . . . . . . . . . . . . . . . . . . . . . . . . . . . . . . . . . . . . . . . . . . . . . . . . .

## In This Chapter

▶ Understanding the psychology of balance

▶ Practicing balancing exercises

. . . . . . . . . . . . . . . . . . . . . . . . . . . . . . . . . . . . . . . . . . . . . . . . . . . . . . . . . .

*B*alance (called *samata* [sah-mah-tah] or *samatva* [sah-mah-tvah] in Sanskrit) is fundamental to Yoga. A balanced approach to life includes being even-tempered and seeing the great unity behind all diversity. Balance translates to being nonjudgmental and treating others with equal fairness, kindness, and compassion.

One way to begin to gain this balance is to practice balancing postures. Remember, according to Yoga, body and mind form a working unit. Imbalances in the body are reflected in the mind, and vice versa. This chapter emphasizes the importance of balance in Yoga and offers six postures that provide you with a *samata* sampling.

## Getting to the Roots of the Posture

When you look at a tree, you see only what is above ground — the vertical trunk, with its crown of branches and foliage, and maybe a few chirping birds. Trees appear to just perch atop the soil, and you wonder how in the world such a top-heavy thing can stay upright.

Well, everyone knows that the secret of the tree's equilibrium is its underground network of roots that anchor the visible part of the plant solidly into the earth. In the balancing postures, you, too, can discover how to grow your "roots" into the earth and stand as steady as a tree.

For us, the balancing postures can be the most fun and the most dramatic of all the postures. Although they're relatively simple, the postures can produce profound effects. As you may expect, they work to improve your overall sense of physical balance, coordination, and grounding. With awareness in these three areas, you can move more easily and effectively, whether you're going about your daily business or are engaged in activities that call for great coordination, such as sports or dance. The yogic balancing postures also have therapeutic applications, such as with back problems or in retraining whole muscle groups.

When you improve your physical balance naturally, you can expect to enjoy improved mental balance. The balancing postures are exceptional seeds for concentration, and when you master them, you earn confidence and a sense of accomplishment.

# Balancing Postures for Graceful Strength

Contemporary life is highly demanding and stressful; if you're not properly grounded, you face a constant risk of being pushed out of balance. *Grounding* means being centered and firm without being inflexible, knowing who you are and what you want, and feeling that you're empowered to achieve your life goals. A good way to begin your grounding work is to improve your physical sense of balance. Improving your balance helps you synchronize the movement of your arms and legs, giving you poise. When you can stand and move in a more balanced manner, your mind is automatically affected. You *feel* more balanced.

A sense of balance is connected with the inner ears. Your ears tell you where you are in space. The ears are also connected with *social space*; if you aren't well balanced, you may feel — or actually *be* — a bit awkward in your social relationships. Balancing and grounding work can remedy this discomfort. Only when you can stand still — in balance — can you also move harmoniously in the world.

The following postures appear in order of ease, starting with simple exercises and moving to more advanced ones. If you try the postures individually instead of as part of a sequence, we recommend that you hold each posture for 6 to 8 breaths. Breathe freely through the nose, and pause briefly after inhalation and exhalation.

# *Warrior at the wall: Vira bhadrasana III variation*

The Sanskrit word *vira* (pronounced *vee-rah*) means "hero." *Bhadra* (pronounced *bhud-rah*) means "auspicious." This posture improves your overall balance and stability. It strengthens the legs, arms, and shoulders, and stretches the thighs — both front and back — and the hips. As with the other one-legged balancing poses, this posture enhances focus and concentration. Check out the following steps:

1. **Stand in the mountain posture (see Chapter 7), facing a blank wall about 3 feet away.**

2. **As you exhale, bend forward from the hips and extend your arms forward until your hands are touching the wall; adjust so that your legs are perpendicular and your torso and arms are parallel with the floor.**

   Depending on your balance, you may prefer to have your palms flat against the wall or touch only with your fingertips.

3. **As you inhale, raise your left leg back and up until it's parallel to the floor (see Figure 8-1).**

4. **Stay in Step 3 for 6 to 8 breaths; repeat with the right leg.**

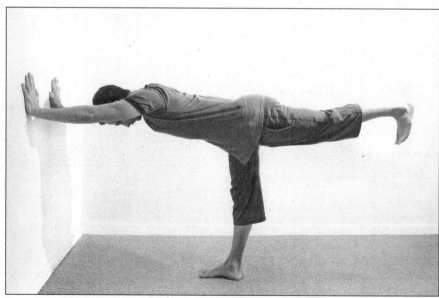

**Figure 8-1:**
A safe balancing posture for beginners.

*Photograph by Adam Latham*

# Balancing cat

The balancing cat posture strengthens the muscles along the spine (the *para-spinals*), as well as the arms and the shoulders, and it opens the hips. The posture enhances focus and concentration and also builds confidence.

1. Beginning on your hands and knees, position your hands directly under your shoulders, with your palms down, your fingers spread on the floor, and your knees directly under your hips; straighten your arms, but don't lock your elbows.

2. As you exhale, slide your left hand forward and your right leg back, keeping your hand and your toes on the floor.

3. As you inhale, raise your left arm and right leg to a comfortable height, as Figure 8-2 illustrates.

4. Stay in Step 3 for 6 to 8 breaths, and then repeat Steps 1 through 3 with opposite pairs (right arm and left leg).

This posture is a variation of *cakravakasana* (pronounced *chuk-rah-vahk-ah-sah-nah*). The *cakravaka* is a particular kind of goose, which, in India's traditional poetry, is often used to convey "love bird." Apparently, when these birds have paired up and then are separated, their heartache causes them to call to each other.

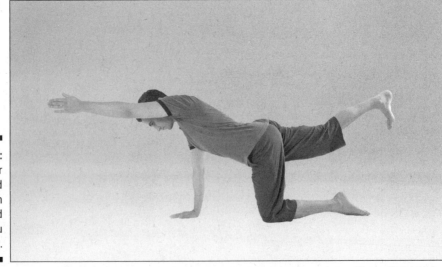

**Figure 8-2:**
Extend your arm and leg fully on the ground before you lift them.

*Photograph by Adam Latham*

# The tree posture: Vrikshasana

The Sanskrit word *vriksha* (pronounced *vrik-shah*) means "tree." The tree posture improves overall balance, stability, and poise. It strengthens your legs, arms, and shoulders, and opens your hips and groin. Like the other one-legged balancing poses, it also enhances focus and concentration and produces a calming effect on your body and mind. Here's how it works:

1. **Stand in the mountain posture (see Chapter 7 for this posture).**

2. **As you exhale, bend your right knee and place the sole of your right foot, toes pointing down, on the inside of your left leg between your knee and your groin.**

3. **As you inhale, bring your arms over your head and join your palms together.**

4. **Soften your arms, and focus on a spot 6 to 8 feet in front of you on the floor (see Figure 8-3).**

5. **Stay in Step 4 for 6 to 8 breaths, and then repeat with the opposite leg.**

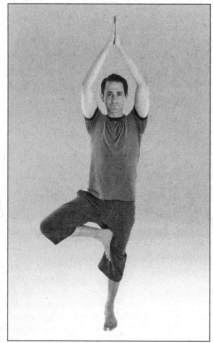

**Figure 8-3:** Focus on a spot 6 to 8 feet in front of you; concentrate and breathe slowly.

*Photograph by Adam Latham*

***Note:*** In the classic (traditionally taught) version of this posture, the arms are straight and the chin rests on the chest.

If you have limited flexibility in your hips and have difficulty getting your foot all the way up to your thigh in Step 2, you can place the foot of your bent leg between your knee and ankle. Just take care not to place your foot directly against your knee joint.

## The karate kid

The karate kid posture improves overall balance and stability. It strengthens the legs, arms, and shoulders, and opens the hips. As with the other one-legged balancing postures, the karate kid enhances focus and concentration.

1. **Stand in the mountain posture, which we describe in Chapter 7.**

2. **As you inhale, raise your arms out to the sides, parallel to the line of your shoulders (and the floor), so that they form a *T* with your torso.**

3. **To steady yourself, focus on a spot on the floor 10 to 12 feet in front of you.**

4. **As you exhale, bend your left knee, raising it toward your chest; keep your right leg straight (see Figure 8-4).**

5. **Stay in Step 4 for 6 to 8 breaths; repeat with the right knee.**

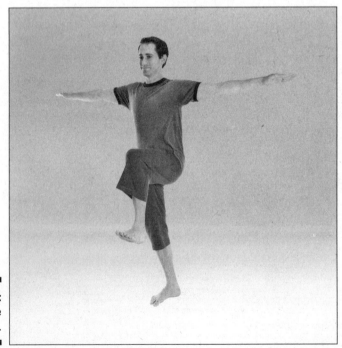

**Figure 8-4:**
The karate kid.

*Photograph by Adam Latham*

The Sanskrit name for this pose is *utthita hasta padangusthasana* variation. I (Larry) called it the "karate kid" based on inspiration from the film *The Karate Kid, Part II.*

# Standing heel-to-buttock

The standing heel-to-buttock posture improves your overall balance and stability. This posture strengthens your legs, arms, and shoulders, and stretches your thighs. As with the other one-legged balancing poses, this posture enhances focus and concentration as well. Here's how it works

1. **Stand in the mountain posture (see Chapter 7).**

2. **As you inhale, raise your left arm forward and overhead.**

3. **To steady yourself, focus on a spot on the floor 10 to 12 feet in front of you.**

4. **As you exhale, bend your right knee and bring your right heel toward your right buttock, keeping your left leg straight; grasp your right ankle with your right hand, as Figure 8-5 illustrates.**

5. **Stay in Step 4 for 6 to 8 breaths; repeat Steps 1 through 5 with your left foot.**

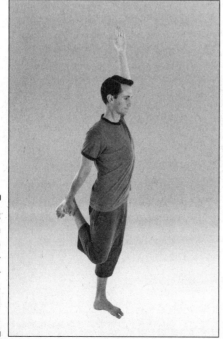

**Figure 8-5:**
This pose can improve your balance for the more advanced postures.

*Photograph by Adam Latham*

# Scorpion

The scorpion posture improves overall balance and stability. This posture, which is a variation of *cakravakasana*, strengthens your shoulders; improves the flexibility of your hips, legs, and shoulders; and enhances focus and concentration.

1. **While on your hands and knees, position your hands directly under your shoulders, with your palms down, fingers spread on the floor, and knees directly under your hips; straighten your arms, but don't lock your elbows.**

2. **Place your right forearm on the floor, with your right hand just behind your left wrist; reach behind you with your left hand, twisting the torso slightly to the left, and grab your right ankle.**

3. **As you inhale, lift your right knee off the floor, raise your chest until it's parallel to the floor, and look up; find a comfortable height for your chest and raised leg, and steady yourself by pressing your right forearm and thumb on the floor (see Figure 8-6).**

4. **Stay in Step 3 for 6 to 8 breaths, and then repeat Steps 1 through 4 on the opposite side (with your left forearm and left foot).**

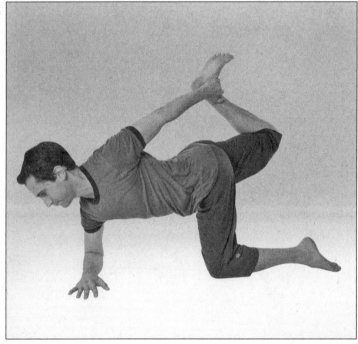

**Figure 8-6:**
Steady yourself by pressing your right forearm and thumb into the floor.

*Photograph by Adam Latham*

# Chapter 9

# Absolutely Abs

*M*any Eastern systems of spiritual exercise and healing consider the lower abdomen to be the vital center of your whole being — body, mind, and spirit. Westerners, on the other hand, think much differently about their bellies, tending to see them as mere food bags or as waste-processing stations.

Many people have a love-hate relationship with their bellies. Although people may be obsessed with having the "perfect" midriff, they tend to neglect or even abuse this area of their bodies. On the inside, they stuff the belly with way too much junk food. On the outside, they let it grow slack. But as the Yoga masters warn, when this area is polluted by impurities, it becomes a seat of sickness.

Apart from diseases, weak bellies (and belly muscles) contribute significantly to lower back problems. Studies indicate that 80 percent of the American population has had, is having, or will have back problems. Back-related problems are the second-leading cause of missed workdays, trailing only respiratory problems or the common cold.

In this chapter, we walk you through some Yoga exercises that focus on the abdomen so that you can keep this vital area of your body strong and healthy.

# Taking Care of the Abdomen: Your Business Center

The abdomen is an amazing enterprise, with its complex food-processing plant (the stomach), several subsidiary operations (liver, spleen, kidneys, and so on), and a 25-foot-long sewer system (the intestines). Poor diets and eating habits lead to annoying and sometimes deadly serious digestive and elimination problems, including constipation, diarrhea, irritable bowel syndrome, and colon cancer. Regular Yoga practice can help you take care of your abdominal organs so they can function well and take care of you without the aid of antacids, digestive enzyme supplements, or laxatives.

In the following section, we describe exercises that work with three sets of abdominal muscles:

✔ The *rectus abdominis*, which is strung vertically along the front of the belly from the bottom of the sternum to the pubis

✔ The internal and external *obliques*, which, as their name suggests, take an "oblique" course along the side of the belly from the lower ribs to the top rim of the pelvis

✔ The *transversalis abdominis*, which lies behind the internal obliques

You may hear these three abdominals called the "stomach muscles," which is really a misnomer. The actual stomach muscles line the baglike stomach and are active only during digestion. Of course, the yogic exercises also positively affect the abdominal organs (stomach, spleen, liver, and intestines). If you take care of your abdominal muscles and the organs they protect — through exercise and proper diet — you have accomplished much of the work to stay healthy.

## Navel secrets, declassified

After a doctor or midwife severs a newborn's umbilical cord, thus creating his navel, no one pays much attention to this birth socket. Yet the navel is a very important feature of your anatomy. According to Yoga, a special psychoenergetic center is located at the navel. This center is known as the *manipura-chakra* (pronounced *mah-nee-poo-rah-chuk-rah*), which means literally "center of the jeweled city." The center corresponds to (but isn't identical with) the *solar plexus*, which is a large network of nerves that has been called the body's second brain. The *manipura-cakra* controls the abdominal organs and regulates the flow of energy through the entire body. The navel center is associated with emotions and the will. You can have "too much navel" (be pushy) or "not enough navel" (be a pushover).

# Exercising Those Abs

Our yogic postures for the abdominal muscles incorporate a team approach that values slow, conscious movement, proper breathing mechanics, and the use of sound. The emphasis here is on the *quality* of the movement rather than sheer quantity. A few movements done with diligent attention are much safer and more effective than dozens and even hundreds of mindless repetitions. Conscious breathing, especially the gentle tightening of the front belly on each exhalation, can encourage and then sustain the strength and tone of the abdominals. The use of sound, which we discuss later in this chapter, further enhances this kind of breathing.

## Exploring push-downs

Push-downs strengthen the abdomen, especially the lower abdomen. In addition to a floor exercise, you can do push-downs in a seated position by pushing your lower back against the back of your chair. You can perform this exercise sitting in a car, on a plane, or at the office.

1. **Lie on your back with your knees bent and your feet on the floor, at hip width.**

   Rest your arms near your sides, palms down.

2. **As you exhale, push your lower back down to the floor for 3 to 5 seconds (see Figure 9-1).**

3. **As you inhale, release your back.**

4. **Repeat Steps 2 and 3 six to eight times.**

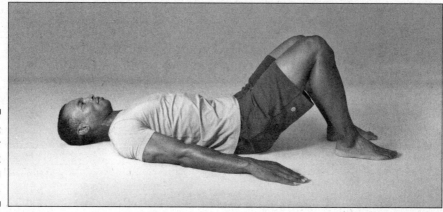

**Figure 9-1:**
Push your lower back down as you exhale.

*Photograph by Adam Latham*

## *Trying yogi sit-ups*

Yogi sit-ups strengthen the abdomen, especially the upper abdomen, the *adductors* (insides of your legs), the neck, and the shoulders.

1. **Lie on your back with your knees bent and your feet on the floor, at hip width.**

2. **Turn in your toes "pigeon-toed," and bring your inner knees together.**

3. **Spread your palms on the back of your head, with your fingers interlocked, and keep your elbows wide.**

4. **As you exhale, press your knees firmly, tilt the front of your pelvis toward your navel, and, with your hips on the ground, slowly sit up halfway.**

   Keep your elbows out to the sides, in line with the tops of your shoulders. Look toward the ceiling. Don't pull your head up with your arms; instead, support your head with your hands and come up by contracting the abdominal muscles, as in Figure 9-2.

5. **As you inhale, slowly roll back down.**

6. **Repeat Steps 4 and 5 six to eight times.**

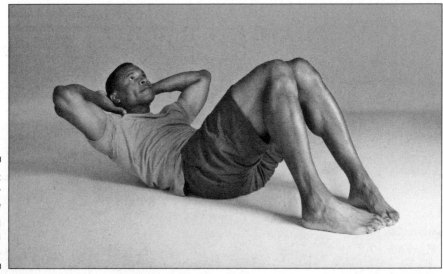

**Figure 9-2:**
Let your eyes follow the ceiling as you sit up.

*Photograph by Adam Latham*

## The sound of Yoga

A very busy, well-known movie producer from Malibu was referred to me (Larry) by his physician. He suffered from a chronic neck and stress condition, and he also had what his girlfriend referred to as a "little jelly belly." Regular sit-ups to tighten his abs just aggravated his neck problem. I gave him a 12-minute, twice-a-day Yoga routine that included the yogi sit-back and the use of sound (both discussed in this chapter). The exercises worked like a charm. His neck problem went away, and his belly firmed up nicely. He liked using sound so much that many members of his movie crew joined him in the afternoon for "a little sound."

## *Strengthening with yogi sit-backs*

Yogi sit-backs strengthen both the lower and upper abdomen. This posture is a variation of *navasana*. The Sanskrit word *nava*, pronounced *nah-vah*, means "boat."

1. **Sit on the floor with your knees bent and your feet on the floor, at hip width.**

2. **Extend your arms and place your hands on the floor, palms down.**

3. **Bring your chin down, and round your back in a *C* curve, as in Figure 9-3a.**

4. **As you inhale, roll slowly onto the back of your pelvis, dragging your hands along on the floor (see Figure 9-3b).**

   Keep the rest of your back off the floor, to maintain the contraction of the abdominals, but don't strain to hold this position; if you have any negative symptoms, don't use this posture.

5. **As you exhale, roll up again, sliding your hands forward.**

6. **Repeat Steps 4 and 5 six to eight times.**

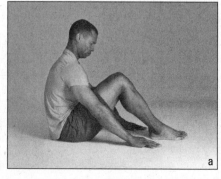 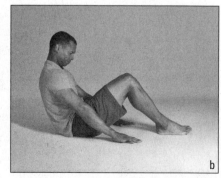

**Figure 9-3:** Bring your chin down, and keep your back rounded in a *C* curve.

a

b

*Photograph by Adam Latham*

Sit-backs are easier on the neck than most sit-ups. However, if you have lower back problems, be cautious with sit-backs. If you notice any pain in your back, just stop and work with the other exercises in this chapter instead.

## Creating variety with extended leg slide-ups

A variation of *navasana*, the extended leg slide-ups strengthen both the upper and lower abdomen, as well as the neck.

If this pose bothers your neck, support your head by putting both hands behind it. If the problem persists, stop.

1. **Lie on your back with your knees bent and your feet flat on the floor, at hip width.**

2. **Bend your left elbow, and place your left hand on the back of your head just behind your left ear.**

3. **Raise the left leg as close to vertical (90 degrees) as possible, but keep your knee slightly bent.**

4. **Draw the top of your foot toward your shin, to flex your ankle, and place your right palm on your right thigh near your pelvis, as Figure 9-4a illustrates.**

5. **As you exhale, sit up slowly halfway and slide your right hand toward your knee.**

   Keep your left elbow back in line with your shoulder, and look at the ceiling. Don't throw your head forward (see Figure 9-4b for the proper positioning).

6. **Repeat Steps 1 through 5 six to eight times, and then repeat Steps 1 through 6 on the other side.**

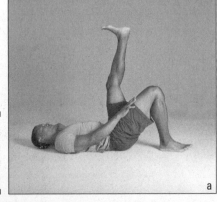
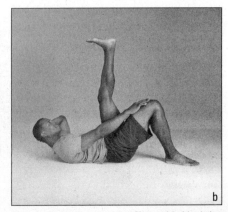

**Figure 9-4:** Work the abs and the hamstrings.

a

b

*Photograph by Adam Latham*

# Arching with the suck 'em up posture

The suck 'em up posture strengthens and tones the abdominal muscles and the internal organs. The posture is especially beneficial for relieving constipation.

1. **Start on your hands and knees, with your hands just below your shoulders and your knees at hip width.**

2. **Inhale deeply through your nose.**

3. **Exhale through your mouth, and hump your back like a camel as you bring your chin down.**

   When you have fully exhaled, don't immediately inhale; hold your breath where it is and then suck your belly up toward your spine (see Figure 9-5).

   Wait 2 to 3 seconds with the belly up and breath restrained, as long as you don't end up gasping for air.

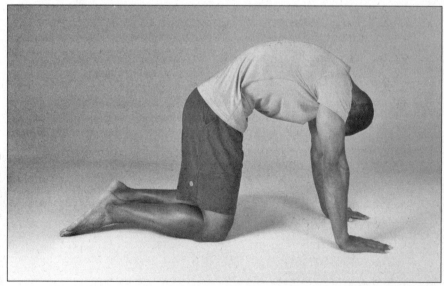

**Figure 9-5:** Make sure you exhale fully before you suck your belly up.

*Photograph by Adam Latham*

4. **As you inhale, return to the starting position and then pause for a breath or two.**

5. **Repeat Steps 2 through 4 four to six times, pausing for a breath or two between each repetition.**

Do this exercise only on an empty stomach, and avoid it if you're having stomach pain or cramps of any kind because it may intensify the symptoms. Also avoid this exercise during menstruation.

## Exhaling "soundly"

The use of sound exercise strengthens and tones the abdomen and its internal organs, in addition to strengthening the muscles of the diaphragm.

1. **Sit in a chair or on the floor, with your spine comfortably upright.**

   If you find yourself slumping, sit on a folded blanket or check out the Yoga props in Chapter 20.

2. **Place the palm of your right hand on your navel so that you can feel your belly contracting as you exhale.**

3. **Take a deep inhalation through your nose and, as you exhale, make the sound *ah, ma,* or *sa.***

   Continue sounding this consonant for as long as you can do so comfortably.

4. **Repeat Steps 2 and 3 six to eight times.**

   Pause for a resting breath or two between each sound.

If you're on a detox program of any kind and the use of sound gives you a headache, work with the other exercises in this chapter instead.

# Chapter 10

# Looking at the World Upside Down: Safe Inversion Postures

*T*housands of years ago, the Yoga masters made an amazing discovery: By tricking the force of gravity with the help of inversion exercises, it's possible to reverse the effects of aging, improve your health, and add years to your life.

To picture how inversions work, take a look at a jug of unfiltered apple juice sitting on the grocery store shelf. Gravity has pulled the solids in the juice to the bottom of the jug, diluting the liquid near the top. If you turn the bottle upside down, gravity pulls the bottom sediment toward the top of the inverted jug, remixing the juice with the pulp of the apples.

In a similar way, when you turn yourself upside down, the sediments — mostly blood and *lymph* (a clear, yellowish fluid similar to blood plasma) — that have collected in your lower limbs during a long day of uprightness sink toward your head and revitalize your entire body and mind, helping you face your fears and reversing the tide of stagnation and mental negativity.

The idea that you must practice the headstand to be a "real yogi" just isn't true. We recommend that you avoid the headstand unless an experienced teacher supervises your efforts. The neck is designed to support the 8 pounds of the head, not the 100 or more pounds of the body. Approach the headstand cautiously and only after proper preparation.

Fortunately, you can practice a variety of inversions other than the headstand. In this chapter, we describe inverted exercises that impart the benefits without the risk. Use yogic breathing (see Chapter 5) to boost their beneficial effect, and grab a prop as necessary to facilitate the postures and ensure easy breathing (see Chapter 20).

# Getting a Leg Up on Leg Inversions

Effective inversions can actually be quite simple. In the next section, we describe four postures that don't require you to literally turn yourself upside down to enjoy the numerous benefits of an inversion.

Avoid all inverted postures if you have an acute headache or if you experience sudden pain while performing the exercise.

Feel free to luxuriate in the two supported inversions; they're both held longer than other poses.

## Legs up on a chair

The legs up on a chair posture improves circulation to your legs, hips, and lower back, and has a calming effect on your nervous system. It also helps alleviate symptoms of PMS in women and prostatitis in men.

To enjoy these benefits, do the following:

1. **Sit on the floor in a simple cross-legged position, facing a sturdy chair, and lean back onto your forearms.**

2. **Slide your buttocks along the floor toward the chair.**

3. **While exhaling, lift your feet off the floor and place your heels and calves on the chair seat.**

   You want your thighs and shins to be at a right angle.

4. **Lie back on the floor with your arms near your sides, palms down or up, as in Figure 10-1.**

5. **Stay in Step 4 for 2 to 10 minutes.**

This posture is a variation of the *classic* (traditionally taught) posture of *urdhva prasarita padasana* (pronounced *oord-hvah prah-sah-ree-tah pahd-ah-sah-nah*), which means "upward extended foot posture."

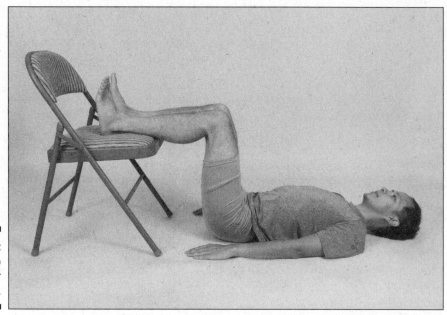

**Figure 10-1:**
The legs up
on a chair
posture.

*Photograph by Adam Latham*

## Legs up on the wall

Legs up on the wall, which is a variation of *urdhva prasarita padasana,* improves circulation to the legs, hips, and lower back, and has a calming effect on the nervous system. It, too, helps alleviate symptoms of PMS in women and prostatitis in men.

Try it for yourself by following these steps:

1. **Sit sideways with your right side as close to the wall as possible, with both legs extended forward (see Figure 10-2a).**

2. **As you exhale, swing both legs up on the wall and lie flat on your back.**

   Extend your legs up as far as possible. Extend your arms comfortably at your sides, palms down, and relax (see Figure 10-2b).

3. **Stay in Step 2 for 2 to 10 minutes.**

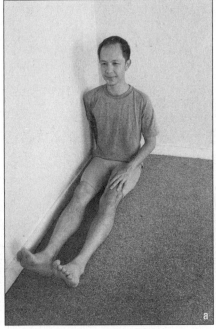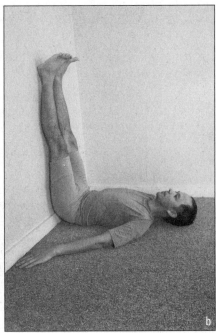

**Figure 10-2:**
The legs up
on the wall
posture.

*Photograph by Adam Latham*

# The happy baby

A variation of *urdhva prasarita padasana*, the happy baby posture improves circulation in the legs, arms, hips, and lower back, and has a calming effect on the nervous system. It also improves the range of motion of the ankles, toes, wrists, and fingers.

Here's how it works:

1. **Lying on your back with your knees bent and feet flat on the floor, place your arms at your sides with your palms down.**

2. **As you exhale, extend your legs and arms up vertically.**

   Keep your limbs relaxed (check out our discussion of Forgiving Limbs in Chapter 3) as you hold them up.

3. **With your feet, toes, hands, and fingers, draw circles in the air both clockwise and counterclockwise, as in Figure 10-3.**

   You can make your hands and feet go in different directions at the same time. Breathe freely. Keep your arms and legs up as long as you feel comfortable, and then return to the starting position.

4. **Repeat Steps 2 and 3 three to five times, but don't hold the limbs up for more than a total of 5 minutes; you don't want to tire yourself out or strain your back.**

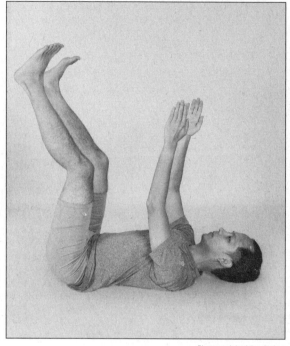

**Figure 10-3:**
Enjoy the freedom of movement in your ankles and wrists.

*Photograph by Adam Latham*

Avoid this posture if you have lower back problems.

## Standing spread-legged forward bend at the wall

The standing spread-legged forward bend at the wall, which is a variation of *prasarita pada uttanasana* (described in Chapter 7), improves circulation in your head and stretches your spine and hamstrings.

Follow these easy steps:

1. **Stand with your back 6 to 12 inches from a sturdy wall, separate your feet to a comfortably wide stance, and then lean your buttocks back against the wall.**

2. **As you exhale, bend forward from the hips and hang your arms and head down.**

   If your hands touch the floor, grasp your elbows with opposite-side hands and let your forearms hang. Keep your knees soft, and relax your neck and head, as in Figure 10-4.

3. **Stay in Step 2 for 2 to 3 minutes; use any of the Yoga breathing techniques we cover in Chapter 5.**

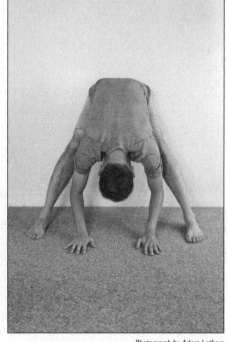

**Figure 10-4:**
The
standing
spread-
legged
forward
bend at the
wall.

*Photograph by Adam Latham*

If you feel light-headed when doing this pose or any other inversion exercise, reduce the duration and then increase the time gradually.

# Trying a Trio of Shoulder Stands

These shoulder stands go from easiest to toughest. Each of these three shoulder stands provides common benefits: improved circulation to your legs, hips, back, neck, heart, and head. The postures all stimulate your endocrine glands and improve your lymphatic drainage, enhance elimination, and produce a calming and rejuvenating effect on your nervous system. The wall provides a useful prop for the easier two variations; when you're ready, you can advance with confidence to *viparita karani*, the half shoulder stand.

Because of the neck's vulnerability, we recommend that you precede these postures with a dynamic (or moving) bridge posture (see Chapter 15), to prepare the neck and follow it with a short rest, and then use a dynamic cobra posture (see Chapter 11) to compensate.

Don't attempt any of these postures if you're pregnant; have high blood pressure or a hiatal hernia; are even moderately overweight; have glaucoma, diabetic retinopathy, or neck problems; or are in the first few days of your period. Also, don't use a mirrored wall — you can injure yourself if you fall.

# Half shoulder stand at the wall

This posture is a variation of *viparita karani* (see "Half shoulder stand: *Viparita karani*," later in this section) and is perhaps the easiest way to pick up the half shoulder stand in a step-by-step manner. The wall provides support as you build experience with the shoulder stand exercises.

Here's how you do it:

1. **Lie on your back with your knees bent, your feet flat on the floor, your toes just touching the base of a sturdy wall, and your arms extended along the sides of your torso, with your palms down.**

2. **Place your soles up on the wall so that your bent knees form a right angle (with your thighs parallel to each other and your shins perpendicular to the wall), as in Figure 10-5a.**

   You may need to slide your buttocks closer to or farther away from the wall to get the angle just right.

3. **As you inhale, press down with your hands, push your feet to the wall, and lift your hips as high as you comfortably can (see Figure 10-5b).**

4. **Bend your elbows and bring your hands to your lower back.**

   Press your elbows and the backs of your upper arms onto the floor for support. Relax your neck (see Figure 10-5c).

5. **As you exhale, take one foot off the wall and extend that leg until you're looking straight up at the tip of your big toe, as in Figure 10-5d.**

   You can use just one leg at a time and switch, or you can raise both legs together. If you alternate legs, divide the time evenly between each leg.

6. **Stay in Step 4 or 5 for as long as you feel comfortable, or up to 5 minutes; use the Yoga breathing techniques we recommend in Chapter 5.**

   When you want to come back down, slowly place one foot and then the other on the wall, and finally lower your pelvis slowly to the floor.

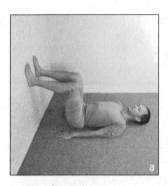
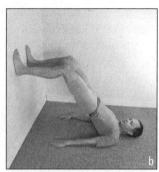
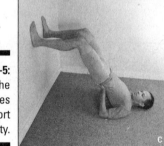
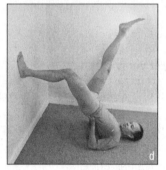

**Figure 10-5:**
Using the wall gives you support and variety.

*Photograph by Adam Latham*

# Reverse half shoulder stand at the wall

The reverse half shoulder stand at the wall (see Figure 10-6b) is also a variation of *viparita karani,* which we discuss in "Half shoulder stand: *Viparita karani,*" later in this chapter. Some people find this exercise easier than the half shoulder stand at the wall. Try them both and see which one is more comfortable for you.

To try this one, follow these steps:

1. **Lie on your back with your head toward the wall at a full arm's distance from the wall. Your legs can be straight (see Figure 10-6a), or you can bend your knees with your feet flat on the floor at hip width, if it feels better for your back. Bring your arms back, and rest your arms along the sides of your body, palms down.**

   Finding the correct distance from the wall depends on the length of your arms. Try these three different measurements: touching the wall with your fingers extended, touching with the knuckles of your fists, and touching with the backs of your hands.

2. **As you exhale, push your palms down, draw your knees in and up, and raise your hips to a comfortable angle of 45 to 75 degrees.**

   Once up, be sure your legs are straight but your knees aren't locked. Your knees, not your feet, should be over your head in this modified shoulder stand.

3. **Bend your elbows and bring your hands to the back of your pelvis; then slide your hands up to your lower back.**

   Press your elbows and the backs of your upper arms onto the floor for support.

4. **Let your toes slowly and gently touch the wall for support; relax your neck (see Figure 10-6b).**

5. **Stay in Step 4 for as long as you feel comfortable, or up to 5 minutes.**

6. **When you want to come down, ease your hips to the floor with the support of your hands, and then bend your knees and lower your feet to the floor.**

**Figure 10-6:**
Another way to use the wall as a prop.

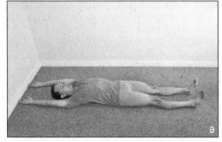 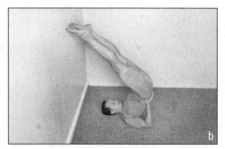

*Photograph by Adam Latham*

## Half shoulder stand: Viparita karani

You can work up to this posture by developing comfort with the half shoulder and reverse half shoulder stands at the wall (see the corresponding sections earlier in this chapter). It lets you enjoy the benefits of inversion without compressing your neck as a full shoulder stand does.

The Sanskrit word *viparita* (pronounced *vee-pah-ree-tah*) means "inverted, reversed," and *karani* (pronounced *kah-rah-nee*) means "action, process." Some authorities call this practice *sarvangasana*, meaning "all limbs posture." The word is composed of *sarva* (pronounced *sahr-vah*) and *anga* (pronounced *ahn-gah*), followed by *asana*.

When you feel you're ready, follow these steps:

1. **Lie on your back with your knees bent and your feet flat on the floor at hip width; rest your arms along the sides of your body, with your palms down.**

2. **As you exhale, push your palms down, draw your bent knees in and up, and then straighten your legs as you raise your hips to a comfortable angle of 45 to 75 degrees (see Figure 10-7a).**

3. **Bend your elbows and bring your hands to the back of your pelvis; then slide your hands up to your lower back.**

   Make sure your legs are straight but your knees aren't locked, and keep your feet directly above your head. Press your elbows and the backs of your upper arms onto the floor for support. Relax your neck. Figure 10-7b shows this portion of the posture.

4. **Stay in Step 3 for as long as you feel comfortable, or up to 5 minutes.**

5. **When you want to come down, first ease your hips to the floor with the support of your hands, and then bend your knees and lower your feet to the floor.**

**Figure 10-7:** The half shoulder stand.

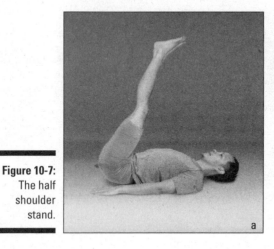 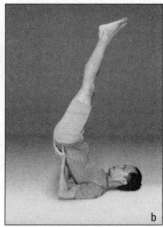

*Photograph by Adam Latham*

# Chapter 11

# Easy 'round the Bends: Classic Bending Floor Postures

This chapter presents a variety of yogic bends. Think of them as simple extensions of the breath. Inhalation takes you naturally into a back bend, and exhalation takes you into a forward bend (for more on breath and movement, flip to Chapter 5). You can perform bending postures from many different positions — standing, kneeling, sitting, lying, or even turned upside-down (see Chapter 10). Because we cover the upright bending postures in Chapter 7 and the most popular bends for warm-up in Chapter 6, this chapter highlights the classic bending postures that you do on the floor.

## Gaining a Strong Backbone (and Some Insight)

Without the spinal column, you'd never experience back pain — but then again, you couldn't walk upright, either! The backbone enables you to bend forward, backward, and sideways, and it also allows you to twist. You perform all these motions every day, but you may do them unconsciously and without adequate muscular support. Yoga uses the natural movements of the spine to train the various muscles supporting it, which contributes to a healthy back and prevents back pain.

## The spine as the axis of your world

According to Yoga symbolism, the spine corresponds to the axis of the universe, which is pictured as a gigantic golden mountain called Mount Meru. At the top of this mountain (that is, in your head) resides heaven, where all the deities are seated.

Although the spinal column's elegant curvature is well designed for the upright position, people aren't always very clever about using it correctly. The 33 vertebrae, or backbones (24 of which comprise the flexible part of the spine), stay in place thanks to a series of powerful muscles and ligaments that require regular exercise to maintain top working order.

Numerous muscles, arranged in several layers in the front, back, neck, and *perineum* (the area between the anus and the genitals), maintain the spine in position. When they become weak or damaged from inadequate or improper use or injury, any one of these can pull the spine out of alignment, leading to discomfort, pain, and inadequate nerve communication to the organs and other parts of the body, possibly leading to further complications.

The spinal column is so important because it protects the spinal cord — a bundle of nerves that runs through the bony tower, your backbone. The nerves feed the trunk and limbs with information from the brain, and the brain returns the favor. If the nerve connection is severed at any point, you lose conscious control of the affected part of your body.

The spine also has psychological significance. A person of integrity and strength of character is said to "have backbone," and a coward is said to be "spineless." Because people believe that outside presentation reflects inside influences, they tend to judge a person's mental state from his bodily demeanor. If you're chronically hunched over, you signal to others that you're weary or sad, or otherwise inwardly collapsed. On the other hand, if you stand straight and tall, you give others the impression of self-assuredness, energy, and courage.

From a yogic point of view, the spine is the physical aspect of a subtle energetic pathway that runs from its base to the crown of the head. This pathway is known as the *central channel*, or *sushumna-nadi* ("gracious conduit," pronounced *soo-shoom-nah nah-dee*). In traditional Hatha Yoga and Tantra Yoga, the awakened "serpent power," or *kundalini-shakti*, rises through this channel. When this power of pure consciousness reaches the crown of the head, you experience a sublime state of ecstasy. We say more about the central channel in Chapter 23.

# Bending over Backward

Daily life entails a lot of forward bending: putting on a pair of pants, tying shoelaces, picking things up from the floor, working at your computer, gardening, playing sports, and so on. A forward bend closes the front of the torso, shortens the front of the spine, and rounds the back. This closing and rounding is exaggerated by the unhealthy habit of bending forward from the waist instead of from the hip joints. Bending forward in the wrong way day in and day out can lead to spinal problems.

To experience the difference between bending from the hips and bending from the waist, sit upright in a chair with your feet flat on the floor, and place your hands on the outside of your hip bones, with your fingers turned inward. As you inhale, move your spine upward, lift your chest, and look straight ahead. As you exhale, keep your chest lifted and bend forward: You're bending forward from the hips. Now sit in the chair and move your hands up a few inches until they're just under your rib cage. As you exhale, bring your chin to your chest and your head down toward your thighs, bowing your spine. This bend is from the waist. Over the years, this waist-bending habit leads to what is often called a *stoop*, characterized by a sunken chest, a forward-leaning head, aches and pains, and shallow breathing.

The antidote for the cumulative effects of forward bending is the regular practice of Yoga back bends, which stretch the front of the torso (and spine). Take a deep inhalation right now and notice how your torso (and spine) naturally extends during this active, opening phase of the breathing cycle, inviting you to bend backward. Back bends are expansive, extroverted postures that can trigger powerful emotions. The major back bends usually come toward the middle of a Yoga routine so that you have plenty of time to prepare for these movements and to compensate afterward (see Chapter 15 for more on preparation and compensation). In this section, we present some of the classic floor back bends.

To make these cobra and locust postures easier, place a small pillow or a folded blanket underneath you between your abdomen and your chest. You can move the blanket a little forward or backward to suit your needs (see Figure 11-4b later in the chapter for an illustration).

When you lie face down on the floor, raise your chest and head, and use your arms in some fashion, you're doing some form of the cobra posture. When you raise just your legs, or a combination of your legs, chest, and arms, you're performing some form of the locust posture.

Move slowly and cautiously in all the cobra and locust postures. Avoid any of the postures that cause pain in your lower back, upper back, or neck.

# Cobra I: Salamba bhujangasana

The cobra posture increases the flexibility and strength of the muscles of the arms, chest, shoulders, and back. Cobra I especially emphasizes the upper back. The cobra opens the chest, increases lung capacity, and stimulates the kidneys and the adrenals.

This first cobra posture is also called the sphinx. It's a variation of *bhujangasana*, which we describe in the next section.

1. **Lie on your abdomen, with your legs spread at hip width and the tops of your feet on the floor.**

2. **Rest your forehead on the floor, and relax your shoulders; bend your elbows and place your forearms on the floor, with your palms turned down and positioned near the sides of your head (see Figure 11-1a).**

3. **As you inhale, engage your back muscles, press your forearms against the floor, and raise your chest and head.**

   Look straight ahead, as in Figure 11-1b. Keep your forearms and the front of your pelvis on the floor, being mindful of relaxing your shoulders.

**Figure 11-1:**
Cobra I
emphasizes
the upper
back and is
easier than
cobra II.

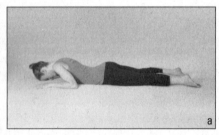 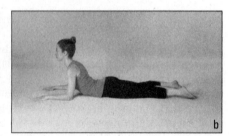

Photograph by Adam Latham

4. **As you exhale, lower your torso and head slowly back to the floor.**

5. **Repeat Steps 3 and 4 three times, and then stay in Step 3 (the last raised position) for 6 to 8 breaths.**

If you have lower back problems, separate your legs wider than your hips, let your heels turn out, and let your toes turn in.

# To clench or not to clench: That is the question

An ongoing controversy in the Yoga world is whether to keep the buttocks firm or soft in the cobra posture. The traditional instruction is to firm the buttocks. However, the work of New Zealand–born physiotherapist Robin McKenzie has revolutionized back care — and ideas about back bends. In his own version of the cobra, called The McKenzie Technique, McKenzie recommends keeping the buttocks soft, to facilitate the healing of numerous lower back ailments. Try the cobra both ways, with the buttocks firm and then soft, and see which feels best to you. **Note:** This discussion applies to cobra only; in all the locust postures, the buttocks are usually tight.

## Cobra II: Bhujangasana

This posture rewards you with most of the same benefits as cobra I, which we describe in the preceding section. In addition, cobra II emphasizes flexibility in your lower back.

1. **Lie on your abdomen, with your legs spread at hip width and the tops of your feet on the floor.**

2. **Bend your elbows and place your palms on the floor, with your thumbs near your armpits; rest your forehead on the floor and relax your shoulders, as in Figure 11-2a.**

3. **As you inhale, press your palms against the floor, engage your back muscles, and raise your chest and head; look straight ahead (see Figure 11-2b).**

Keep the top front of your pelvis on the floor, and relax your shoulders. Unless you're very flexible, keep your elbows slightly bent.

**Figure 11-2:**
Cobra II emphasizes flexibility in the lower back.

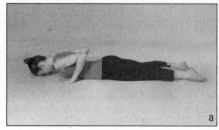
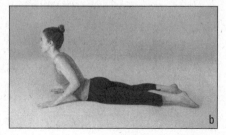

*Photograph by Adam Latham*

4. **As you exhale, slowly lower your torso and head back to the floor.**

5. **Repeat Steps 3 and 4 three times, and then stay in Step 3 (the last raised position) for 6 to 8 breaths.**

*Note:* In the classic (traditionally taught) posture, the inner legs are joined and the knees are straight. The head is in alignment with the spine, and the eyes look forward. The palms are on the floor close to the sides of the torso near the navel, the elbows are slightly bent, and the shoulders are relaxed.

If you move your hands farther forward, you make the cobra less difficult; if you move your hands farther back, you increase the difficulty.

The Sanskrit word *bhujangasana* consists of *bhujanga* (pronounced *bhooj-ahng-gah*), meaning "serpent," and *asana*, or "posture."

# Cobra III

Cobra III, which is another version of the classic *bhujangasana*, is unique because it doesn't ask you to place your hands on the floor. The emphasis is on strengthening both the lower and upper back.

1. **Lie on your abdomen, with your legs spread at hip width and the tops of your feet on the floor; rest your forehead on the floor.**

2. **Extend your arms back along the sides of your torso, with your palms on the floor, as in Figure 11-3a.**

3. **As you inhale, raise your chest and head, and sweep your arms like wings out to the sides and then all the way forward; your palms can touch or face each other a few inches apart.**

Keep your legs on the floor, as in Figure 11-3b.

4. **As you exhale, sweep your arms back, and lower your torso and your head slowly to the floor.**

5. **Repeat Steps 3 and 4 three times, and then stay in Step 3 (the last raised position) for 6 to 8 breaths.**

**Figure 11-3:**
Cobra III strengthens the lower and upper back and the neck.

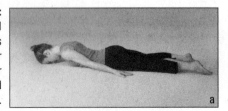
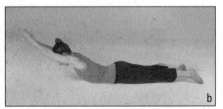

*Photograph by Adam Latham*

# Locust I: Shalabhasana

The locust posture strengthens the entire torso, including the lower back and the neck. In addition, it strengthens the buttocks and the legs, and it improves digestion and elimination.

1. **Lie on your abdomen, with your legs spread at hip width and the tops of your feet on the floor; rest your forehead on the floor.**

2. **Extend your arms along the sides of your torso, with your palms on the floor.**

   To make the pose easier, try turning the palms up

3. **As you inhale, raise your chest, head, and one leg up and away from the floor as high as is comfortable for you (see Figure 11-4a).**

   Consider trying this posture with blankets for more personal comfort. Figure 11-4b shows you the basic blanket positioning, although you can shift it as necessary.

**Figure 11-4:**
Raise your chest, head, and leg on an inhale, using a blanket, if necessary.

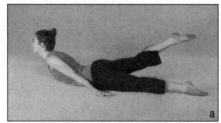
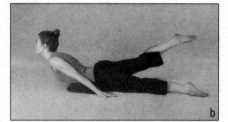

*Photograph by Adam Latham*

4. **As you exhale, lower your chest, head, and leg together slowly to the floor, and repeat Steps 3 and 4 with the other leg.**

5. **Repeat Steps 3 and 4 three times, and then stay in Step 3 (the last raised position) for 6 to 8 breaths.**

You can increase the level of difficulty by raising both legs at the same time in Step 3.

*Note:* In the classic posture, the inner legs are joined and the knees are straight.

# Locust II

This posture, which is another variation of *shalabhasana*, also teaches the two sides of the body how to work independently of one another. Many back problems result from imbalances in the muscle system on each side of the spine. Health professionals often call this situation an *asymmetrical problem*. Locust II helps bring your back into symmetry again and also improves your coordination.

1. **Lie on your abdomen, with your legs spread at hip width and the tops of your feet on the floor; rest your forehead on the floor.**

2. **Extend your right arm forward, with your palm resting on the floor; bring your left arm back along the left side of your torso, with the back of your hand on the floor (see Figure 11-5a).**

3. **As you inhale, slowly raise your chest, head, right arm, and left leg up and away from the floor as high as is comfortable for you; try to keep your upper right arm and ear in alignment, and raise your left foot and right hand to the same height above the floor (see Figure 11-5b).**

4. **As you exhale, slowly lower your right arm, chest, head, and left leg to the floor at the same time.**

5. **Repeat Steps 3 and 4 three times, and then stay in Step 3 for 6 to 8 breaths.**

6. **Repeat Steps 1 through 5 with opposite pairs (left arm and right leg).**

**Figure 11-5:**
This posture balances the muscles on each side of your back.

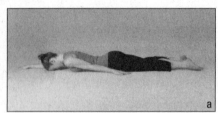 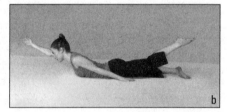

*Photograph by Adam Latham*

Locust II features some interesting biomechanics. When you raise your chest and your right arm, you strengthen the right side of your upper back. When you raise your left leg, you strengthen the right side of your lower back. So even though this posture uses opposite arms and legs, it strengthens one side of the upper and lower back at a time.

Be careful with locust variations that lift just the legs. Lifting the legs alone increases interabdominal and chest pressure, heart rate, and tension in the low back and neck.

## Locust III: Superman posture

This posture, a further variation of *shalabhasana*, gets its name from the image of Superman flying through the air at warp speed, with his arms extended out in front leading the way. It's the most strenuous back bend because fully extending your arms and legs as in Figure 11-6 puts quite a load on your entire back. Use this pose only when you're comfortable with locust I and II.

This posture is physically challenging. Don't attempt it if you have back or neck problems.

1. **Lie on your abdomen, with your legs spread at hip width and the tops of your feet on the floor; extend your arms back along the sides of your torso, with your palms on the floor, and rest your forehead on the floor (see Figure 11-6a).**

2. **As you inhale, raise your chest, legs, and head; sweep your arms like wings out to the sides and then all the way forward, as Figure 11-6b illustrates.**

   In the beginning, try sweeping your arms only halfway forward in a *T* position; it allows your back muscles to gradually become accustomed to the posture's physical demands.

3. **As you exhale, sweep your arms back and slowly lower your torso, legs, and head to the floor at the same time.**

4. **Repeat Steps 2 and 3 three times, and then stay in Step 2 (the last raised position) for 6 to 8 breaths.**

**Figure 11-6:** Make sure you're ready for this "super" posture.

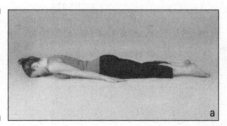 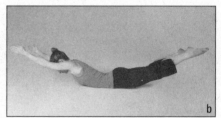

*Photograph by Adam Latham*

# Bending from Side to Side

The spinal column can move in four basic ways: forward *(flexion)*, backward *(extension)*, sideways *(lateral flexion)*, and twist *(rotation)*. The side bend is often the least practiced in Yoga. This missed opportunity is unfortunate because side bends help stretch and tone the muscles along the sides of the abdomen, ribcage, and spine, to keep your waist trim, your breathing full, and your spine supple.

A true side bend fully contracts one side of the body while expanding the other. To experience the effects of a side bend right now, simply lean to your right (or left) side as you exhale and reach the same-side arm downward. To realize the full effect of the stretch, reach the opposite-side arm up toward the ceiling. In this section, we cover some safe, creative ways to use side bends on the floor.

## Seated side bend

This seated side bend is a great way to ease into the position if you're not used to bending from side to side. Just follow these steps:

1. **Sit comfortably in a simple cross-legged position; place your right palm on the floor, near your right hip.**

   Check out Chapter 6 for some appropriate seated positions.

2. **As you inhale, raise your left arm out to the side and above your head beside your left ear.**

3. **As you exhale, slide your right hand across the floor out to the right, letting your torso, head, and left arm follow as you bend to the right (see Figure 11-7).**

   Don't let your buttocks come off the floor as you bend.

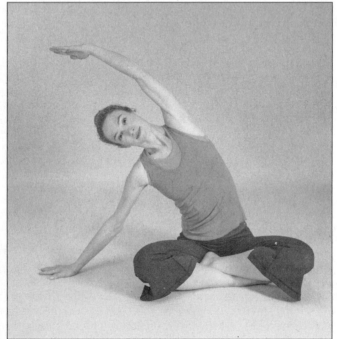

**Figure 11-7:**
Slide your hand across the floor as you bend.

*Photograph by Adam Latham*

4. **As you inhale, return to the upright position (as you were at the start of Step 2).**

5. **Repeat Steps 2 through 4 three times, and then stay in the bent position (Step 3) for 6 to 8 breaths.**

6. **Repeat Steps 1 through 5 on the other side.**

## All-fours side bend

Many people with back or hip problems have a hard time sitting upright on the floor. The all-fours position gives the spine more freedom and is an easier side bend from the floor.

1. **Start on your hands and knees, with your knees below your hips and your hands below your shoulders, with your palms on the floor.**

   Straighten your elbows, but don't lock them. Look straight ahead.

2. **As you exhale, bend your head and torso sideways to the right, and look toward your tailbone (see Figure 11-8).**

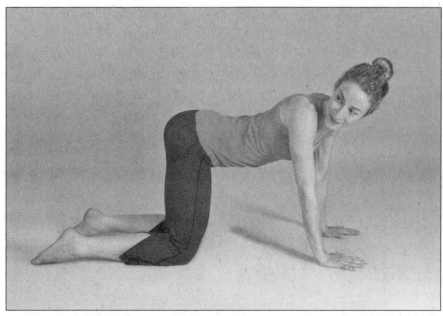

**Figure 11-8:**
Look back
as you bend.

*Photograph by Adam Latham*

3. As you inhale, return to the starting position in Step 1.

4. Repeat Steps 2 and 3 three times, and then stay in Step 2 for 6 to 8 breaths.

5. Repeat Steps 2 through 4 on the other side.

## Folded side bend

The Sanskrit word *bala* (pronounced *bah-lah*) means "child." This practice was inspired by a baby's folded position in the womb. The benefits of this side bend, which is a variation of *balasana*, the child's posture (see Chapter 15 for this posture), are the same as for the seated side bend.

1. Sit on your heels with your toes pointing back, and fold forward by laying your abdomen on your thighs and your forehead on the floor; extend your arms forward with your palms on the floor, as in Figure 11-9a.

2. As you exhale, stay in the folded position and slide your upper torso, head, arms, and hands to the right as far as possible, as in Figure 11-9b; wait for a few seconds and, again, with another exhalation, slide farther to the right if you can do so without straining.

3. Return to center and repeat the sequence to the left side, staying in Step 2 for 6 to 8 breaths on each side.

**Figure 11-9:**
Wait a few moments before you stretch farther on each side.

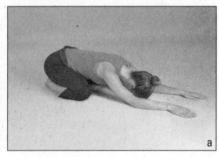
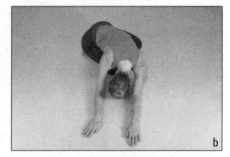

a

b

*Photograph by Adam Latham*

## Bending Forward

Of all the ways the human torso (and spine) can move, bending forward is the maneuver folks most commonly use. A tucked or fetal position is inherently comforting to most people, perhaps because they spend their first 9 months positioned like that in their mothers' wombs.

Forward bends are usually a good way to begin any movement routine (unless you're dealing with spinal disc injuries or certain other back problems). Back bends are the lively extroverts of the *asana* family, and forward bends are the retiring introverts; you always perform them with an exhalation — the passive, contracting phase of the breathing cycle.

Constantly bending forward from the waist tends to put stress on the lower back and neck. Yogic forward bends call for movement from the hip joints, a switch that can help you maintain a healthy, stress-free spine as you correct the poor forward-bending habits we discuss earlier in this chapter.

Be very careful of all the seated forward bends if you have disc-related back problems.

If you have a problem sitting upright on the floor in the seated forward bend or in any of the following forward-bending postures, raise your hips with folded blankets or firm pillows, as in Figure 11-10c.

## Seated forward bend: *Pashcimottanasana*

The seated forward bend intensely stretches the entire back side of the body, including the back of the spine and legs. It also tones the muscles and organs of the abdomen and creates a calming and quieting effect.

1. **Sit on the floor, with your legs at hip width and comfortably stretched out in front of you; bring your back up nice and tall, and place your palms on the floor near your thighs.**

2. **As you inhale, raise your arms forward and overhead until they're beside your ears, as in Figure 11-10a.**

   Keep your arms and legs soft and slightly bent in Forgiving Limbs, which we describe in Chapter 3.

3. **As you exhale, bend forward from the hips; bring your hands, chest, and head toward your legs; rest your hands on the floor or on your thighs, knees, shins, or feet.**

   If your head isn't close to your knees, bend your knees more until you feel your back stretching (see Figure 11-10b).

4. **Repeat Steps 2 and 3 three times, and then stay folded (Step 3) for 6 to 8 breaths.**

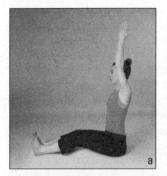 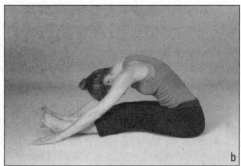

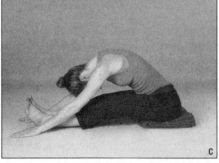

**Figure 11-10:** If your head isn't close to your knees, bend your knees more.

*Photograph by Adam Latham*

*Note:* In the classic posture, the inner legs are joined, the knees are straight, and the ankles are extended so that the toes point up. The chin rests on the chest, the hands hold the sides of the feet, the back is extended forward, and the forehead is pressed against the legs.

In Sanskrit, *pashcimottanasana* (pronounced *pash-chee-moh-tah-nah-sah-nah*) translates to the "extension of the West posture." In yogic jargon, the West refers to the back, and the East stands for the front. The symbolism refers to both the physical and psychological effects of this posture: It stretches the back of the body, especially the back of the spine and legs, and just as the sun sets in the West, the "light" of your consciousness draws inward as you fold upon yourself.

## Head-to-knee posture: Janushirshasana

The head-to-knee posture keeps your spine supple, stimulates the abdominal organs, and stretches your back, especially on the side of the extended leg. It also activates the central channel *(sushumna-nadi)*. As we explain in Chapter 5, the *central channel* is the pathway for the awakened energy of pure consciousness (called *kundalini-shakti*), which leads to ecstasy and spiritual liberation.

Follow these steps to achieve this posture:

1. **Sit on the floor, with your legs stretched out in front of you, and then bend your left knee and bring your left heel toward your right groin.**

2. **Rest your bent left knee on the floor (but don't force it down), and place the sole of your left foot on the inside of your right thigh.**

   The toes of the left foot point toward the right knee.

3. **Bring your back up nice and tall; as you inhale, raise your arms forward and overhead until they're beside your ears, as Figure 11-11a shows.**

   Keep your arms and your right leg soft and slightly bent in Forgiving Limbs, which we describe in Chapter 3.

4. **As you exhale, bend forward from the hips, bringing your hands, chest, and head toward your right leg; rest your hands on the floor or on your thigh, knee, shin, or foot.**

   If your head isn't close to your right knee, bend your knee more until you feel your back stretching on the right side (see Figure 11-11b).

**Figure 11-11:**
The head-
to-knee
posture.

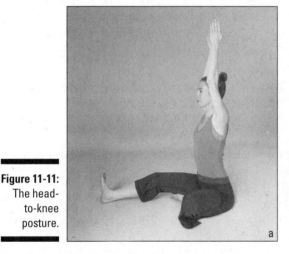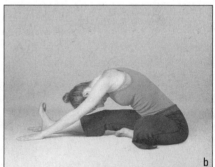

a b

*Photograph by Adam Latham*

5. **Repeat Steps 3 and 4 three times, and then stay in Step 4 (the final forward bend) for 6 to 8 breaths.**

6. **Repeat Steps 1 through 4 on the opposite side.**

Keep your back muscles as relaxed as possible.

The Sanskrit word *janu* (pronounced *jah-noo*) means "knee," and *shirsha* (pronounced *sheer-shah*) means "head."

## The great seal: Mahamudra

Ancient Hatha Yoga texts give high praise to the volcano posture. It strengthens the back, stretches the legs, and opens the hips and chest. This posture is unique, in that has qualities of both a forward bend and a back bend. When used with special locks *(bandhas)* that contain and channel energy in the torso, this technique has both cleansing and healing effects.

1. **Sitting on the floor, with your legs stretched out in front of you, bend your left knee and bring your left foot toward your right groin.**

2. **Rest your bent left knee on the floor to the left (but don't force it down), and place the sole of your left foot on the inside of your right thigh, with your heel in your groin.**

    The toes of the left foot point toward the right knee.

3. **Bring your back up nice and tall; as you inhale, raise your arms forward and overhead until they're beside your ears.**

    Keep your arms and the right leg soft and slightly bent in Forgiving Limbs, as we describe in Chapter 3. Refer to Figure 11-11a in the preceding section, if necessary.

4. **As you exhale, bend forward from the hips, lift your chest forward, and extend your back without letting it round; place your hands on your right knee, shin, or toes, and look straight ahead (see Figure 11-12).**

5. **Repeat Steps 3 and 4 three times, and then stay in Step 4 for 6 to 8 breaths.**

6. **Repeat the same sequence on the opposite side.**

*Note:* In the classic posture, the front leg and the arms are straight, and the hands are holding the toes of the front leg. The back is extended, and the chin is pressed onto the chest. The abdominal muscles are pulled up into the abdominal cavity, and the anal sphincter is tightened.

The Sanskrit term *mahamudra* (pronounced *mah-hah-mood-rah*) means "great seal." Here it applies to a Yoga posture, but in other contexts, *mahamudra* is a mental exercise that allows your mind to flow out into the open sky. Try combining this inner "attitude" with the physical pose.

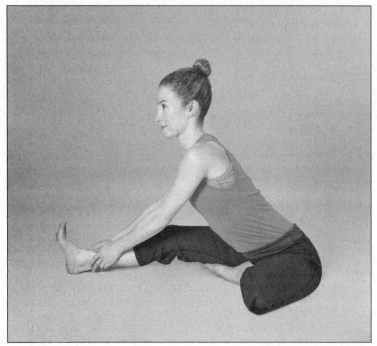

**Figure 11-12:**
The volcano is a great all-inclusive posture.

*Photograph by Adam Latham*

# Wide-legged forward bend: Upavishta konasana

The wide-legged forward bend stretches the backs and insides of the legs (hamstrings and adductors) and increases the flexibility of the spine and hip joints. It improves circulation to the entire pelvic region, tones the abdomen, and has a calming effect on the nervous system. Note, though, that muscle density may make this posture difficult for most men.

1. **Sit on the floor, with your legs straight and spread wide apart (but not more than 90 degrees).**

   Because this posture is challenging, give yourself an advantage by pulling the flesh of the buttocks (you may know them as "cheeks") out from under the *sits bones* (the bones directly under that flesh; they're also known as the *ischial tuberosities*) and bending your knees slightly. Alternatively, sit on some folded blankets.

2. **As you inhale, raise your arms forward and overhead until they're beside your ears.**

   Keep your elbows soft and your legs slightly bent in Forgiving Limbs, as we describe in Chapter 3. Bring your back up nice and tall (see Figure 11-13a).

3. **As you exhale, bend forward from the hips and bring your hands, chest, and head toward the floor.**

   Rest your extended arms and hands palms down on the floor. If you have the flexibility, place your forehead on the floor as well, as in Figure 11-13b.

4. **Repeat Steps 2 and 3 three times, and then stay in Step 3 (the folded position) for 6 to 8 breaths.**

**Figure 11-13:**
The wide-legged forward bend.

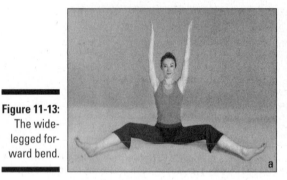 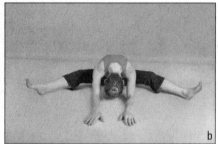

*Photograph by Adam Latham*

***Note:*** In the classic posture, the legs are straight, with the toes vertical; the chin and chest are on the floor; and the arms are extended forward, with the palms joined.

The wide-legged forward bend is also called the *lifetime posture* because it can take a whole lifetime to master. But don't worry if you don't quite reach mastery. Some Yogis believe that if you don't master the pose in this lifetime, you can try again in the next lifetime.

The Sanskrit term *upavishta* (pronounced *oopah-vish-tah*) means "seated," and *kona* (pronounced *koh-nah*) means "angle."

# Chapter 12

# Several Twists on the Yoga Twist

. . . . . . . . . . . . . . . . . . . . . . . . . . . . . . . . . . . . . . . . .

*In This Chapter*

▶ Enjoying spinal fitness — with a yogic twist

▶ Introducing six simple twists

. . . . . . . . . . . . . . . . . . . . . . . . . . . . . . . . . . . . . . . . .

*I*magine you're cleaning the kitchen with a wet sponge. After you mop up some spills, the sponge gets dirty. You hold it under the kitchen faucet, turn on the water, and squeeze out the dirty water. As you release the pressure on the sponge, it sucks up some clean water. You're ready to start again.

This description is a lot like how yogic twists work on the spine. The pulpy pads *(discs)* between the individual bones have no direct blood supply of their own after about age 20, so they depend on your everyday movements to help them wring out the accumulated wastes and soak up a fresh supply of blood and other reviving fluids. Over time, if you don't continually squeeze and soak your discs, they tend to harden and dry out, like a sponge left unused for a few days. Consequently, your spine stiffens up and shrinks.

Twists are an important component of any Yoga practice. They clean out the discs and help keep them firm and supple; massage the internal organs, such as your intestines and kidneys; stoke the inner fire of digestion; and stretch and strengthen the muscles of your back and abdomen.

This chapter features seated twists, which emphasize the upper spine, and reclining twists, which emphasize the lower spine. For standing twists, see Chapter 8.

Approach all twists with caution if you're suffering from disc problems anywhere in your spine. Consult your physician, chiropractor, or physical therapist, or work with a reputable Yoga therapist after you have a diagnosis.

# Trying Simple Upright Twists

When done properly, Yogic twisting postures strengthen your body, especially the weak spots (notably the lower back). While twisting is part of your everyday movements, unless your muscles are well trained, you can easily injure yourself. The exercises in this section can help you get your back in tip-top shape as you look forward to enjoyment and enlightenment along the way.

## Easy chair twist

This seated posture is an excellent way for a beginner to safely achieve a good twist before moving on to more complex methods of twisting. And you can use this simple, effective posture to liberate your spine while at the office without drawing too much attention to yourself. Your spine will thank you!

Twist mainly from your shoulders; the head and neck come along for the ride.

1. **Sit sideways on a chair, with the chair back to your left, your feet flat on the floor, and your heels directly below your knees.**

2. **Exhale, turn to the left, and hold the sides of the chair back with your hands.**

3. **As you inhale, extend or lift your spine upward.**

4. **As you exhale, twist your torso and head farther to the left, as in Figure 12-1.**

5. **Repeat Steps 1 through 4, gradually twisting farther with each exhalation, for 3 breaths (don't force it); then hold the twist for 6 to 8 breaths.**

6. **Repeat Steps 1 through 5 on the opposite side.**

If your feet aren't comfortably on the floor for the easy chair twist, elevate them with a folded blanket or a phone book.

## Easy sitting twist

When you can twist comfortably while seated on a chair (see the preceding section), you can transfer your newly gained skill to the floor and try the following exercise. Its effect is similar to that of the easy chair twist, and it fits nicely into a regular Yoga practice, a large part of which you can do on the floor.

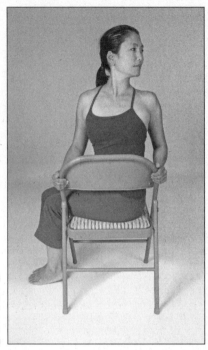

**Figure 12-1:**
Easy chair
twist.

*Photograph by Adam Latham*

1. **Sit on the floor with your legs in a simple cross-legged position, and extend your spine upward, nice and tall.**

2. **Place your left hand palm down on top of your right knee.**

3. **Place your right hand palm down on the floor behind your right hip, to prop yourself up.**

4. **As you inhale, extend your spine upward.**

5. **As you exhale, twist your torso and head to the right (see Figure 12-2).**

6. **Repeat Steps 4 and 5 for 3 breaths, gradually twisting farther with each exhalation (don't force it); then hold the twist for 6 to 8 breaths.**

7. **Repeat Steps 1 through 6 on the opposite side.**

If you have difficulty sitting upright in this seated twist, use blankets or pillows under your bottom to make your hips even with your knees.

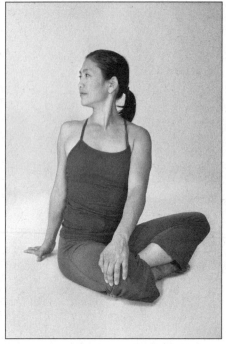

*Photograph by Adam Latham*

## The sage twist

The easy chair twist and the easy sitting twist (in the preceding sections) are the simplest yogic twists. By changing the position of your legs, you alter the level of difficulty and also enhance the overall benefit. The sage twist does so, to give you extra rewards for your investment.

1. **Sit on the floor with both legs extended forward; bend your right knee and place your right foot on the floor just inside your left thigh, with your toes facing forward.**

2. **Place your right hand, palm down, on the floor behind you; wrap the palm of your left hand around the side of your right knee.**

3. **As you inhale, extend or lift your spine upward.**

4. **As you exhale, twist your torso and head to the right, as in Figure 12-3.**

5. **Repeat Steps 3 and 4, gradually twisting farther with each exhalation, for 3 breaths (don't force it); then hold the twist for 6 to 8 breaths.**

6. **Repeat Steps 1 through 5 on the opposite side.**

If you have difficulty sitting upright in this seated twist, sit on blankets or pillows until your hips are even with your knees.

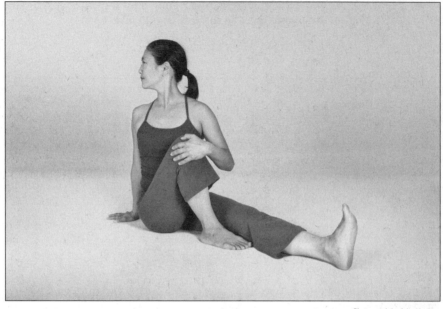

**Figure 12-3:**
Beginners
can enjoy
benefits
from this
sage twist
variation.

*Photograph by Adam Latham*

This posture is a variation of the classic posture *maricyasana*. The Sanskrit word *marici* (pronounced *mah-ree-chee*) means "ray of light" and is the name of an ancient sage.

# Twisting while Reclining

The remaining exercises in this chapter call for you to lie down. You can harvest all kinds of benefits from them, including a delicious feeling of release in your spine.

## Bent leg supine twist

The bent supine twist is a variation of the classic posture known as *parivartanasana*. The Sanskrit word *parivartana* (pronounced *pah-ree-vahr-tah-nah*) means "turning."

This posture has a calming effect on the lower back. Here's how you do it:

1. **Lie on your back with your knees bent and feet on the floor at hip width, and extend your arms from your sides like a *T* (in line with the top of your shoulders), with your palms down.**

2. **As you exhale, slowly lower your bent legs to the right side while turning your head to the left (see Figure 12-4).**

   Keep your head on the floor.

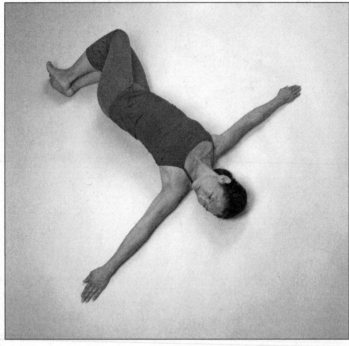

Photograph by Adam Latham

**Figure 12-4:**
Turn your head in the opposite direction of your legs.

3. **As you inhale, bring your bent knees back to the middle.**

4. **As you exhale, slowly lower your bent knees to the left while turning your head to the right.**

5. **Repeat Steps 1 through 4, alternating three times slowly on each side; then hold one last twist on each side for 6 to 8 breaths.**

## The Swiss army knife

This posture, a variation of the classic *jathara parivritti*, tones the abdominal organs and intestines and also stretches the lower back and hips. *Jathara parivritti* (pronounced *jat-hah-rah pah-ree-vree-tee*) means "belly twisting." Just follow these steps:

1. **Lie flat on the floor with your legs straight down, and extend your arms out from your sides like a *T* (in line with the top of your shoulders), with your palms up.**

2. Bend your right knee, and draw your thigh into your abdomen.

3. As you exhale, slowly lower your bent right leg to the left side and extend it a comfortable distance.

4. Extend your left arm on the floor along the left side of your head (palm up), and then turn your head to the right, as in Figure 12-5.

   Keep your head on the floor, and try to visualize lines of energy going out through your arms and legs.

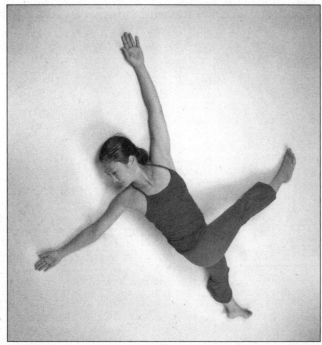

**Figure 12-5:** Extend your arm and turn your head the opposite way.

*Photograph by Adam Latham*

5. Follow Steps 1 through 4; then relax and stay in Step 4 for 6 to 8 breaths.

6. Repeat Steps 1 through 5 on the opposite side.

## Extended legs supine twist: Jathara parivritti

If you enjoy practicing the Swiss army knife (see the preceding section), you're likely to enjoy this slightly more demanding exercise. This variation of *jathara parivritti* gives you the same benefits as the Swiss army knife but creates an even more pronounced stretch of the lower back and hips. Of course, stretching is good for your muscles and your spine, too. The following steps show you how it works:

1. **Lie on your back with your knees bent and your feet on the floor at hip width, and extend your arms out from your sides like a *T* (in line with the top of your shoulders), with your palms down.**

2. **Bend your knees and draw both thighs into your abdomen.**

3. **As you exhale, slowly lower your bent legs to the right side.**

4. **Extend both legs a comfortable distance, and then turn your head to the left, as Figure 12-6 illustrates.**

    Keep your head on the floor. If this posture is difficult, try bending both legs a little more.

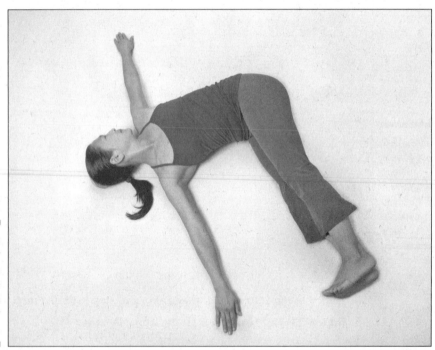

**Figure 12-6:**
Keep your head on the floor as you turn it and extend your legs.

*Photograph by Adam Latham*

5. **Follow Steps 1 through 4; then relax and stay in Step 4 for 6 to 8 breaths.**

6. **Repeat Steps 1 through 5 on the opposite side.**

*Note:* In the classic (traditionally taught) version of this posture, the knees are straight and the joined legs are resting on the floor. The arms are straight and extended to the sides at right angles to the torso. The hand on the same side of the extended legs holds the top foot.

# Chapter 13

# Dynamic Posture: The Rejuvenation Sequence and Sun Salutation

*T*he sun has long captured humanity's attention for its life-giving power. Sun worship is one of humankind's first and most natural forms of spiritual expression: Just think of the Sumerians, Egyptians, and Mayans. But nowhere has this homage to the solar spirit been as well preserved as in India's 10,000-year-old civilization: To this day, millions of people there pay respects to the sun as a part of their daily rituals.

You don't have to be a sun worshiper, though, to benefit from Yoga's sun salutation (*surya namaskara*, pronounced *soor-yah nah-mahs-kah-rah*). This exercise — a special sequence of postures — is considered so profound that many people practice it on its own.

The sun salutation helps you remember the yogic idea that your body is condensed sunlight. The saluting gesture, called *namaskara mudra* in Sanskrit (pronounced *nah-mahs-kah-rah mood-rah*), is a salute to the highest aspect within yourself — the spirit.

The actual technique for and number of steps in the sun salutation vary somewhat among the different Yoga schools and organizations. In this chapter, we focus on the best-known form of sun salutation — a 12-step sequence that the late Swami Vishnu Devananda, a disciple of the great Swami Shivananda of Rishikesh, India, introduced to the U.S. in the early 1960s. First, though, we introduce a modified 7-step version you do from a kneeling position; it's ideally suited for anyone who hasn't yet developed enough flexibility, muscle strength, and fitness for the 12-step version.

## The dawn of the sun salutation

No one knows how old the sun salutation is, but at the beginning of the 20th century, the Raja of Oudh, representing a small state in Northern India, encouraged all his subjects to learn and practice this exercise sequence. He personally practiced the sun salutation for health and happiness.

# *Warming up for the Sun: Rejuvenating in 9 Steps*

Do you need a more user-friendly version of the sun salutation? Do you have a hard time kneeling (as the 7-step sun salutation requires later in this chapter) or stepping through (as the 12-step sun salutation requires later in this chapter)? Then try the 9-step rejuvenation sequence, direct from California, using the focus breathing technique from Chapter 5:

1. **Stand in the mountain posture, with your feet at hip width and arms at your sides (see Figure 13-1a).**

2. **As you inhale, slowly raise your arms out from the sides and overhead (see Figure 13-1b); then pause.**

3. **As you exhale, bend forward from the waist and bring your head toward your knees; bring your hands forward and down toward the floor in the standing forward bend (see Figure 13-1c).**

   Keep your arms and legs soft (see Chapter 3 for an explanation of Forgiving Limbs); then pause.

4. **Bend your knees quite a bit and, as you inhale, sweep your arms out from the sides, but come only halfway up with your arms in a *T* (half forward bend), as in Figure 13-1d; then pause briefly.**

5. **As you exhale, fold all the way down again and hang your arms in the standing forward bend (see Figure 13-1e).**

6. **As you inhale, sweep your arms from the sides like wings, and bring your torso all the way up again, standing with your arms overhead in the standing arm raise (see Figure 13-1f).**

7. **As you exhale, bend your knees and squat halfway to the floor.**

   Soften your arms, but keep them overhead; look straight ahead (see Figure 13-1g).

8. **As you inhale, bring your torso all the way up again, standing with your arms overhead in the standing arm raise (see Figure 13-1h).**

9. **As you exhale, bring your arms back to your sides, as in Step 1 (see Figure 13-1i).**

Repeat the entire sequence six to eight times slowly.

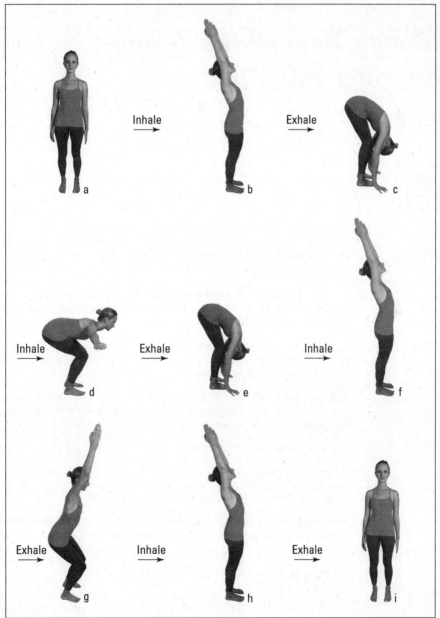

**Figure 13-1:** The 9-step rejuvenation sequence.

To make it harder on the last round, stay for 6 to 8 breaths in the half forward bend (Step 4), the standing forward bend (Step 5), and the half squat or half chair (Step 8).

To make it much harder, do the entire sequence standing on your toes.

# Gliding Through the 7-Step Kneeling Salutation

If you aren't quite ready to tackle the 12-step sun salutation, the following 7-step variation can give you many benefits and also help you get in shape for the standing variety. Use focus, chest-to-belly, or belly-to-chest breathing techniques from Chapter 5, and follow these steps.

Just follow your breath — inhale when you're opening, exhale when you're folding. Move slowly, pausing after each inhalation and exhalation.

1. **Sit on your heels in a bent-knee position, bring your back up nice and tall, and place your palms together in the prayer position, with your thumbs touching the sternum (breastbone) in the middle of your chest (see Figure 13-2a).**

2. **As you inhale, open your palms and slightly raise your arms forward and then overhead; raise your buttocks away from your heels, arch your back, and look up at the ceiling, as in Figure 13-2b.**

3. **As you exhale, bend forward slowly from the hips, placing your palms, forearms, and then forehead on the floor; pause, relaxing your hips, as Figure 13-2c shows.**

4. **Slide your hands forward on the floor until your arms are extended; slide your chest forward, bending your elbows slightly, and arch up into cobra II (see Figure 13-2d).**

   Flip to Chapter 11 for instructions on cobra II.

5. **As you exhale, turn your toes under, raise your hips, extend your legs, and bring your chest down, keeping both hands on the floor for the downward-facing dog (see Figure 13-2e).**

6. **As you inhale, bend your knees to the floor, with your gaze toward the floor, slightly in front of you, as in Figure 13-2f.**

7. **As you exhale, sit back on your heels and return your hands to the saluting position, as in Step 1 (see Figure 13-2g).**

Repeat the entire sequence 3 to 12 times.

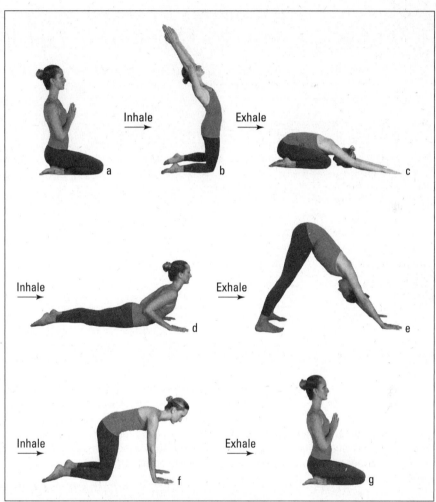

*Photograph by Adam Latham*

**Figure 13-2:**
The
7-step sun
salutation.

If you're not able to sit on your heels in Steps 1 and 7, simply keep your palms in the prayer position and stand on your knees instead. You can also fold a blanket under your knees for comfort.

If you find this 7-step salutation too difficult for you, head to the following section and try Steps 1 through 3 only of the 12-step version until you're ready to do more.

## Shedding light on the benefits of sun saluting

Respected for its excellent effects, the sun salutation reputedly provides an array of benefits, including the following:

- Stretching your spine and strengthening the muscles that support it

- Strengthening and stretching your arms and legs

- Improving your posture, coordination, and endurance

- Complementing the delicate balance between muscle tension and muscle relaxation

- Linking body, breath, and mind

- Granting (in most of its forms) aerobic benefits

- Improving your lung function and the delivery of oxygen to your muscles (including the heart)

- Working well (with modifications) for people of all ages, from children to seniors

The Yoga masters claim that the sun salutation has deeper psychological and spiritual implications because it stimulates subtle vital energies leading to states of higher awareness. No wonder so many Yoga DVDs on the market today include the sun salutation!

# Advancing to the 12-Step Sun Salutation

To enjoy the greatest benefit from this sequence (as well as all your Yoga postures), execute each part with full participation of your mind. When you stand, really stand; plant your feet firmly on the ground. When you bend or stretch, bend or stretch with complete attention. Your mind makes your practice not only elegant, but also potent. Use any of the Yoga breathing techniques from Chapter 5, and follow these steps:

1. **Start in a standing position, with your feet at hip width, and place your palms together in the prayer position, with your thumbs touching the sternum (breastbone) in the middle of your chest (see Figure 13-3a).**

2. **As you inhale, open your palms slightly and raise your arms forward and overhead; arch your back and look up toward the ceiling without throwing your head back (see Figure 13-3b).**

3. **As you exhale, bend forward from the hips, soften your knees (as in Forgiving Limbs, which Chapter 3 covers), and place your hands on the floor; bring your head as close as possible to your legs, as Figure 13-3c shows.**

4. **As you inhale, bend your left knee and step your right foot back into a lunge.**

Make sure that your left knee is directly over your ankle and your thigh is parallel to the floor so that your knee forms a right angle. Your gaze should be downward, a few inches in front of you on the floor, keeping your neck in a long and neutral position. Figure 13-3d gives you a visual of this step.

5. **As you exhale, step your left foot back beside the right and hold a push-up position; if your arms tire, bend your knees to the floor and pause on your hands and knees (see Figure 13-3e).**

6. **Inhale and then, as you exhale, lower your knees (from the push-up), chest, and chin to the floor, keeping your buttocks up in the air (see Figure 13-3f).**

7. **As you inhale, slide your chest forward along the floor, and then arch back into cobra II, as in Figure 13-3g.**

8. **As you exhale, turn your toes under, raise your hips, extend your legs, and bring your chest down, keeping both hands on the floor (see Figure 13-3h).**

   This pose is the same downward-facing dog position from Chapter 7.

9. **As you inhale, step your right foot forward between your hands and, again, point your gaze toward the floor a few inches ahead of you (see Figure 13-3i).**

10. **As you exhale, step your left foot forward, parallel to and even with your right foot; soften your knees and fold into a forward bend, as in Step 3 (see Figure 13-3j).**

11. **As you inhale, raise your arms either forward and overhead from the front, or out and up from the sides like wings; then arch back and look up, as in Step 2 (see Figure 13-3k).**

If you have back problems, lifting up from the forward bend with your arms to the front or sides may cause you some discomfort. If so, you can try the roll-up: Keep your chin on your chest and roll up, stacking the vertebrae one at a time, with your arms hanging at your sides and your head coming up last. When you're fully upright, bring your arms forward, up, and overhead from the front; arch your back just a little; and look up.

12. **As you exhale, return your hands to the prayer position, as in Step 1 (see Figure 13-3l).**

Repeat the entire sequence 3 to 12 times. First lead with the right foot, and then alternate with the left foot, for an equal number of repetitions (each side counts as half a sequence).

If you're ready for greater challenges, consider the advanced sun salutations in *Power Yoga For Dummies*, by Doug Swenson (Wiley), from the Ashtanga Yoga system, or check the Internet for the Iyengar sun salutation or various "flow" sequences.

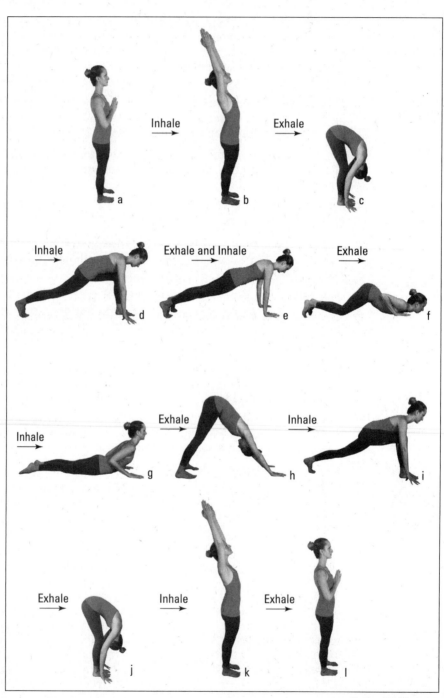

Inhale → Exhale →

Inhale → Exhale and Inhale → Exhale →

Inhale → Exhale → Inhale →

Exhale → Inhale → Exhale →

**Figure 13-3:**
The
12-step sun
salutation.

*Photograph by Adam Latham*

# Chapter 14

# A Recommended Beginners' Routine for Men and Women

• • • • • • • • • • • • • • • • • • • • • • • • • • • • • • • • • • • • • • • • • • • • • • • • • • • •

## In This Chapter

▶ Keeping current on basic Yoga principles

▶ Presenting a basic Yoga routine for beginners

• • • • • • • • • • • • • • • • • • • • • • • • • • • • • • • • • • • • • • • • • • • • • • • • • • • •

*T*he Yoga routine in this chapter is a tried-and-true sequence from Larry Payne's Prime of Life Yoga and is an excellent way for a beginner to get started. Taught around the world, this sequence has helped thousands of people — including the staff at the J. Paul Getty Museum in Los Angeles and, slightly farther from home base, 100 members of the World Presidents Organization (a diverse and successful international organization of CEOs), which meets all the way up at the North Pole. The routine is safe and doable and includes segments that reduce stress and increase strength, flexibility, and overall pep and vitality.

## Starting Slowly and Wisely

Most people find that they can successfully incorporate 15 to 20 minutes of practicing a new endeavor into their day on a regular basis. This chapter provides you with a short *asana* routine about that length that's designed to jump-start your Yoga practice. If you practice this routine three to six times per week, you'll notice improvements in your flexibility, muscle tone and strength, and concentration. You'll likely notice a number of other benefits as well, such as better stamina, digestion, and sleep.

When practicing the postures we describe in the following section, either follow the directions for breath and movement or simply stay in each posture for six to eight breaths.

Because this may be your first Yoga experience — and you may have turned directly to this chapter — following is a quick trip through some basic Yoga principles you want to keep in mind:

✔ **Yoga isn't competitive.** Be patient. If you follow the directions, you'll improve over time, regardless of your starting level.

✔ **Move slowly into and out of the postures.** Never rush your Yoga session. Remember that coming into a posture and moving out of a posture are integral parts of the posture itself.

✔ **Use yogic breathing throughout the routine, and pause briefly after each inhalation and exhalation.** Chapter 5 gives you more info on yogic breathing.

✔ **Challenge yourself, but don't strain yourself.** Yoga must never hurt or cause you pain. Check out Chapters 2 and 3 for more on the proper Yoga attitude.

✔ **Move smoothly into and out of a posture several times before holding the posture.** Doing so prepares your body for a deeper stretch and helps you concentrate on linking the body, breath, and mind, as we discuss in Chapter 5.

✔ **Don't change the order of the sequence and just randomly pick the postures you want.** All the routines have a special order or sequence, to give you the maximum benefits. (For details on how to put together your own routines, see Chapter 15.)

# Trying out a Fun Beginner Routine

As you perform the postures in this short routine, notice how you start by giving your body and mind a chance to transition from your previous activity, how you move your body in several different directions, and how you end the routine with rest. These activities are some of the fundamental elements of a well-balanced Yoga routine, regardless of its length. Use focus breathing (which we cover in Chapter 5) throughout the routine.

## Corpse posture

1. **Lie flat on your back, with your arms relaxed along the sides of your torso, your palms up, and your feet open out toward the sides of the room (see Figure 14-1).**

2. **Inhale and exhale through your nose slowly for 8 to 10 breaths.**

   Pause briefly after each inhalation and exhalation.

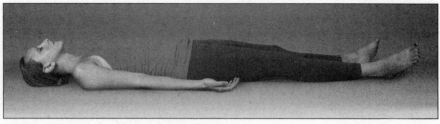

**Figure 14-1:**
Corpse
posture.

*Photograph by Adam Latham*

## Lying arm raise

1. **Lie in the corpse posture (see the preceding section), with your arms relaxed at your sides and your palms down (see Figure 14-2a).**

2. **As you inhale, slowly raise your arms overhead and touch the floor behind you, as in Figure 14-2b; pause briefly.**

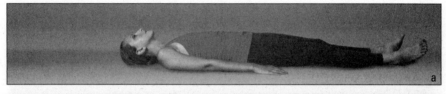

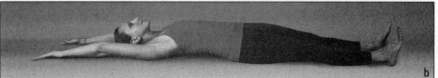

**Figure 14-2:**
Lying arm
raise.

*Photograph by Adam Latham*

3. **As you exhale, bring your arms back to your sides, as in Step 1.**

4. **Repeat Steps 2 and 3 six to eight times.**

## Knee-to-chest posture

1. **Lie on your back with your knees bent and your feet flat on the floor.**

2. **As you exhale, bring your right knee into your chest and extend your left leg down; hold your shin just below your knee (see Figure 14-3).**

   If you have knee problems, hold the back of your thigh instead.

3. **Stay in Step 2 for 6 to 8 breaths, and then repeat on the left side.**

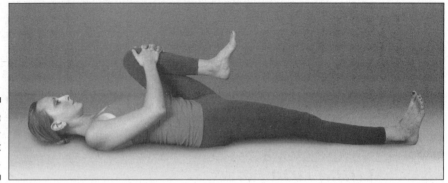

*Photograph by Adam Latham*

**Figure 14-3:**
Knee-
to-chest
posture.

# Downward-facing dog

1. **Beginning on your hands and knees, place your hands directly under your shoulders, with your palms spread on the floor and your knees directly under your hips.**

   Straighten your arms, but don't lock your elbows. Figure 14-4a shows an example.

2. **As you exhale, lift and straighten (but don't lock) your knees; as your hips lift, bring your head down to a neutral position so that your ears are between your arms (see Figure 14-4b).**

   If possible, press your heels to the floor and your head toward your feet (stop if doing so strains your neck).

**Figure 14-4:**
Downward-
facing dog.

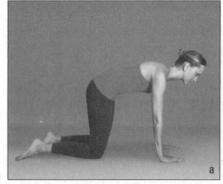

a

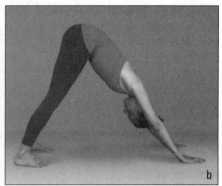

b

*Photograph by Adam Latham*

3. As you inhale, come back down to your hands and knees, as in Step 1.

4. Repeat Steps 1 through 3 three times, and then stay in Step 2 for 6 to 8 breaths.

## Child's posture

1. **Starting on your hands and knees, place your knees about hip width apart, with your hands just below your shoulders.**

   Keep your elbows straight but not locked.

2. **As you exhale, sit back on your heels; rest your torso on your thighs and your forehead on the floor.**

   You don't have to sit all the way back.

3. **Lay your arms back on the floor beside your torso, with your palms up, or reach your relaxed arms forward, with your palms on the floor.**

4. **Close your eyes and stay in the folded position for 6 to 8 breaths (see Figure 14-5).**

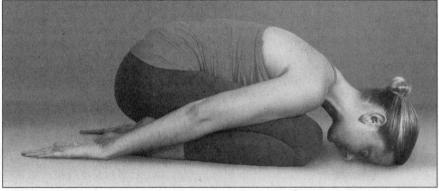

**Figure 14-5:**
Child's
posture.

*Photograph by Adam Latham*

## Warrior 1

1. **Stand in the mountain posture (see Chapter 7 for this pose). Turn your left foot out to about 45 degrees, and raise your right arm out in front of your right shoulder. Take a big step forward (about 3 to 3½ feet, or the length of your arm) with your right foot as you exhale.**

2. **Place your hands on the top of your hips, and square the front of your pelvis; release your hands and hang your arms, as in Figure 14-6a.**

3. **As you inhale, raise your arms forward and overhead, and bend your right knee to a right angle so that it's directly over your ankle and, ideally, your thigh is parallel to the floor (see Figure 14-6b).**

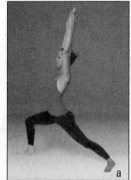 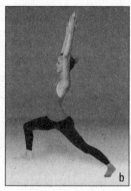

**Figure 14-6:**
Warrior I.

Photograph by Adam Latham

4. **Soften your arms (see Chapter 3 for a description of Forgiving Limbs) and face your palms toward each other; look straight ahead.**

   If your lower back is uncomfortable, lean your torso slightly over the forward leg until your back releases any tension that may be present.

5. **Repeat Steps 3 and 4 three times, and then hold once on the right side for 6 to 8 breaths.**

6. **Repeat Steps 1 through 5 on the other (left) side.**

## Standing forward bend

1. **Start in the mountain posture (refer to Chapter 7), and raise your arms forward and then up overhead as you inhale (see Figure 14-7a).**

2. **As you exhale, bend forward from the hips; when you feel a pull in the back of your legs, soften your knees (see Chapter 3 for more on Forgiving Limbs) and hang your arms as in Figure 14-7b, and relax your head and neck downward.**

   If your head isn't close to your knees, bend your knees more. If you have the flexibility, straighten your knees while keeping them soft.

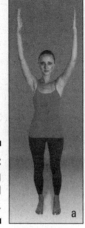 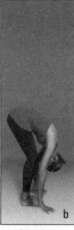

**Figure 14-7:**
Standing
forward
bend.

a            b

*Photograph by Adam Latham*

3. **Exhaling, roll your body up like a rag doll, stacking your vertebrae one at a time.**

   Flip to Chapter 8 for more advanced ways to come up from a forward bend.

4. **Repeat Steps 1 through 3 three times, and then stay down in Step 2 for 6 to 8 breaths.**

## Reverse triangle posture variation

1. **Stand in the mountain posture (check out Chapter 7 for a description), and step out to the right about 3 to 3½ feet (or the length of one leg) with your right foot as you exhale.**

2. **As you inhale, raise your arms out to the sides, parallel to the line of your shoulders (and the floor), so that your shoulders form a *T* with your torso (see Figure 14-8a).**

3. **As you exhale, bend forward from your hips and place your right hand on the floor near the inside of your left foot.**

4. **Raise your left arm toward the ceiling and look up at your left hand (see Figure 14-8b).**

   Soften your knees and arms. Bend your left knee or, if you experience strain or discomfort, move your right hand away from your left foot and more directly under your torso.

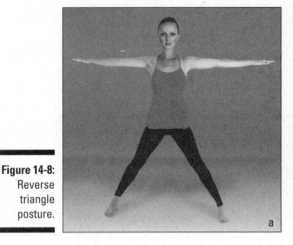
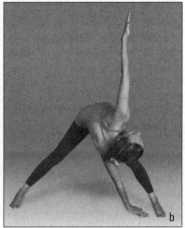

**Figure 14-8:**
Reverse
triangle
posture.

a

b

*Photograph by Adam Latham*

5. **Repeat Steps 2 through 4 on the same side three times, and then stay down in Step 4 for 6 to 8 breaths.**

6. **Repeat Steps 1 through 5 on the right side.**

You can strengthen or strain your neck in this posture, so turn your neck down if you're uncomfortable.

## Standing wide-legged forward bend

1. **Stand in the mountain posture (see Chapter 7), and step out to the right about 3 to 3½ feet (or the length of one leg) with your right foot as you exhale.**

2. **As you inhale, raise your arms out to the sides, parallel to the line of your shoulders (and the floor), so that your shoulders form a *T* with your torso (see Figure 14-9a).**

3. **As you exhale, bend forward from the hips and soften your knees.**

4. **Hold your bent elbows with the opposite-side hands, and hang your torso and arms.**

5. **Stay folded in this posture (see Figure 14-9b) for 6 to 8 breaths.**

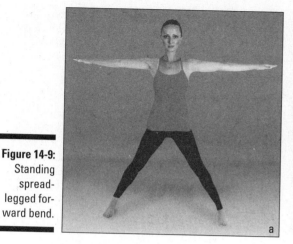 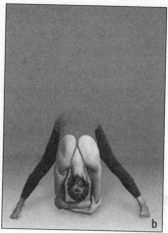

**Figure 14-9:**
Standing spread-legged forward bend.

*Photograph by Adam Latham*

# The karate kid

1. Stand in the mountain posture (see Chapter 7), and raise your arms out to the sides, parallel to the line of your shoulders (and the floor), so that your shoulders form a *T* with your torso as you inhale.

2. Steady yourself and focus on a spot on the floor 10 to 12 feet in front of you.

3. As you exhale, bend and raise your left knee toward your chest, keeping your right leg straight (see Figure 14-10); hold for 6 to 8 breaths.

4. Repeat Steps 1 through 3 with your legs reversed.

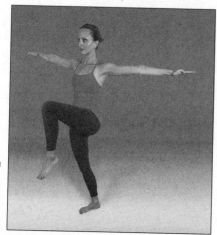

**Figure 14-10:**
The karate kid.

*Photograph by Adam Latham*

When you become stable in the karate kid posture, try extending your bent left leg forward and up. Gradually work toward fully extending your left leg parallel to the floor — take your time! Try this added step on both sides.

### Corpse posture redux

Repeat the corpse posture exercise as the earlier section "Corpse posture" describes (see Figure 14-1 for an illustration). Stay in this posture for 8 to 12 breaths, or choose one of the relaxation techniques in Chapter 4.

## Reaching Beyond the Beginning

When you become comfortable with the beginners' routine in this chapter, you can expand it and add variety by following the guidelines we present in Chapter 15; we walk you through designing your own Yoga program in that chapter. If you're young and fit, you may want to try the routines in Chapter 18. If you're midlife or older, or if you haven't exercised for a while, Chapter 19 provides less strenuous (but equally beneficial) routines.

Of course, with a taste of Hatha Yoga, you may want to take private lessons or go to a group class for feedback, to boost your morale or simply to practice — with new confidence — in the company of others.

Practicing on your own is fine, but nothing replaces working with a teacher. Before you get into too much of a Yoga groove, we recommend that you ask a Yoga teacher to check for any bad postural habits and, if you like, to give you some suggestions for taking the next step.

# Part III
# Creating and Customizing Your Yoga Routine

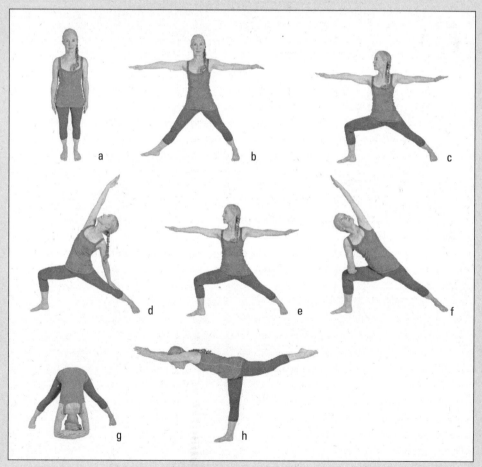

Photograph by Adam Latham

The joys and benefits of your Yoga practice need not be restricted to the Yoga studio or even your Yoga mat. See how you can take your Yoga to go at www.dummies.com/extras/yoga.

# In this part . . .

✔ Mix up your routine with the elements of Yoga session design, using postures you're already familiar with

✔ Pair up and explore the essentials of Partner Yoga

✔ Incorporate any desired adaptations for pregnant women, children, teens, and anyone in the prime of life and beyond

✔ Get the scoop on helpful props, including items you already have in your own home

✔ Explore how your own walls give you a great way to add variety and spice to your Yoga routines

# Chapter 15

# Designing Your Own Yoga Program

### In This Chapter

▶ Understanding posture sequencing

▶ Warming up to your session

▶ Exploring main and compensation postures

▶ Taking a rest during your routine

▶ Using the Classic Formula to create routines that suit your time frame

*T*he art and science of sequencing in Yoga is called *vinyasa-krama* (pronounced *veen-yah-sah-krah-mah*). In the Sanskrit language, the word *vinyasa* means "placement" and *krama* means "step" or "process." This concept is often called flow. The flow of postures is important, and paying attention to proper sequencing can help you derive maximum benefit from your Hatha Yoga session.

Before you experiment with various Yoga postures, you need to know how to combine postures correctly. The more you know about sequencing, the better. Understanding sequencing is like figuring out how to unlock the door of a bank vault. You may have a list of all the correct numbers, but if you don't know the correct combination, you can never open the door to the treasures hidden in the vault. In this chapter, we give you the secret combination, the essential rules for postural sequencing, so that you can create a Yoga program that's just right for you.

If you're dealing with a specific health challenge, you need to work one on one, under the guidance of your doctor, with a Yoga therapist or other health professional. This chapter focuses on "do-it-yourself" Hatha Yoga for general conditioning and stress reduction. Our emphasis is on prevention rather than therapy.

# *Applying the Rules of Sequencing*

The sequence of postures depends on the overall format of your Yoga session, which, in turn, depends on your specific goals. What do you have in mind for your Yoga practice? What do you expect to accomplish? Are you interested in a simple stress-reduction program, or do you want to put together a routine for general conditioning? After you establish your goal, you need a plan that can bring you safely and intelligently to your goal. A good plan includes these considerations:

- ✔ Your starting point
- ✔ Your next activity
- ✔ Your available time

Taking these factors into consideration helps you remain in the moment during your practice session.

After you establish your goals, you're ready to apply the rules of sequencing to achieve the best possible flow of exercises. Sequencing has many approaches, and we encourage you to consult a qualified teacher. (See Chapter 2 for more on setting goals and picking a teacher.) However, you can't go wrong when you bear in mind the following four basic categories:

- ✔ Warm-up or preparation
- ✔ Main postures
- ✔ Compensation
- ✔ Rest

## Know thy schedule

Early in my teaching career, before I (Larry) had learned sequencing, I received a call from a high-level, highly stressed executive at a major corporation to arrange a private Yoga session in his office. I taught him a 30-minute routine and then asked him to lie on the floor with his feet up on a chair. I covered his eyes, recommended long exhalations, and then gave him a long, guided relaxation. He became so relaxed and looked so comfortable that I didn't want to disturb him when it was time for me to leave.

He had already paid me, so I left thinking he'd appreciate continuing the relaxation on his own. What I didn't know was that he was giving a presentation shortly after the class. His secretary had to wake him in a hurry, and he was so spaced out for his presentation that he was even accused of being on drugs. The moral of the story: Never pay your Yoga instructor ahead of time. Just kidding. The true moral is that you always need to take your next activity into account when designing your Yoga session.

Follow each step-by-step instruction carefully, to avoid injuring yourself and also to enjoy maximum benefits. Always move into and out of the posture slowly, and pause after the inhalation and exhalation; we give you the details on correct breathing in Chapter 5.

The first part of this chapter includes some sample warm-up, compensation, and rest postures. We cover the main postures earlier in the book and refer to them throughout the chapter. The latter part of the chapter gives you a recipe to design your own Yoga routine using these concepts.

# Getting Started with Warm-ups

Any physical exercise requires adequate warm-up, and Yoga is no exception. Warm-up exercises increase circulation to the parts of your body you're about to use and make you more aware of those areas of your physical self. What's different about the Yoga warm-up (called *preparation postures*) is that you do it slowly and deliberately, with conscious breathing and awareness. It's integral to the Yoga session.

Consider some of the benefits of yogic warm-up:

- ✔ Brings awareness and presence of mind
- ✔ Allows you to test your body before executing the postures
- ✔ Increases the temperature and blood supply to your muscles, joints, and connective tissue
- ✔ Prepares your body for more challenging demands and reduces the possibility of muscle tear or strain
- ✔ Enhances the supply of oxygen and nutrients, thus providing more stamina for the practice
- ✔ Prevents muscle soreness

You typically perform warm-up postures *dynamically*, which means you move in and out of them. In general, the safest Yoga warm-ups are simple forward bends and easy sequences that fold and unfold the body. Figure 15-1 shows some of our recommended warm-up exercises. You may select from the various reclining, sitting, and standing positions in this chapter. Normally, two or three postures make for an adequate warm-up.

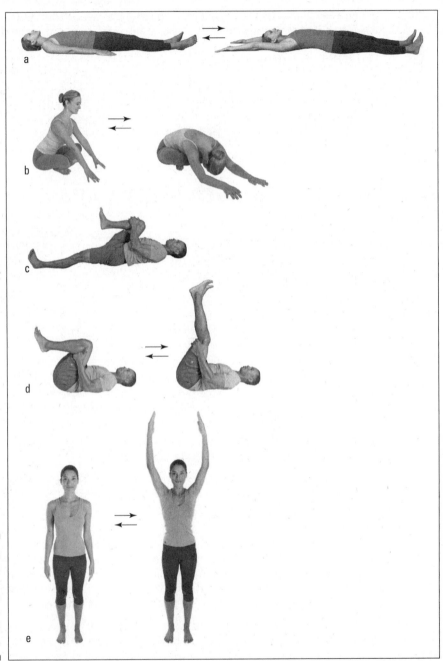

**Figure 15-1:**
Warm-ups usually include gentle bending and extending.

If you have disc problems in your lower back, forward bends may not be a good way to warm up. Check with your medical or chiropractic doctor.

Warm-up or preparation postures are also used throughout a given routine to precede and enhance the effect of the main postures. (See Figure 15-2 for some samples.) For example, you do the leg lift just before a seated forward bend to stretch the hamstrings; you do the bridge posture just before a shoulder stand.

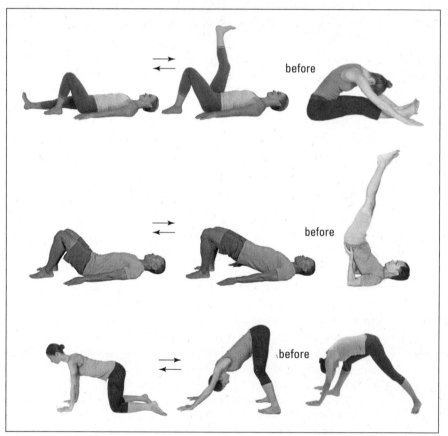

**Figure 15-2:** Warm-up postures help you prepare for specific main postures.

*Photograph by Adam Latham*

Avoid warming up with more complex postures such as shoulder stands (see Figure 15-3a), advanced back bends (see Figure 15-3b), or deep twists (see Figure 15-3c). Also, we recommend avoiding a heavy cardiovascular workout before a strenuous Yoga practice because you can experience muscle cramps.

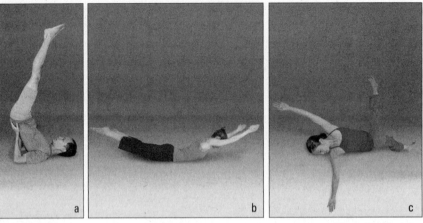

*Photograph by Adam Latham*

**Figure 15-3:**
Avoid using
complex
postures as
warm-ups.

## *Reclining warm-up postures*

Most Yoga practitioners enjoy reclining *(supine)* exercises because the postures are intrinsically relaxing. When you pair them with warm-ups, the combination effectively allows you to warm up specific muscles or muscle groups while keeping the other muscles at rest. You're having your cake and eating it, too.

The following warm-up exercises require you to start with the corpse posture, which we describe in Chapter 4. These exercises help revive you even when you start your Yoga session dead tired.

### *Lying arm raise*

Many of the muscles that go to the neck start between your shoulder blades. Raising the arms brings circulation to frequent sights of tension. You can see an illustration in Figure 15-1a.

1. **Lie flat on your back, with your arms relaxed at your sides and your palms turned down.**

2. **As you inhale, slowly raise your arms over your head and touch the floor.**

3. **As you exhale, bring your arms back to your sides, as in Step 1.**

4. **Repeat Steps 1 through 3 six to eight times.**

### *The double breath*

If you want to double your pleasure, the double breath enhances tension release in your body and prepares your muscles for the main postures.

1. **Repeat Steps 1 and 2 of the lying arm raise in the preceding section.**

2. **After you raise your arms overhead on the inhalation, leave them on the floor above your head and fully exhale.**

   Your arms remain where they are for another inhalation while you deeply stretch your entire body from the tips of your toes to your fingertips.

3. **On the next exhalation, return your arms to your sides and relax your legs; repeat three to four times.**

### Knee-to-chest posture

Use this exercise for either warm-up or compensation. The knee-to-chest posture is also a classic in lower back programs (see Chapter 24 for more on Yoga therapy for the low back). Figure 15-1c shows you what it looks like.

1. **Lie on your back, with your knees bent and your feet flat on the floor.**

2. **As you exhale, bring your right knee into your chest and hold your shin just below your knee.**

   If you have knee problems, hold the back of your thigh instead of your shin.

3. **If you can do so comfortably, straighten your left leg on the floor.**

   If you have back problems, though, keep your left knee bent.

4. **Repeat Steps 1 through 3 on the other side, holding each side for 6 to 8 breaths.**

### Double leg extension

This exercise, which uses both legs simultaneously, has a dual function: It prepares the lower back and gently stretches the hamstrings. Check it out in Figure 15-1c.

1. **Lie on your back, and bring your bent knees toward your chest.**

2. **Hold the backs of your thighs at arm's length.**

3. **As you inhale, straighten both legs perpendicular to the floor; as you exhale, bend both legs again.**

4. **Repeat Steps 2 and 3 six to eight times.**

### Hamstring stretch

Without your hamstrings (the muscles and the associated tendons), you'd have to let your fingers do all the walking. You can injure the hamstrings quite easily, especially if you overwork them, so you want to prepare them properly for exercise. Refer to Figure 15-4 for a visual.

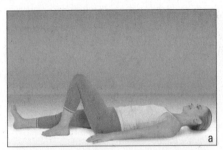
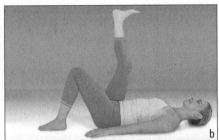
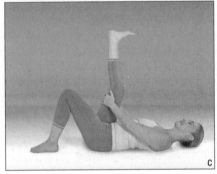

**Figure 15-4:**
Unlock your hamstrings, and you open the door to many Yoga postures.

Photograph by Adam Latham

1. **Lying on your back with your legs straight, place your arms along your sides, with your palms down.**

2. **Bend just your left knee, and put that foot on the floor (see Figure 15-4a).**

3. **As you exhale, bring your right leg up as straight as possible (see Figure 15-4b); as you inhale, return your right leg to the floor.**

   Keep your head and your hips on the floor.

4. **Repeat Steps 3 and 4 three times, and then, with your hands interlocked on the back of your raised thigh just above your knee, hold your leg in place for 6 to 8 breaths (see Figure 15-4c).**

5. **Repeat Steps 1 through 4 on the other side.**

Support your head with a pillow or folded blanket if the back of your neck or your throat tenses when you raise or lower your leg.

### Dynamic bridge: Dvipada pitha

You can use this exercise for warm-up and compensation, and also as a main posture. The Sanskrit term *dvipada* means "two-footed," and *pitha* means "seat," which is a synonym for *asana*. (The pronunciation is *dvee-pah-dah peet-hah*.)

1. **Lie on your back, with your knees bent, your feet flat on the floor at hip width, and your arms at your sides, with your palms turned down (see Figure 15-5a).**

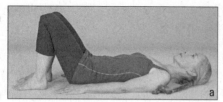 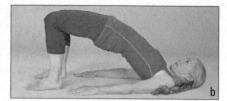

**Figure 15-5:**
The dynamic bridge.

*Photograph by Adam Latham*

2. **As you inhale, raise your hips to a comfortable height (see Figure 15-5b).**

3. **As you exhale, return your hips to the floor.**

4. **Repeat Steps 3 and 4 six to eight times.**

### Bridge variation with arm raise

This posture is another good candidate for both warm-up and compensation.

1. **Lie on your back, with your knees bent, your feet flat on the floor at hip width, and your arms at your sides, with your palms turned down (refer to Figure 15-5a).**

2. **As you inhale, raise your hips to a comfortable height and, at the same time, raise your arms overhead to touch the floor (see Figure 15-6).**

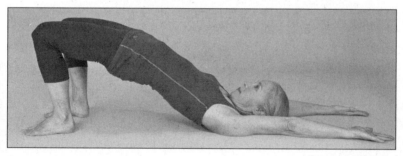

**Figure 15-6:**
Bridge variation with arm raise.

*Photograph by Adam Latham*

3. **As you exhale, return your hips to the floor and your arms to your sides.**

4. **Repeat Steps 3 and 4 six to eight times.**

### Dynamic head-to-knee

The dynamic head-to-knee posture is a nice warm-up before a slightly more physical routine.

Dynamic head-to-knee is a little more vigorous kind of warm-up. Don't perform this sequence if you're having neck problems.

1. **Lie flat on your back, with your arms relaxed at your sides and your palms turned down, as in Figure 15-1a, earlier in the chapter.**

2. **As you inhale, raise your arms slowly overhead and touch the floor.**

3. **As you exhale, draw your right knee toward your chest, lift your head off the floor, and then grasp your right knee with your hands.**

   Keep your hips on the floor. Bring your head as close to your knee as possible, but don't force it. Figure 15-7 shows you what this position looks like.

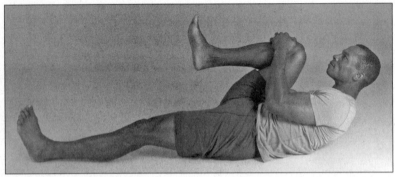

**Figure 15-7:**
The dynamic head-to-knee.

*Photograph by Adam Latham*

4. **As you inhale, release your knee and return your head, arms, and straightened right leg to the floor as they are in Step 2.**

5. **Repeat Steps 2 through 4 six to eight times on each side, alternating right and left.**

To make the sequence a little easier, keep your head on the floor in Step 3.

## Standing warm-up postures

The standing postures are probably the most versatile of all the groups. Use them for warm-up/preparation, for compensation, or as main postures. As a warm-up, use standing postures when you also plan to perform the next part of your routine from a standing position.

### Standing arm raise

You can perform this versatile warm-up (see Figure 15-1e) almost anywhere you want to enjoy a complete break from sitting. Try it at the office, and start a new trend.

1. Stand tall but relaxed, with your feet at hip width.

2. Hang your arms at your sides, with your palms facing in; look straight ahead.

3. As you inhale, raise your arms forward and then up overhead.

4. As you exhale, bring your arms down and back to your sides.

5. Repeat Steps 3 and 4 six to eight times.

### The head-turner

Sequences like the head-turner combine breath and movement in parts of the upper body to stretch, strengthen, and heal your entire wingspan. This breath and movement sequence for the upper back and neck is great for minor stiff necks.

1. Stand tall but relaxed, with your feet at hip width.

2. Hang your arms at your sides, with your palms turned back; look straight ahead.

3. As you inhale, raise your right arm forward and overhead as you turn your head to the left, as Figure 15-8 illustrates.

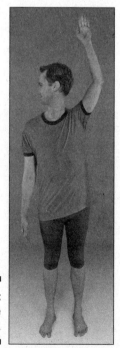

**Figure 15-8:**
The
head-turner.

*Photograph by Adam Latham*

4. As you exhale, bring your arm down and turn your head forward.

5. As you inhale, raise your left arm forward and overhead while turning your head to the right.

6. Repeat Steps 3 through 5 six to eight times on each side, alternating right and left.

### Shoulder rolls

Shoulder rolls crop up in many types of exercise routines. When you do them in Yoga, you move slowly and with awareness, coordinating with the breath.

1. Stand tall but relaxed, with your feet at hip width.

2. Hang your arms at your sides, with your palms turned back; look straight ahead.

3. As you inhale, roll your shoulders up and back, as in Figure 15-9; as you exhale, drop your shoulders.

4. Repeat Step 3 six to eight times, reversing the direction of the rolls.

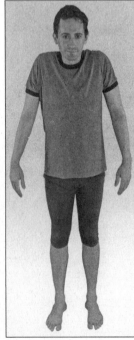

**Figure 15-9:**
Move slowly in the shoulder rolls, coordinating breath and movement.

*Photograph by Adam Latham*

### Dynamic standing forward bend

As with many other warm-ups, you can also use this exercise for compensation.

1. **Stand tall but relaxed, with your feet at hip width.**

2. **Hang your arms at your sides, with your palms turned back.**

3. **As you inhale, raise your arms forward and overhead (see Figure 15-10a).**

4. **As you exhale, bend forward; when you feel a pull in the back of your legs, bend your legs and arms slightly (see Figure 15-10b).**

   This position is called Forgiving Limbs, and we cover it in Chapter 3.

5. **As you inhale, roll up slowly, stacking the bones of your spine one at a time from bottom to top; then raise your arms overhead and, finally, release your arms back to your sides.**

6. **Repeat Steps 3 through 5 six to eight times.**

Rolling up is the safest way to come up in Step 5. If you don't have back problems, you may want to try two more advanced techniques after a few weeks: As you come up, sweep your arms out and up from the sides like wings, then overhead. Alternately, as you inhale, extend your slightly bent arms forward and up until they're parallel with your ears. Then raise your upper back, your midback, and then your lower back until you're all the way up and your arms are overhead.

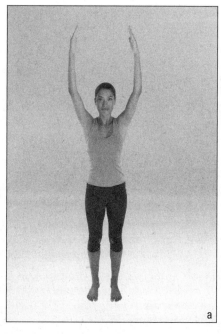
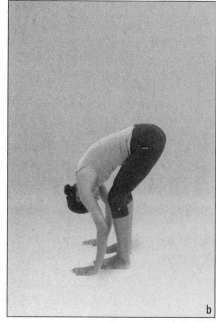

**Figure 15-10:**
Feel free to soften your knees in the dynamic standing forward bend.

a

b

*Photograph by Adam Latham*

## Seated warm-up postures

Yoga postures provide a broad spectrum of possibilities. You can do an entire routine from a seated position, including forward bends, back bends, side bends, and twists. In this section, we show you how to prepare for main postures from a seated position. (***Note:*** Most of the postures here utilize the easy posture, *sukhasana*. Check out that discussion in Chapter 6.)

### Seated fold

The seated fold is a simple way to warm up your back for forward bends or to compensate after seated twists.

1. **Sit on the floor with your legs crossed in the easy posture, and place your hands on the floor in front of you, with your palms down (refer to Figure 15-1b for a visual).**

2. **As you exhale, slide your hands out along the floor and bend forward at the hips.**

   If possible, bring your head down to the floor; otherwise, just come as close as you comfortably can.

3. **As you inhale, roll your torso and head up and return to the starting position in Step 1.**

4. **Repeat Steps 2 and 3 four to six times; then switch your legs and repeat four to six times.**

If you have a disc-related back problem, exercise caution with forward bends.

### Rock the baby

This series prepares you for advanced sitting postures and forward bends.

1. **Sit on the floor, with your legs stretched out in front of you.**

   Press your hands on the floor behind you for support

2. **Shake out your legs.**

3. **Bend your right knee and place your right foot just above your left knee, with your right ankle to the outside of the left knee (see Figure 15-11a).**

4. **Stabilize your right foot with your left hand and your right knee with your right hand; swing your right knee up and down six to eight times by gently pressing and then releasing your inner right thigh.**

5. **Carefully lift your right foot, and cradle it in the crook of your left elbow or support it with your left hand; cradle your right knee in the crook of your right elbow or cradle it with your right hand and, if you can, interlock your fingers (see Figure 15-11b).**

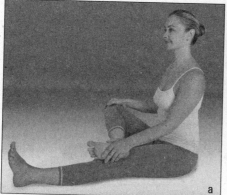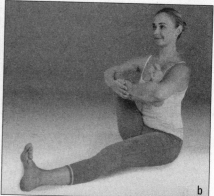

Figure 15-11:
Rock the
baby.

a      b

*Photograph by Adam Latham*

6. **Lift your spine and rock your right leg gently side to side six to eight times.**

7. **Repeat Steps 1 through 6 with your left leg.**

8. **Shake out your legs to finish.**

If you can't do this sequence without pain, don't try the more advanced seated postures in Chapter 6. Moreover, we don't recommend the rock the baby sequence if you have knee or hip problems.

# Selecting Your Main Postures and Compensation Poses

When your body is warmed up, you can move into what we refer to as the *main postures*, the central part of the routine. Interspersed among the main postures are *compensation postures*, which allow your body to come back into balance after each main posture and prevent discomfort and injury.

## Getting stronger with standard asanas

The main postures are the standard *asanas* you find featured in the classical Yoga texts and modern manuals. These *asanas* are the stars of your routine, requiring you to work a little harder. The chapters of Part II describe many of the main postures we recommend for beginners. Figure 15-12 shows you some examples. Whichever *asanas* you select, remember to match them with your specific goals.

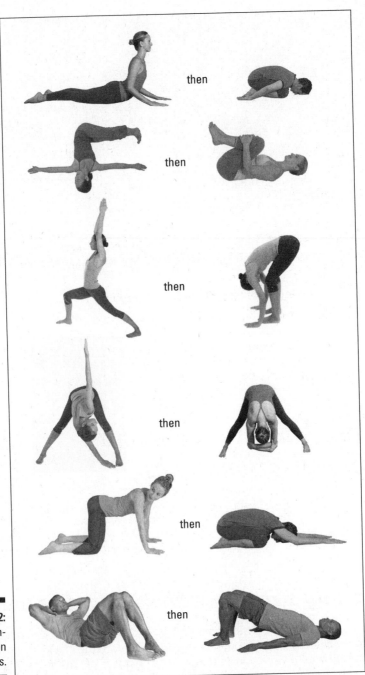

then

then

then

then

then

then

**Figure 15-12:**
Compen-
sation
postures.

Photograph by Adam Latham

Whenever possible, a warm-up posture precedes and a compensation posture follows each category of main postures.

The number of postures you select for your Yoga session depends on your available time and your goals. Later in this chapter, we provide you with a framework for selecting postures for varying lengths of time, as well as guidelines to create routines that focus on general conditioning, stress reduction, preparation for meditation, and a quick pick-me-up.

## Bringing balance with compensation postures

*Compensation* is part of bringing you back into balance, which is a key concept in Yoga. Use compensation postures to unwind or bring your body back into neutral, especially after strenuous postures.

Some basic guidelines are useful with compensation postures:

- Use one or two simple compensation postures to neutralize tension you feel in any area of the body after a Yoga posture or sequence.

- Always use the conscious breathing we describe in Chapter 5.

- Perform compensating postures that are simpler or less difficult than the main posture right after the main posture. Do them dynamically.

- Don't follow a strenuous posture with another strenuous posture in the opposite direction. Some Yoga instructors teach the fish posture as compensating for the shoulder stand. However, this combination can cause problems, especially for beginners, so we recommend the less strenuous cobra posture instead.

- Use compensation postures even when you feel no immediate need for them, especially after deep back bends, twists, and inverted postures.

- Gentle forward bends typically compensate back bends, twists, and side bends.

- Many forward bends are self-compensating. However, we follow with gentle back bends after doing a lot of forward bending.

- Rest after strenuous postures, such as inverted postures or deep back bends, before beginning the compensation postures.

Following are some great compensation postures.

### The dynamic cat

The dynamic cat is a nice compensation posture for twists, but you can also use it as a warm-up.

1. **Starting on your hands and knees, look straight ahead.**

2. **Place your knees at hip width, with your hands below your shoulders (see Figure 15-13a).**

   Straighten but don't lock your elbows.

3. **As you exhale, sit back on your heels and look at the floor (see Figure 15-13b).**

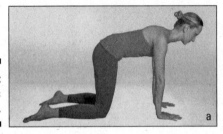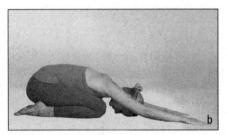

**Figure 15-13:** Dynamic cat.

*Photograph by Adam Latham*

4. **As you inhale, slowly return to the starting position in Step 1.**

   Again, look straight ahead.

5. **Repeat Steps 3 and 4 six to eight times.**

### Dynamic knees-to-chest

You can find many variations of knees-to-chest (including the regular version later in this chapter), but this variation is especially good after back bends.

1. **Lie on your back, and bend your knees toward your chest.**

2. **Hold your legs just below your knees, with one hand on each leg (see Figure 15-14a).**

   If you have any knee problems, be sure to hold the backs of your thighs.

3. **As you exhale, draw your knees toward your chest (see Figure 15-14b).**

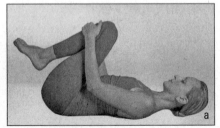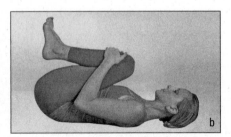

**Figure 15-14:** Dynamic knees-to-chest.

*Photograph by Adam Latham*

4. **As you inhale, move your knees away from your chest.**

5. **Repeat Steps 3 and 4 six to eight times.**

### *Thunderbolt posture: Vajrasana*

This exercise is useful for compensation or warm-up. *Vajra* (pronounced *vahj-rah*) means both "diamond/adamantine" and "thunderbolt."

1. **Kneel on the floor, with your knees and feet at hip width.**

2. **Sit back on your heels, and bring your back up nice and tall. Hang your arms close to your sides.**

3. **As you inhale, lift your hips back up and sweep your arms up over your head (see Figure 15-15a); lean back and look up.**

4. **As you exhale, sit on your heels again, fold your chest to your thighs, and bring your arms behind your back (see Figure 15-15b).**

   Get into a nice flow: Inhale when you open, exhale when you fold.

5. **Repeat Steps 3 and 4 six to eight times.**

Don't perform the thunderbolt if you have knee problems.

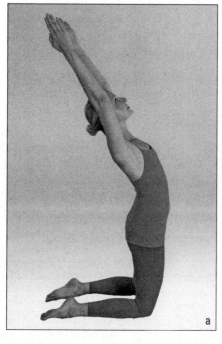 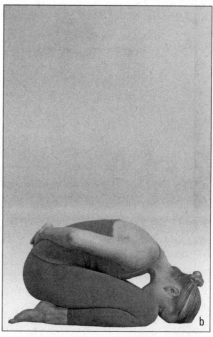

**Figure 15-15:**
The thunderbolt posture.

a

b

*Photograph by Adam Latham*

# Including Plenty of Rest and Relaxation

Rest periods are an indispensable part of any good Yoga routine. Rest isn't just zoning out at the end of a session. In Yoga, a quiet interval is an active tool for enhancing the quality of your practice at the following times:

- ✔ Before the beginning of a class, to shift gears and establish a union with your body, breath, and, mind
- ✔ Between postures, to renew and prepare for the next posture
- ✔ As part of compensation after strenuous postures
- ✔ To restore proper breathing
- ✔ For self-observation
- ✔ To prepare for relaxation techniques

## Knowing when to rest and when to resume

The two best indicators of your need to rest are your breath and your energy level. Monitor yours throughout the session: If your breath is loud and uneven, rest. If you feel a little tired after a posture, rest.

No formula can prescribe how long you need to rest. Simply rest as needed until you're ready for the next posture. Don't cheat yourself out of well-deserved rest periods between the postures and at the end of a session.

## Mastering rest postures

Figure 15-16 shows you some recommended rest postures.

Stay in any rest posture for 6 to 12 breaths or as long as it takes to feel rested, which may depend on how much time you have and where you are in the sequence of the routine. Yoga must never feel like you're in a hurry.

### Corpse posture: Shavasana

The word *shava* (pronounced *shah-vah*) means "corpse," and *asana* means "posture." Refer to Figure 15-16a and Chapter 4 for a full description of the posture.

### Shavasana variation with bent legs

Follow the steps for *shavasana* in Chapter 4, but keep your knees bent, with your feet on the floor at hip width, as in Figure 15-16b.

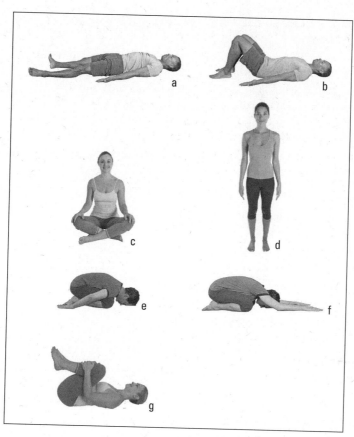

*Photograph by Adam Latham*

If your back is uncomfortable, place a pillow or blanket roll under your knees. If your neck or throat is tense, place a folded blanket or small pillow under your head.

### Easy posture: Sukhasana

The word *sukha* means "easy" or "pleasant" — indeed, this posture is as its name suggests. You can keep your eyes open or closed in this posture. Check out Figure 15-16c and Chapter 6 for more details.

### Mountain posture: Tadasana

The Sanskrit word *tada* (pronounced *tah-dah*) actually means "palm tree"; hence, this exercise is also called the palm tree posture.

1. **Stand tall but relaxed, with your feet at hip width; keep your arms at your sides, with your palms turned toward the sides of your legs.**

2. **Visualize a vertical line connecting the hole in your ear, your shoulder joint, and the sides of your hip, knee, and ankle.**

3. **Look straight ahead, with your eyes open or closed, as Figure 15-16d illustrates.**

### Child's posture: Balasana

The Sanskrit word *bala* (pronounced *bah-lah*) means "child." This classic version of the child's posture is a nurturing pose.

1. **Start on your hands and knees.**

2. **Place your knees about hip width, with your hands just below your shoulders.**

   Keep your elbows straight but not locked.

3. **As you exhale, sit back on your heels; rest your torso on your thighs and your forehead on the floor.**

4. **Lay your arms on the floor beside your torso, with your palms up, as in Figure 15-16e.**

5. **Close your eyes and breathe easily.**

### Child's posture with arms in front

This variation of the child's posture gives you more stretch in your upper back. Follow the steps for the child's posture in the preceding section, but extend your arms forward at Step 4, spreading your palms on the floor, as Figure 15-16f illustrates.

### Knees-to-chest posture: Apanasana

The Sanskrit word *apana* (pronounced *ah-pah-nah*) refers to the downward-going life force or exhalation.

1. **Lie on your back, and bend your knees in toward your chest.**

2. **Hold your shins just below the knees, as in Figure 15-16g.**

   If you have any knee problems, hold the backs of your thighs instead.

# Cooking Up a Creative Yoga Routine with the Classic Formula

When you create your own Yoga program with our Classic Formula, you have to think about these components:

✔ Determine how long you want the routine to be.

✔ Select the main postures from the range of postures in Chapters 6 through 13 (or, of course, from any source you consider reliable).

> ✔ Decide how you want to prepare and/or compensate for each main category of postures.
>
> ✔ Allocate time for rest and relaxation at the end so you can digest the nutritious meal of Yoga exercises that you prepared for yourself.

What we call the Classic Formula consists of the following 12 categories:

1. Attunement (integrating body, breath, and mind)
2. Warm-up/preparation (also used between main exercises wherever necessary)
3. Standing postures
4. Balance postures (optional)
5. Abdominals
6. Inversions (optional)
7. Back bends
8. Forward bends
9. Twists
10. Rest (to be inserted between main exercises whenever you feel the need)
11. Compensation (to be inserted after main exercises)
12. Final relaxation

You don't have to use every category, as long as you follow the proper sequence from 1 to 9 and always conclude with 12. Depending on your available time, you may choose to omit number 4 or 6 and continue, or even stop the asanas after number 5 if time is short and jump to step 12. You can repeat the categories of rest, warm-up/preparation, and compensation wherever appropriate. Balancing postures and inversions are optional because their inclusion depends on your available time, your wall space, and your skill level.

The Classic Formula is optimal for 30- to 60-minute general conditioning programs, but we also refer to it in the 15- and 5-minute programs. The beauty of our formula is that, as your Yoga practice grows over the years, you can explore safe postures from any book or system and then insert them into their appropriate slots within our 12-category module.

# *Enjoying a postural feast: The 30- to 60-minute general conditioning routine*

Most beginning Yoga students find sustaining more than a 30-minute practice on their own difficult; however, if your appetite increases, we want you to have the tools to be a 60-minute gourmet. Simply follow the recipes in each of the categories to create your own great custom routine.

Plan for an average of about 2 minutes for each posture you select. Some postures take more time, some take less. Doing both sides of an *asymmetrical*, or one-side-at-a-time (right and left), posture like the warrior (see Chapter 7) counts as one exercise or posture. If you choose our sun salutation or a similar dynamic series from Chapters 13 and 15 or another source, double or triple the time allotted, depending on the series and the number of repetitions.

*Note:* As we indicate throughout this chapter, you can use many of these postures in more than one category when developing a general conditioning routine.

The simplest way to expand a 30-minute routine into a 45-minute routine is to do two sets of your chosen standing postures and add one extra posture to the abdominal, back bend, and forward bend categories.

### *Attunement*

*Attunement* helps you establish the conscious link with your body, your breath, and your mind or awareness. If you forget about the attunement stage, you miss much of what makes Yoga, Yoga.

First, for routines of any length, select a style of breathing from Chapter 5. If you're a beginner, choose something simple, like focus breathing or belly breathing. Later you can try either the classic three-part breathing or chest-to-belly breathing or adopt the *ujjayi* technique.

Be sure not to confuse these styles of breathing with the traditional techniques of breath control (*pranayama*) that we also describe in Chapter 5.

Next, select one of the resting postures from earlier in this chapter, or opt for a seated posture from Chapter 6, depending on your frame of mind, your physical condition, and what you have planned for the rest of your routine. The corpse posture (lying flat on your back) is always a good starting point for beginners. It's a great way to shift gears from a hectic lifestyle and slow things down before beginning your postural exercises. Lying flat on your back definitely shifts your mood toward relaxation. However, sitting in the easy posture and standing in the mountain posture are also great starting points. Figure 15-16 shows some examples of rest postures you can use to help achieve attunement.

Use 8 to 12 breaths to achieve attunement. The more you pay attention to your breath and attunement, the more benefit you can expect to derive from your program. Think of the benefits you receive as "mileage plus."

### Warm-up

You may notice that almost all the warm-ups we describe earlier in this chapter are folding and opening motions (flexion and extension). Either motion provides the easiest way for your body to prepare for breath and movement. Select a warm-up posture or sequence that's a similar position to your attunement posture.

 Make your Yoga practice as smooth as possible. Flow like a gentle river. For example, do both the attunement and the warm-up on the floor; then stand for the next series of postures. Avoid getting up and down like a yo-yo. Economy of movement is one of the principles of good Hatha Yoga practice.

 In a routine of 30 minutes or more, you usually have time for at least two warm-up postures. Because the neck is a frequent site of tension, we recommend using a warm-up posture that incorporates moving the arms. In addition to stretching the spine, arm movement prepares your neck and shoulders and helps you release tension. Also, warm-ups that move the legs and prepare the lower back are helpful for the standing postures that usually follow. Check out "Getting Started with Warm-ups," earlier in the chapter, for some examples of common warm-ups in the lying, sitting, and standing positions.

### Standing postures

The standing postures tend to be the most physical part of a program. If you're doing a 30-minute routine, you usually have time for three or four standing postures. In a 60-minute program, you may have as many as six or seven standing *asanas*. You can choose any of the standing postures from Chapter 7 for this portion of your routine.

 As a general rule, back bends, twists, and side bends (the hallmarks of many standing postures) come before forward bends. Therefore, you want to include standing forward bends after most of the standing postures you choose.

Figure 15-17 shows you examples of standing postures for a 30- or 60-minute program. As an alternative, you can choose the dynamic kneeling or standing sequence (sun salutation) or the standing rejuvenation sequence for beginners from Chapter 13. The dynamic postures take the place of three to six standing postures, depending on which sequence you choose and how many rounds you do. When you select a dynamic sequence, try to allow time at the end for one twist and one compensating forward bend. We mention this note because all our dynamic sequences are forward and backward bends only.

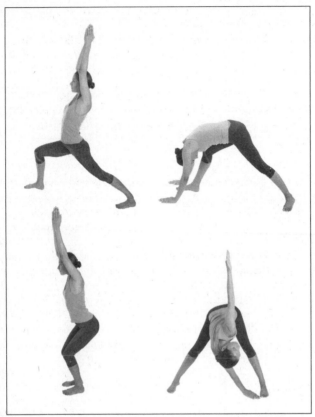

*Photograph by Adam Latham*

**Figure 15-17:**
Examples
of popular
standing
postures.

If you want your routine to be more physically challenging, simply do two sets of the standing postures.

### Balancing postures (optional)

Balancing postures are optional and depend on your time and stamina. They're often the most athletic postures and require overall coordination. Balancing postures are rewarding because you can see your progress immediately. They fit nicely after the standing postures because, at this point in your routine, you're fully warmed up. All our recommended balancing postures are either standing or kneeling, which means they fit smoothly into the sequence. Choose one balancing posture from Chapter 8 for a 30- to 60-minute routine; Figure 15-18 shows you some options.

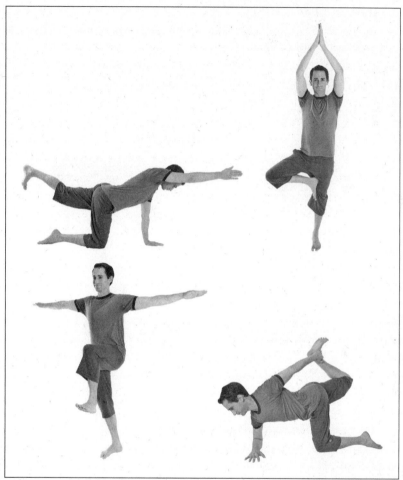

*Photograph by Adam Latham*

**Figure 15-18:**
You can
practice
balance
from many
different
positions.

## Rest

Most people usually welcome a rest at this point of the routine. Resting is usually done lying, sitting, or kneeling. We emphasize the importance of not feeling rushed during your Yoga session. At least for the short duration of your routine, believe that you have all the time in the world. In a 30- or 60-minute routine, the first rest usually comes at the halfway point. This resting period gives you the opportunity for inward observation of any physical, mental, or emotional feedback resulting from your Yoga practice so far.

Remember that you need to rest until you feel ready to move on. If you're really pinched for time, this first major rest is also a logical place to end a session. Choose from any of our recommended resting postures in Figure 15-16, or any of the sitting postures you're comfortable with from Chapter 6.

### Abdominals

We recommend that you include one or two abdominal postures in any program lasting 30 minutes or more. Think of your abdomen as the front of your back — a very important place. Choose one of the abdominal postures we describe in Chapter 9 for a 30-minute routine, or select one or two for a 60-minute routine. You can check out some examples in Figure 15-19.

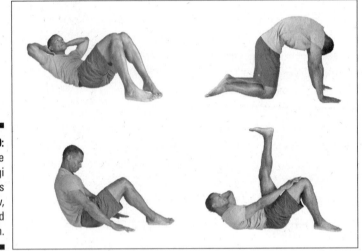

**Figure 15-19:**
Practice your yogi ab postures with a slow, coordinated breath.

*Photograph by Adam Latham*

### Compensation and preparation

Take a short rest when you finish the abdominal exercises, and then do 6 to 8 repetitions of the dynamic bridge or bridge variation (both discussed earlier in the chapter and shown in Figure 15-5) or the lying arm raise (also covered earlier). The action of the dynamic bridge plays a dual function here because it compensates the abdomen, returning it to neutral, and also warms up or prepares the back and the neck if you choose to include an inversion posture or move on to back bends next.

### Inversion (optional)

Indian Yoga teachers often teach inverted postures toward the beginning or at the end of a class. For Westerners, we prefer to introduce inverted postures closer to the middle of the routine, when they've properly prepared their backs and necks and have plenty of time for adequate compensation. Inverted postures like the ones in Figure 15-20 are optional, and we recommend that beginners avoid the half shoulder stand and the half shoulder stand at the wall until they've practiced Yoga for 6 to 8 weeks.

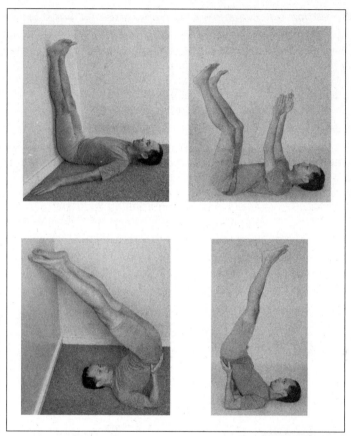

**Figure 15-20:**
Inversions are powerful postures that deserve respect.

*Photograph by Adam Latham*

Attempt inversions only if you have no neck problems. Inverted postures are worthy of a healthy respect. They're powerful postures that demand a sense of balance and strong muscles. We offer you several easy and safe inversion postures in Chapter 10. Select just one for your 30- to 60-minute routine, assuming that you're ready and want to include an inversion in your practice.

Even if you're ready for an inversion, we advise against practicing the shoulder stand or the half shoulder stand at the wall if any of the following conditions applies to you: glaucoma, retinopathy, high blood pressure, a history of heart attacks or stroke, hiatal hernia, the first few days of menstruation, pregnancy, or 40 or more pounds of excess weight.

### Compensation for inversions and preparation for back bends

Be sure to rest after the simpler inverted postures, normally in the corpse posture (see Chapter 4). After the half shoulder stand, rest and then compensate further with any one of the cobra postures (see Chapter 11) or the thunderbolt posture (covered earlier in the chapter). Cobra I and the thunderbolt posture also prepare you for further back bends.

### Back bends

You can use back bends as a compensation for inversion, but cobra I and II also are gentle back bends that serve as good preparation for more physical back bends, such as the locust posture. Westerners bend forward far too much, which makes back bends a vital part of your Hatha Yoga practice. Whenever possible in general conditioning Yoga routines, select one back bend from Chapter 11; in programs longer than 30 minutes, use two. Figure 15-21 shows some common back bends you can try.

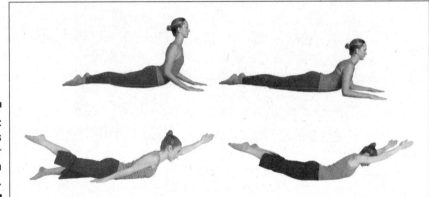

**Figure 15-21:** Examples of four common back bends.

*Photograph by Adam Latham*

### Compensation for back bends

The compensation for *prone* (lying face down) back bends is usually some form of a bent-knee forward bend (shown in Figure 15-22). We often recommend the knees-to-chest posture or the child's posture, discussed earlier in the chapter. After more strenuous back bends, such as any of the varieties of the locust postures, we recommend a short rest followed by one of the bent-knee forward bends and then the dynamic bridge posture as a second compensatory posture. This sequence helps neutralize the upper back and neck.

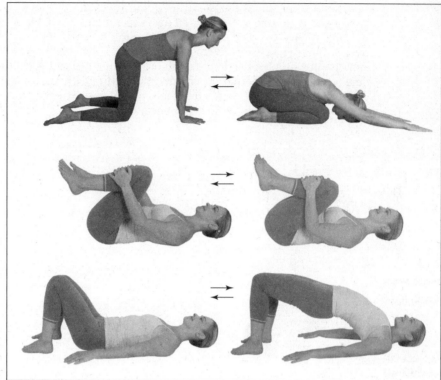

**Figure 15-22:**
Compensating for back bends is an important part of your Yoga program.

*Photograph by Adam Latham*

### Preparation for forward bends

Preparation is particularly critical for extended leg forward bends. Stretching the hamstrings or the hips just before doing a seated forward bend (refer to Chapter 11) not only improves the posture, but is also safer for your back. Use the hamstring stretch or the double leg stretch for a 30-minute routine (see Figure 15-4). For a longer routine, use both or the rock the baby sequence (see Figure 15-11).

### Forward bends

The seated forward bends normally come toward the end of an exercise program because they have a calming effect. Of all the postures in this book, the seated extended-leg forward bends divide the sexes the most. Because of their higher muscle density, especially in the hip and groin area, men are usually tighter in the hamstrings. Preparation of the hamstrings is particularly important for them in these postures. If you have a hard time with this category, bend your knees more and, if necessary, place some blankets under your hips to give yourself a better angle for the forward bends (which we cover in Chapter 11). For a 30-minute routine, choose just one forward bend from Chapter 11; pick two for a 60-minute routine. Figure 15-23 shows you some possibilities. Alternately, you may substitute with one kneeling or seated side bend from Chapter 11, and one seated or kneeling forward bend from earlier in this chapter for compensation.

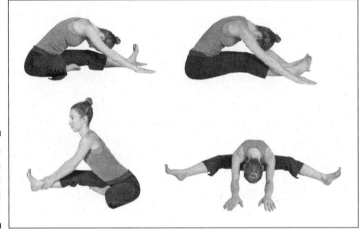

**Figure 15-23:**
Some forward bend options.

*Photograph by Adam Latham*

### Compensation for forward bends

The forward bends are usually self-compensating. However, sometimes you may want to use a gentle back bend like the dynamic bridge as a counter pose.

### Preparation for twists

The preparation for all twists is a forward bend, so moving from forward bends to twists flows naturally. Check out the earlier section "Forward bends" for guidance on choosing a bend.

### Twists

Twists, like forward bends, have an overall calming effect; the floor twists are the dessert in our program because, at the end of the routine, they feel so good. Choose one floor twist from Chapter 12 for a 30-minute routine, and pick one or two for a 60-minute routine. Figure 15-24 shows some common twists.

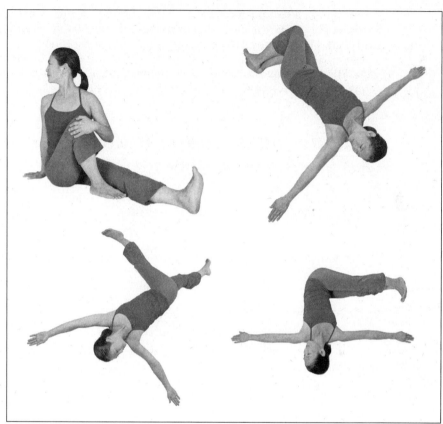

*Photograph by Adam Latham*

**Figure 15-24:**
Twists are calming postures, and they just plain feel good.

### Compensation for twists

Compensation for twists is always flexion, or a forward bend. After a floor twist, we usually recommend choosing one of the lying knees-to-chest or the regular knees-to-chest postures in Figure 15-13 and Figure 15-4, earlier in the chapter.

### Relaxation

No matter how short your program, remember to include some form of relaxation. Rest provides a place where you digest all the marvelous energy your Yoga exercises unleash. It's like receiving "mileage plus" from your Yoga practice.

This final category in our classic formula can take several forms: a relaxation technique (see Chapter 4), *pranayama* yogic breathing (see Chapter 5), or meditation (see Chapter 23).

First, choose a rest posture or one of the seated postures from Chapter 6. Next, select one of the breathing or *pranayama* techniques from Chapter 5, a relaxation technique from Chapter 4, and/or a meditation technique from Chapter 23. In a 60-minute routine, you may choose both a breathing and a relaxation technique. Whichever technique you choose, use it for at least 2 to 3 minutes, and not more than 15 minutes.

## Making the most of a little: A 15-minute routine

Sometimes you have only 15 minutes, but even 15 minutes of Hatha Yoga can put you back on an even keel and refresh you.

When you opt for a 15-minute program, you need to be specific about your goals. Consider some of the more common uses for a short routine:

- ✔ A quick general conditioning program
- ✔ A stress-reduction and relaxation program
- ✔ A preparation program for Yoga breathing or meditation

### General conditioning

For the purposes of general conditioning, choose the following categories and do them in the order listed. You can also use the illustrations earlier in this chapter as a reference point.

Some of the postures appear in this chapter; you can also find information in the listed chapters.

- ✔ Either a standing or a seated rest posture for attunement (flip to "Mastering rest postures," earlier in this chapter, as well as Chapters 6 and 7) and a Yoga breathing technique from Chapter 5

- ✔ A dynamic series, such as either kneeling or standing sun salutation (Chapter 13); the rejuvenation sequence, which counts as three or four postures (also in Chapter 13); or three to four standing postures (see "Standing postures," earlier in this chapter, plus Chapter 7) for 6 to 8 minutes

- ✔ A lying twist (see "Twists," earlier in this chapter, as well as Chapter 12)

- ✔ Compensation with knees- or knee-to-chest postures (check out Figure 15-13, earlier in the chapter)

✔ A lying or seated rest posture from the "Mastering rest postures" section, earlier in the chapter

✔ A breathing exercise from Chapter 5 and/or a relaxation technique from Chapter 4

### Preparation for meditation and Yoga breathing

If you're looking for a routine to help you reduce stress, just plain relax, or prepare for meditation and Yoga breathing, choose the following elements in the order listed:

✔ A lying or seated posture from this chapter's "Mastering rest postures" section or Chapter 6 or 7 for attunement, and a Yoga breathing technique from Chapter 5. Repeat this posture or a similar one at the end of the routine.

✔ Two lying warm-up postures from "Getting Started with Warm-ups," earlier in the chapter — one that moves the arms and another that moves the legs.

✔ A prone back-bending posture, such as cobra I or locust I (see this chapter's "Back bends" section and Chapter 11), or a lying back bend such as the bridge.

✔ A bent-knee compensation exercise, such as the child's posture or knees-to-chest posture, covered in "Compensation for back bends," earlier in the chapter.

✔ A lying hamstring posture, such as rock the baby, earlier in the chapter.

✔ A lying twist (see this chapter's "Twists" section, as well as Chapter 12).

✔ A lying bent-knee compensation exercise, which Figure 15-14 shows earlier in the chapter.

## Satisfying an appetite for a quick pick-me-up: A 5-minute routine

A 5-minute program is the easiest to create. For a busy person, even 3 to 5 minutes once or twice a day can provide beneficial effects. Settle into a rest posture or a seated posture from this chapter's "Mastering rest postures" section or Chapter 6, and then employ a yogic breathing or *pranayama* technique (see Chapter 5) for 3 to 5 minutes. You can come up with many possible combinations for a quick, relaxing, and enjoyable routine.

# Chapter 16

# Partnering Up for Yoga

**Y**oga need not be a solitary practice. *Yoga* means "union," and partner Yoga fosters unity. Partner Yoga is a modern American development of the late 20th century, although some people trace its roots back to ancient Yoga lineages. Its modern expression may even have developed independently by different practitioner-teachers, but clearly, it's an idea whose time has come. As with other varieties of Yoga postures, partner Yoga is suitable for all levels of complexity and challenge. In this chapter, we present the many benefits and joys of practicing partner Yoga and illustrate several safe postures you and a partner can try.

# Defining Partner Yoga

Partner Yoga is a joyful practice that brings two people together to create a new posture. In contrast to what's referred to as assisted Yoga, in partner Yoga, each person gives support and receives benefits as the two create a posture together. When you and your partner try this, you discover and enjoy one of the requirements and lessons of partner Yoga: dialogue and clear communication.

Consider the benefits of partner Yoga:

✔ Can be practiced by two strangers in a class

✔ Extends Yoga's emphasis on experimentation and personal discovery to an experience shared with another person

✔ Utilizes traction, leverage, and kinesthetic awareness

✔ Involves engaging physically with another person, yet is not sexual

✔ Can add an element of delight when practiced by romantic couples

Partner Yoga is best practiced with someone your same size, but differences in height and weight can stimulate creativity to make the postures work.

# Enjoying the Benefits of Partner Yoga

Partner Yoga can be good for your health. By its very nature, partner Yoga is a playful practice and can even evoke laughter. Laughter can be a very healing experience, as Norman Cousins has taught the world.

Partner Yoga fosters your ability to trust and feel secure with another person. It gives you the opportunity to surrender to another individual and feel supported. That experience of trust on the mat can spill over to your life *off* the mat.

How comfortable are you with being touched? Partner Yoga isn't sexual, but it involves touching. Because of differences in personality, personal experience, upbringing, and culture, the idea of touching another person during your Yoga routine may be more or less comfortable than the practice of going solo. Although partner Yoga can help you address issues with intimacy, only you know your limits and what's right for you. As with all other aspects of your Yoga practice, listen to and respect your inner voice.

---

## Partner Yoga as a metaphor for how we live in the world

According to Cain Carroll and Lori Kimata, authors of *Partner Yoga,* the first axiom of partner Yoga is, "All things are interdependent." Partner Yoga gives you immediate feedback on how you interact with your partner and, by extension, with others in your life. For instance, if one person pushes too far, both will fall over. Now how's that for immediate feedback?

Consider the opportunities for feedback that partner Yoga offers:

✔ Do you communicate your needs?

✔ Do you listen when your partner communicates his needs?

✔ Are you sensitive to the subtle adjustments and movements of your partner?

✔ Do you give support when needed?

✔ Are you flexible enough to allow your partner to move with ease yet maintain your own integrity?

✔ Can you find that healthy medium between rigidity and flexibility?

What new shapes can you and your significant other make if you pair up for partner Yoga? For a totally unique and personal holiday greeting card, enlist the help of a friend with a camera or a smartphone, bend and blend yourselves, and shoot away. The partner tree pose is often a favorite holiday shot.

# Exploring Twelve Ways to Pose with a Partner

In this section, we illustrate and describe 12 safe and fun Yoga postures that you can practice with a partner. Feel free to mix and match, and sprinkle them within a more traditional practice session in which you each practice on your own.

## Partner suspension bridge

The partner suspension bridge decompresses the entire spine, provides traction, and stretches the hamstrings. It also builds strength in the arms and shoulders. You can see it illustrated in Figure 16-1 and watch trust and leverage in action at www.dummies.com/go/yoga.

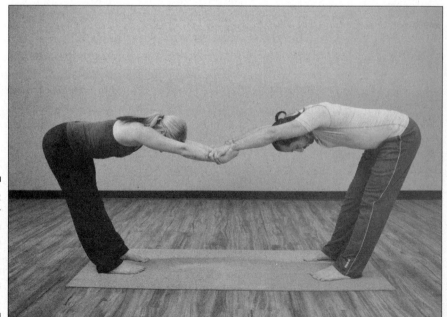

**Figure 16-1:** The partner suspension bridge gives both partners a delicious stretch.

© John Wiley & Sons, Inc.

1. **Face your partner standing, and hold on to one another's wrists with corresponding right and left hands (known as the fireman's grip).**

2. **Begin to bend forward, and walk backward until you're both parallel to the floor.**

3. **Lean back with your hips, and communicate with your partner to arrive at a stretch that's a comfortable maximum for you both.**

4. **Stay for 6 to 8 breaths.**

5. **To come out of the pose, walk back toward one another and release one another's wrists.**

When you're comfortable in the partner suspension bridge, try wiggling your hips a few times to stretch your hips and lower back.

Avoid the partner suspension bridge if you have back or shoulder problems, or if you feel pain in your lower back or shoulders when executing the posture.

## Partner teeter-totter

The partner teeter-totter decompresses the lower back and builds strength in the arms and shoulders. Take a peek at Figure 16-2 to see what it looks like: You start as in the suspension bridge and add a flourish.

1. **Face your partner standing, and hold on to one another's wrists with corresponding right and left hands.**

2. **Begin to bend forward, and walk backward until you're both parallel to the floor.**

3. **Lean back with your hips, and communicate with your partner to arrive at a stretch that's a comfortable maximum for you both.**

4. **Now one partner bends at the knees and goes down into a half or full squat.**

   Communicate to decide who goes first.

   Squat only as far as you feel comfortable. Stay focused on your partner for the best communication.

5. **When you're ready to come out of the pose, let your partner know. When you're both standing, step forward and release each other's wrists.**

6. **After 6 to 8 breaths, switch and have the other partner move into a squat for another 6 to 8 breaths.**

It's perfectly fine if only one partner wants to squat.

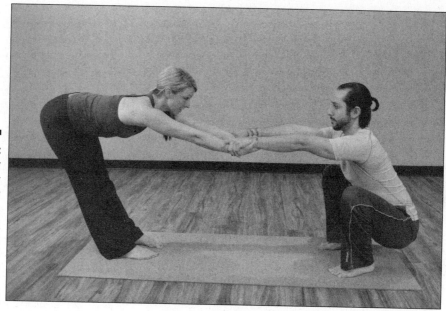

**Figure 16-2:** The partner teeter-totter is nearly everyone's favorite on the Yoga mat (as well as in the playground).

Avoid the partner teeter-totter if you have back or knee problems, or if you feel pain in your lower back, knees, or shoulders.

## Hugasana

Hugs teach us how to give and receive. And if that's not enough, research suggests that touch (and what is a hug, if not touch?) can contribute to healing sickness, disease, loneliness, depression, anxiety, and stress.

1. **Stand and face your partner; move close to one another.**

2. **Open your arms wide, and each of you wrap them around your partner in a nice embrace, as in Figure 16-3.**

3. **Stay for 4 to 5 breaths.**

Smiling and laughter are also good for your health, so let loose and go with the flow as you perform the hugasana with your partner.

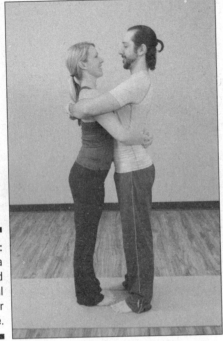

**Figure 16-3:**
A hug is a simple and delightful partner posture.

## Partner warrior II

Warrior II as a partner pose blends the many benefits of this powerful posture — especially improvements in strength, stamina, and balance — with the interpersonal benefits of partner Yoga. You can see its final expression in Figure 16-4.

1. **Stand sideways with your partner, facing the same forward direction.**

2. **Touch the insides of your feet together.**

3. **Reach with your inside hand, and place it on your partner's upper arm.**

4. **Turn your outside foot out and away from your partner about 90 degrees, and raise your outside arm so it's parallel to the floor.**

5. **Inhale deeply and, as you exhale, bend your outside leg to a right angle as your back hand slides along your partner's arm toward his wrist.**

6. **Stay in the final posture, firmly gripping your partner's wrist, for 6 to 8 breaths.**

7. **When you're finished, straighten your legs, release your hands, switch places, and repeat on the other side.**

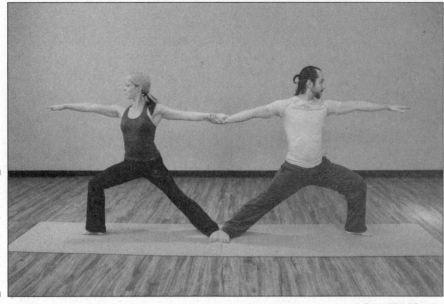

Figure 16-4:
What's
mightier
than a
warrior?
Two
warriors!

© John Wiley & Sons, Inc.

When you're holding the posture in step 6, try tucking your tail, to allow your hips to open. Also think of lengthening through the top of your head and widening with your arms.

## Partner table pose

The partner table pose stretches the upper back and shoulders, relieving neck tension. It also stretches the hamstrings. It differs from the partner suspension bridge (see Figure 16-1), in that it doesn't decompress and provide traction to the lower back. You can see it illustrated in Figure 16-5.

1. **Standing, face your partner; move toward one another, and place your hands on your partner's opposite shoulders.**

2. **Bend forward from the hips until you're both parallel to the floor; soften your knees, if necessary, and let your neck and head relax downward to a comfortable position.**

3. **Stay for 6 to 8 breaths.**

4. **When you're ready to come out of the pose, let your partner know and step forward as you release your hands from one another's shoulders.**

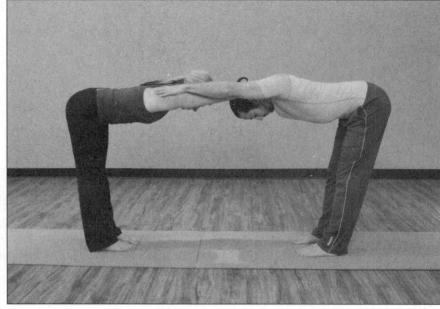

**Figure 16-5:**
You form a table with a friend in the aptly named partner table pose.

© John Wiley & Sons, Inc.

## Double triangle

The double triangle provides an excellent side stretch to the body and the spine. It strengthens the legs and helps the digestive system, and also improves stability and balance. You can see it illustrated in Figure 16-6.

1. **Turn back to back with your partner as both of you spread your legs to a comfortable distance, about 3 to 5 feet apart; open one foot on the same side, and turn in the back foot about 45 degrees or less.**

2. **Place your bottom hand on your forward thigh, bring your top arm up, and entwine your arm with your partner's top arm and hand.**

3. **Lean back gently, and slide your bottom hand down your forward leg as far as you feel comfortable.**

4. **Stay for about 6 to 8 breaths, and then repeat on the other side.**

Avoid this pose if you're suffering from a back condition, migraines, high blood pressure, or neck injuries.

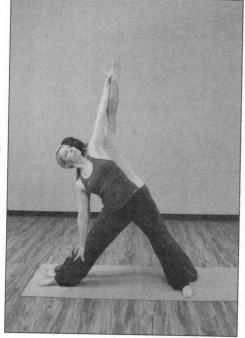

**Figure 16-6:**
The double triangle delivers all the benefits of the triangle, plus the fun of practicing with a partner.

© John Wiley & Sons, Inc.

## Partner tree pose

This simple-looking posture brings a bounty of benefits. It creates stability and balance, improves concentration, opens the hips, and strengthens the ankles. You can see it illustrated in Figure 16-7.

1. **Stand side to side with your partner, facing the same way, about 1 to 2 feet from each another.**

2. **Bring your inside arms straight up, with your hands extended, and touch your partner's palms (or anywhere on the inside of the arms, depending on your size matchup).**

3. **Bend your outside leg and bring your outside heel into your groin, or to a comfortable spot between your groin and your knee.**

   If you can't reach that high, place your heel between your ankle and your knee — but not on the knee joint, which can cause injury.

4. **Bring your outside arms to the middle, and touch palms in the prayer, or Namaste, position.**

   If you're feeling unstable, entwine your inside extended arms.

5. **Focus on a spot on the floor about 6 to 8 feet in front of you, to help your balance.**

6. **Stay for 6 to 8 breaths; then get out of the pose by first taking down the outside bent leg and placing that foot on the floor, then releasing the inside palms that are touching, and finally, releasing the outside arms and hands that are touching or entwined.**

7. **Switch places, and repeat on the other side.**

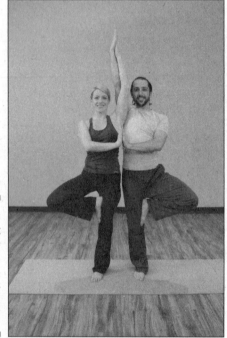

**Figure 16-7:**
The elegant partner tree pose creates stability and builds strength.

© John Wiley & Sons, Inc.

The partner tree pose makes a great photograph of you and your partner for your next holiday card!

## *Yoga Miracle pose*

This pose gives a deep stretch to the hamstring muscles, which helps you with the rest of your practice. After all, the hamstrings are the most influential muscle group for all Yoga postures. You can see this pose in Figure 16-8.

1. **Start with one partner lying face up, with one leg bent and the other leg straight up.**

2. **The other partner kneels in a lunge position, with the forward leg bent and close to the extended leg of the partner on the floor.**

3. **The kneeling partner places a hand at the back of the extended leg and provides resistance; the lying partner pushes steadily and comfortably for 10 seconds.**

   Just a steady medium push of your heel against your partner's hand is fine. This pose isn't competitive!

4. **At the end of 10 seconds, the lying partner releases the push and allows the kneeling partner to push the extended leg to a new flexibility point; do both legs.**

5. **Switch positions, and repeat Steps 1 through 4.**

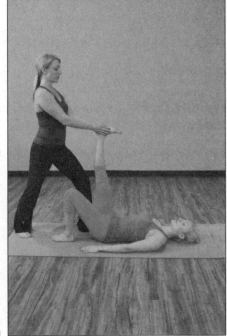

**Figure 16-8:** The hamstring stretch you get in the Yoga Miracle pose benefits the rest of your practice.

© John Wiley & Sons, Inc.

## Seated straddle pose

This pose improves hip and hamstring flexibility and stretches the entire back, as well as the arms and shoulders. You and your partner first rotate together to warm up, and then you alternate leaning forward and back. You can see it illustrated in Figure 16-9.

**Figure 16-9:**
The seated straddle pose focuses on the hips and hamstrings, but it benefits the upper body, too.

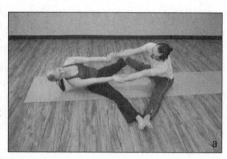 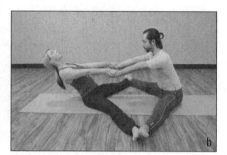

© John Wiley & Sons, Inc.

1. **Sit on the floor, facing your partner, with your legs wide and your feet touching your partner's feet or ankles.**

2. **Reach forward with both hands and hold your partner's corresponding wrists.**

3. **Slowly circle your torsos together, taking turns leaning forward and backward as you rotate in your comfort zone; circle three times in each direction (see Figure 16-9a).**

4. **After the rotation, sit up straight while one partner slowly leans back, gently pulling the other partner forward for 4 or 5 breaths (see Figure 16-9b); then repeat in the other direction.**

Communication is the key here: Convey to your partner how you're doing with something along the lines of "Stop, that's enough" or "More, more."

Avoid this pose if it causes back pain.

## *The partner diamond*

The partner diamond opens the hips, hamstrings, and inner thighs. Figure 16-10 shows this posture.

1. **Sit on the floor and face your partner, with your legs open wide.**

2. **On the same side as your partner, bend one leg and bring that foot into your groin; let the inside of your foot touch the inner part of your extended leg.**

3. **Bring the hand closest to your extended leg up to your partner's shoulder on the side that's closest to your partner's extended leg.**

4. **Raise your outside arms straight up, and touch hands.**

5. **As you exhale, lean together sideways toward your extended legs; inhale back up, and repeat this step three times. Then stay in the folded sideways position for 4 to 5 breaths.**

   When you're in the final step and are leaning together toward your extended legs, think of twisting gently away from your partner.

6. **Repeat Steps 1 through 3 on the other side.**

Avoid this pose if it causes back pain.

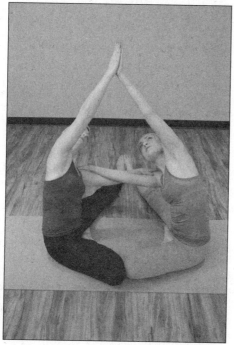

**Figure 16-10:**
The partner diamond is good for opening and stretching.

© John Wiley & Sons, Inc.

## Partner seated twist

The partner seated twist rejuvenates the spine and stimulates the abdominal organs and digestion. Figure 16-11 shows you how it looks.

1. **Sit on the floor in a comfortable position, back to back with your partner (see Chapter 6 for more on sitting).**

2. **Both of you raise your right hands and put them on your own left knees, palm down.**

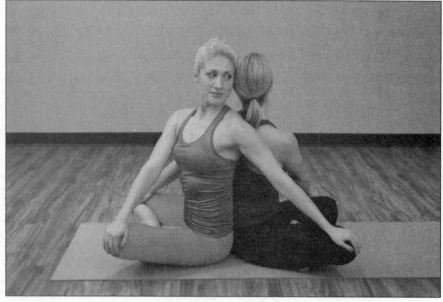

**Figure 16-11:**
A seated twist with a partner doubles the fun.

3. **Both of you move your left arms out to the left as far possible, and then place that arm palm down on your partner's right knee.**

4. **Take a deep breath together and, as you exhale, twist to your left as far as you comfortably can.**

5. **Stay for 4 to 5 breaths, and then repeat Steps 1 through 4 on the other side.**

As you perform the partner seated twist pose, think of lengthening through the top of your head and then rotating your spine and shoulders.

Avoid this pose if it causes back pain.

## Easy partner camel

The easy partner camel extends the back and stretches the abdomen, chest, and throat. It also stimulates the organs in the abdomen and neck. You can see it in Figure 16-12.

1. **Sit on the floor in a comfortable posture, back to back with your partner (see Chapter 6 for more on sitting).**

2. **One partner places her hands on the floor in front of her, while the other partner places her hands on her own knees.**

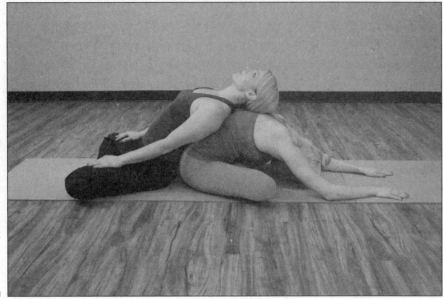

**Figure 16-12:**
The easy
camel
gives you
a stretch
while it
stimulates
your internal
organs.

© John Wiley & Sons, Inc.

3. **The partner with her hands on her knees simply leans backward while the other partner bends forward, sliding her hands forward on the floor.**

4. **Communicate about how far you each want to bend, and then stay in the final posture for 4 to 5 breaths.**

5. **Repeat Steps 1 through 4, switching direction and hand positions.**

Avoid this pose if it causes back or neck pain.

You can make this pose more challenging by hooking bent elbows with your partner.

# Chapter 17

# It's Never Too Soon: Pre- and Postnatal Yoga

The value of regular exercise doesn't dissipate just because you're pregnant. In fact, the American College of Obstetrics and Gynecology (ACOG) recommends that pregnant women become physically active to help alleviate some of the common discomforts associated with pregnancy, prepare for childbirth, and get back into shape afterward.

In this chapter, we discuss the benefits of Yoga practice during pregnancy, go through the best poses for a pregnant body, and provide a quick and easy routine to try.

## Partnering Yoga with Pregnancy

Taking a gentle approach to Yoga during pregnancy can be just what the doctor ordered. It may be just what the midwife ordered as well because it helps you cultivate a sense of confidence in your own body and your ability to give birth. Of course, each woman needs to consult her physician about her own situation, just to be certain she doesn't have any high-risk conditions that require special precautions.

We think the best way to take full advantage of Yoga is to start your practice well before you're pregnant, or at least as soon as you receive the good news. Your Yoga practice can build a strong, healthy body and a stable mind, not only helping you conceive a child (by making you fit and relaxed), but also supporting you during the pregnancy, at birth, and afterward. Many of our students continue their Yoga practice during their entire pregnancies, using the conservative principles we outline in this book.

## Womb with a (yogic) view

One of the unsung benefits of Yoga may be conceiving a baby when stress is the root cause of infertility. One memorable example of this idea is my (Larry's) students Dave and Adrian Lopez. Immersed in busy, demanding careers, they gave up Yoga. When they later decided to start a family, they tried unsuccessfully for 3 years to conceive, despite repeated attempts and the best medical methods available to them. Their physician finally suggested that perhaps their fertility problems were stress related and that they practice Yoga together — which they did. Sounds hard to believe, but after 30 days of practice, which included my weekly class and general conditioning DVD (flip to the appendix), Adrian became pregnant. She continued her Yoga practice until her eighth month and later gave birth to a big, beautiful baby boy.

ACOG recommends that pregnant women get a physical check-up before beginning an exercise program, Hatha Yoga included. They also recommend that pregnant women seek out a Yoga instructor specifically trained in prenatal Yoga. Conscious yogic relaxation and meditation, on the other hand, are right regardless of your physical cautions and imitations and may be helpful tools for labor as well. Your body, mind, and baby will be grateful to you!

## *Enjoying Yoga support as you — and the baby — grow*

Pregnancy entails major physiological and psychological changes. Apart from modifying your shape and weight, it also alters your body chemistry. Thus, you may experience a range of discomforts in addition to the welcome feelings of anticipation, excitement, and joy.

Yoga can make a major difference in your pregnancy experience. The increased self-awareness Yoga brings is helpful during this time when your body is continually undergoing change. Yogic practice provides the many benefits during this special time in your — and your baby's — life:

- Relaxes your whole body
- Helps with back problems
- Relieves nausea
- Reduces swelling and leg cramps

✔ Opens the hips and tones the pelvic floor

✔ Improves mood

✔ Provides focusing and breathing techniques for labor

✔ Provides a sense of community and social support through prenatal and postnatal Yoga classes

When seeking out prenatal Yoga classes, talk to the teacher beforehand. Ask about her training and experience, and assure yourself that she's knowledgeable about modifications that are safe and helpful during pregnancy.

## Exercising caution during pregnancy

Because pregnancy is a time when your actions directly and immediately affect you and your developing baby, we recommend that you keep the following cautions in mind as you exercise:

✔ Always do a little less than you're used to doing, and never hold your breath.

✔ Stay away from extremes in all the postures, especially deep forward or back bends. Don't strain.

✔ Avoid lying on your stomach for any postures.

✔ Steer clear of sit-ups and postures that put pressure on the uterus.

✔ Skip the postures that focus solely on tightening the abs; instead, work on strengthening your core in the context of more gentle postures.

✔ When a posture calls for a twist, twist from the shoulders, not the belly, to avoid compressing the internal organs.

✔ Avoid inverted postures other than putting your feet up on the wall or a chair.

✔ Pass up breathing exercises that are jarring, such as the shining skull (*kapalabhati*) or breath of fire *(bhastrika)*.

✔ Don't jump or move quickly into and out of postures.

✔ Be careful not to overstretch, which you can easily do in pregnancy because of increased hormone levels that cause your joints to become very limber.

ACOG recommends that a pregnant woman avoid lying on her back during exercise after the first trimester — and that includes with Yoga.

# Finding Perfect Pregnancy Postures

Practicing Yoga during pregnancy calls for the same consideration as putting together a yogic plan to manage back problems — no single posture or routine works the same way for everyone. Plus, what feels right during one trimester may not be appropriate during the next. In general, postures that allow you to gently increase flexibility in your hips can be useful as you prepare for giving birth, and many postures achieve that safely. We recommend that you seek out a qualified Yoga teacher to guide you in either a prenatal Yoga class or one-on-one instruction.

In the following sections, we describe three of the most recommended and useful Yoga postures for you to use any time during pregnancy and postpartum. We also describe a safe 15- to 20-minute Yoga routine that helps relieve discomforts and prepare your body for childbirth.

## Side-lying posture

Use the side-lying posture as an alternative to the corpse posture (*shavasana*) in your practice. You may also want to use the posture on its own to relieve feelings of general fatigue or nausea during pregnancy, labor, and the postpartum period, or as a good position for nursing. You need four or five blankets or three large pillows.

1. **Lie on your side on a comfortable surface.**
2. **Place one of the pillows or blankets under your head and the other just in front of you on the floor between the top of your thighs and the bottom of your chest; hang your top arm over the pillow in front of you.**
3. **Bend your knees, and place two blankets between your feet and your knees (see Figure 17-1).**

Stay and breathe naturally for as long as you feel comfortable. Repeat as often as you need to.

## The cat and cow

This posture, a variation of the cat (*chakravakasana*), extends the lower back and helps relieve symptoms of general back pain resulting from pregnancy.

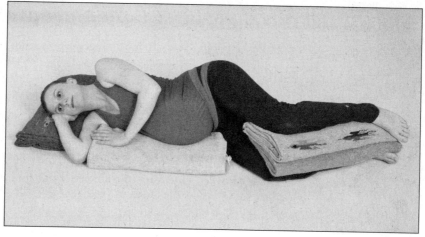

**Figure 17-1:**
Side-lying
posture.

*Photograph by Adam Latham*

Don't exaggerate or force your lower back down in Step 4. Don't practice this pose if you experience any negative symptoms.

1. **Starting on your hands and knees, look straight ahead.**

2. **Place your knees at hip width and your hands below your shoulders; straighten your elbows, but don't lock them.**

3. **As you exhale, arch your back like a cat; turn your head down and look at the floor (see Figure 17-2a).**

4. **As you inhale, slowly look up toward the ceiling and drop your lower back so that the shape of your back resembles that of a cow, as in Figure 17-2b.**

5. **Repeat Steps 3 and 4 six to eight times.**

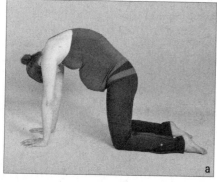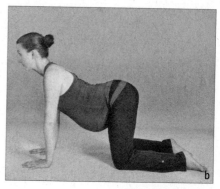

**Figure 17-2:**
The cat
and cow.

a

b

*Photograph by Adam Latham*

# The cobbler's posture: Badda konasana

The cobbler's posture helps you prepare for delivery by opening your groin and hips. It also improves alignment and provides a sitting posture for advanced breathing (remember, no holding your breath) and meditation techniques.

1. **Sit on the floor with your legs straight out in front of you; place your hands palms down at your sides, with your fingers forward.**

2. **Shake out your legs in front of you a few times.**

3. **Bend your knees outward, and slide the soles of your feet toward each other until they touch; hold the sides of your feet and lift gently from the chest (see Figure 17-3).**

**Figure 17-3:** The cobbler's posture.

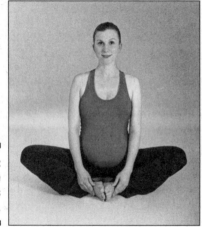

*Photograph by Adam Latham*

Sit in the posture for 30 seconds to a minute; as you progress, you can gradually increase to 3 to 5 minutes.

If your knees aren't close to the floor, you can sit on blankets or place the blankets under your knees.

# A safe, quick prenatal routine

The short routine in this section focuses on the areas of the body that you want to strengthen as you prepare your body for giving birth. Chapter 7 gives you more information on these postures.

### Mountain posture: Tadasana

One of the benefits of the mountain posture during pregnancy is that it directs your attention to your posture during this period when your weight and balance have gradually but steadily changed.

After you find your center of balance, begin the process of making a mental shift (which we discuss in Chapter 14), using the breathing style of your choice from Chapter 5. Stay in mountain posture (see Figure 17-4) for 6 to 8 breaths.

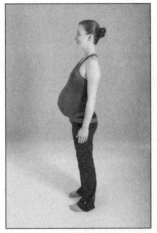

**Figure 17-4:** Mountain posture.

*Photograph by Adam Latham*

### Warrior I: Vira bhadrasana I

As its name suggests, warrior I strengthens the legs and improves stamina and balance. It's especially beneficial during pregnancy because it stretches your hips and helps with tension in your neck and swelling in your fingers.

Move into and out of the posture three to four times, and then stay for 6 to 8 breaths on each side. Figure 17-5 illustrates.

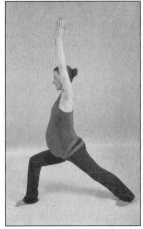

### Warrior II: Vira bhadrasana II

Another variation in the warrior family, this powerful posture opens your hips as it builds stamina and strengthens your arms. Move into and out of the posture three to four times, and then stay for 6 to 8 breaths on each side. Check out Figure 17-6.

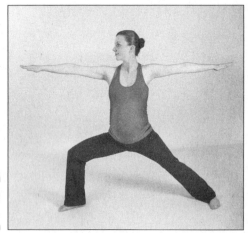

### Standing wide-legged forward bend: Prasarita pada uttanasana

This modified forward bend improves circulation in the head and lengthens the spine, hamstrings, and adductor muscles on the inside of the thighs. Just hang in this posture (shown in Figure 17-7) for 6 to 8 breaths.

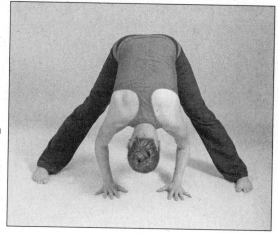

**Figure 17-7:** Standing wide-legged forward bend.

*Photograph by Adam Latham*

You can also try this standing posture with your hips at a wall or door.

### Triangle posture: Utthita trikonasana

The triangle posture stretches the sides of the spine, the back of the legs, and the hips while it opens the chest. Move into and out of the posture three to four times, and then stay for 6 to 8 breaths on each side. Figure 17-8 gives you a visual.

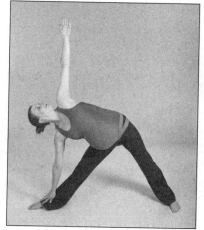

**Figure 17-8:** Triangle posture.

*Photograph by Adam Latham*

### Supported chair squatting posture: Modified ardha utkatasana

The supported chair squatting posture builds overall stamina while it strengthens your back, legs, shoulders, and arms. Move into and out of the posture three to four times, and then stay for 6 to 8 breaths.

Use an actual chair, as in Figure 17-9, unless you feel comfortable without it. Use a wide stance to maintain your center of balance.

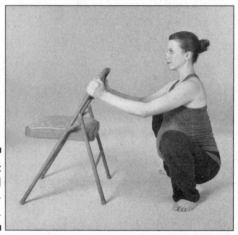

**Figure 17-9:**
Supported chair squatting posture.

*Photograph by Adam Latham*

### Cobbler's posture

This posture (flip to "The cobbler's posture" and Figure 17-3, earlier in this chapter) is a wonderfully relaxing way to end this short routine. Use an advanced breathing technique from Chapter 5 that doesn't require breath retention, such as alternate nostril breathing, and/or a meditation technique from Chapter 21.

## Use your Yoga tools to ease your labor — and have a healthier child

In their pure and hybrid forms, all the various methods of childbirth preparation — Lamaze, The Bradley Method, Birthing from Within, Birthworks, and Hypnobirthing — draw upon techniques that are integral to Yoga. In its own way, each method teaches the laboring woman to focus on her breath, breathe into a focal point, and/or utilize relaxation and meditation techniques. Your Yoga practice can help you more effectively apply whichever method of childbirth preparation you choose. Why is this connection important when the pain of childbirth can be controlled pharmacologically? Because babies born through nonmedicated births are better able to breastfeed, and breastfed babies are healthier, as are their mothers. You and your baby may continue to reap the benefits of your prenatal Yoga practice through your lifetimes.

# Continuing Yogic Exercise after Pregnancy (Postpartum)

Many traditional cultures honor a period of rest for the newly delivered mother, to give her time to recover from childbirth and bond with her newborn. This break typically lasts about 4 to 6 weeks; in Spanish, it's known as *la cuarentena*, or "the 40-day quarantine." Not surprisingly, physicians generally recommend that new mothers wait about 6 weeks before resuming their usual exercise routines — and a couple weeks longer if they had a Caesarean section.

When you return to your Yoga mat, avoid all inverted postures for at least 6 weeks postpartum because of uterine blood flow (called *lochia*). Also be careful with sit-ups because the groin area is fragile from its recent stretch. A good way to get started is with short walks and the side-lying corpse posture (see "Side-lying posture" and Figure 17-1, earlier in the chapter). All women have postnatal bleeding for a few weeks after pregnancy. Watch your flow, and slow your Yoga practice a little if the bleeding becomes heavier or turns bright red. If in doubt, consult your physician.

If you can, seek out a postpartum class with other new mothers. A skilled and experienced Yoga teacher can focus on those areas of your body that are likely to need extra attention during this transitional period — neck, shoulders, and upper back from the stress of carrying your baby and leaning over to attend to him; gentle belly toners to help you get back into shape; and so on. And don't underestimate the value of connecting with other new mothers. Few new mothers are fully prepared for the feelings of isolation and lack of control over their daily lives that are so common in the early postpartum period, especially among women who are used to being in the world and getting things done. The company of other new mothers who are feeling similar is often comforting and grounding.

Expect your life to change radically after the baby is born. Your Yoga practice will seem like an oasis, even if your practice sessions are short, as you handle the joyful but exhausting responsibilities of caring for your new baby. Don't feel guilty about making taking time for yourself. You need to recharge. Your hormone levels may make you feel emotional and a little unstable, and your Yoga practice can help you find balance. Final relaxation after your postures also can help you feel more rested, even though the enjoyment of a full night's sleep may be but a sweet and distant memory.

Your child took 9 months to grow inside your body, so give yourself 9 months to get back into shape. Set your clock to "mommy time" and enjoy the ride.

# Chapter 18

# Yoga for Kids and Teens

*Y*oung people have a natural affinity for Yoga. You can introduce even the youngest children to Yoga through play. As the names of common Yoga postures reveal, the postures were inspired by animals — the cat, the cow, the dog, the bear, and so on. The focused coordination of movement and breath that makes these movements Yoga and not just physical exercise easily lends itself to child's play. When combined with play — for example, imitation of animal sounds, a magic box of plush animal toys, balls of various sizes — voilà! You have the beginnings of kid-friendly Yoga.

For the "young and restless," also known as teens, Yoga offers tools to cultivate health in body, mind, and spirit. It provides a noncompetitive way for young people to develop strength and confidence and to manage stress — the plague of the times.

Classroom teachers are catching on to how Yoga can help their students gather up their boundless energy and focus on their academic tasks. Parents and Yoga teachers alike are finding that Yoga can also play a therapeutic role for children with challenges such as autism and ADHD.

In this chapter, we offer pointers, sample postures, and kid-friendly ways for parents or caregivers to introduce Yoga to children. Teachers reading this book can find information here to whet their appetites for incorporating Yoga into their classrooms. Teens and adults with energy to spare also get a guide to a classical routine that challenges the body while focusing the mind.

# Kid Stuff: Making Yoga Fun for Youngsters

The sense of calm, focus, and balance that draws adults to the practice of Yoga is also available to children, even ones as young as 3, as long as you introduce them to it in a playful, child-friendly fashion. When guided with a developmentally appropriate approach, preschoolers and the primary school set alike can reap Yoga's numerous benefits, such as improved concentration skills, an ability to calm and center themselves, and greater self-esteem and self-confidence. In many ways, young children are naturals for Yoga because they can participate without the physical and mental tightness that adults have acquired. Afi Kobari, creator of the Yogamama program in Los Angeles, describes a palpable energy and joy in her young students when she guides them through postures with a playful approach. The following sections give you some tips on engaging your child in Yoga, as well as several poses to try.

## Engaging the imagination: Approaching poses in a child-friendly way

Child's play, when slowed and joined with consciousness, can provide a platform for kid-friendly Yoga practice. Yoga postures (originally derived from and often named for animals) and concepts lend themselves to play in a variety of ways:

- Try having your child vocalize a posture's animal's call, to draw attention to the breath.

- Let your child pick from a selection of animal cards and then strike the pose of the chosen animal.

- Incorporate balance into any number of children's games that involve running and stopping at a specified moment by directing your child to be still and balance on one leg after stopping.

- Adding a children's Yoga book or idea with a story also helps to keep kids focused and share more philosophy with them, in addition to asana.

- Add rolling a ball with one hand while the child's other hand is engaged in a seated posture, to encourage right/left brain development.

## Bring balance to children with special needs

According to the Mayo Clinic, growing evidence suggests that Yoga may help alleviate symptoms of ADHD. On its physical level, Yoga encourages focus on breath before, during, and between postures; physical exertion through the asanas; and a focused winding-down period afterward — all of which can help calm hyperactive tots. Yoga helps hyperactive children get in touch with their bodies in a relaxed and noncompetitive way, and its cumulative effects for your little yogi or yogini may result in improved capacity for schoolwork and creative play. Seek out a Yoga teacher who can create a strong bond with your child, to gain his trust and attention.

Yoga can also help children with autism gain new motor, communication, and social skills — and thus enjoy an overall improvement in their quality of life. Structure and repetition are key for Yoga sessions for a child with autism. By gradually adding subtle modifications to the postures one at a time, Yoga can help children practice becoming comfortable with change. Over time, children develop a greater capacity to handle the stress that so often accompanies autism, along with greater body awareness and concentration.

The right Yoga teacher for your child with autism is someone who respects his abilities as well as his challenges. This special teacher must be willing to meet your child where he is and gain his trust.

Be flexible when introducing your child to Yoga. Keep the following pointers in mind:

- ✔ Short, happy practice sessions that your child wants to come back to are better than a longer session that loses her attention.

- ✔ Be willing to adjust the Yoga session to your child's mood. A tired child may enjoy sitting poses. Cooling breathing exercises help a cranky child calm down. On a rainy day, active poses bring physical release of pent-up energy.

## *Finding Yoga postures kids love*

Children need to skip the headstand and shoulder stand. Although their bodies are flexible, they lack the strength and stability to do those postures safely.

We designed the postures in the following sections to be kid-friendly and wrote the accompanying text to be parent-friendly, to help you guide your child. You can find more detail about each of the postures in other chapters throughout the book, as we note in each section; when done in sequence, this set of postures forms a well-balanced routine. In addition to providing you with instructions to give your child as he gets into the posture, the sections suggest sounds he can make while in the pose. The sounds serve a dual purpose: They inspire your child's imagination while he's holding the pose (keeping him engaged) and also guide him to breathe instead of hold his breath.

*Note:* In these sections, we sometimes refer to *yummy poses.* The term *yummy pose* is just a kid-friendly description of a resting pose, in which you allow your body and mind to release. Afi Kobari, a specialist in Yoga for children, coined the phrase.

Children have short attention spans. You know your child best, so do only as many postures as he has attention for. In time, he'll be able to do more.

Find a special spot to practice Yoga with your child. Does he gravitate to a certain spot in your house or apartment for play? That area may be the perfect place to begin to share your love of Yoga.

### The mountain posture

Figure 18-1 gives you and your child a visual of this kiddie posture; flip to Chapter 7 for more info on the adult version. Give your child the following instructions:

1. **Stand tall like a mountain.**

2. **Breathe through your nose, and imagine you're in a very, very quiet place.**

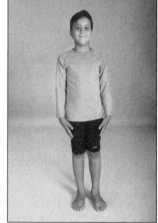

**Figure 18-1:**
The mountain posture for kids.

*Photograph by Adam Latham*

# How long does your child need to hold a posture?

Younger children may want to stay for only a few seconds before they're ready to move. Older children can stay longer. Adults usually hold a position for 6 breaths, after first having moved into and out of it a few times. Ask your child to hold the position only as long as you feel she will be comfortable. If she starts to get squirmy, have her come out of the position.

## *Warrior I*

See the preceding section for instructions to get your child into mountain posture. Figure 18-2 and Chapter 7 give you more guidance on warrior I.

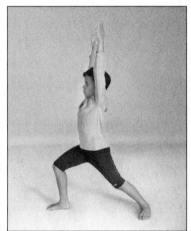

**Figure 18-2:**
Warrior I
for kids.

*Photograph by Adam Latham*

If your child's knee bends so much that you see it extending farther than the ankle, tell him to bend the knee a little bit less. The following instructions can lead your little yogi to warrior I success:

1. **Start in the mountain posture, and take a big step forward with one leg.**

2. **Bend your front knee and raise your arms overhead by your ears.**

3. **Feel how powerful and strong you are in this posture; next time, as you bend your knee and raise your arms, say, "Yes! I can!"**

4. **Keeping your knee bent and your arms raised, stay in this position and really feel like a warrior.**

5. **Try the same movements on the other side.**

### Bear posture

Check out Figure 18-3 and the following instructions to direct your child into bear posture.

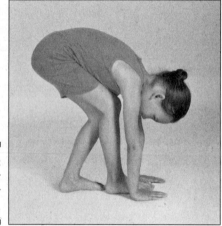

**Figure 18-3:**
Bear
posture for
kids.

_Photograph by Adam Latham_

1. **Start in the mountain posture, and then bend forward and hang down.**

2. **Staying bent, walk around, dragging your arms and hands as you growl and imagine you're a bear.**

### Cat and cow

The following directions help you walk your child through cat and cow; kids usually have a lot fun with this sequence, especially when you do it with them.

1. **Get down on your hands and knees as if you're going to crawl, but stay in one place.**

2. **Make your back round so you can look down and back at your legs (see Figure 18-4).**

3. **Imagine you're a cat, and make the sound of a cat: meow.**

4. **Move your back so that your belly goes down toward the floor, your chest goes up, and you look ahead.**

   Show your child Figure 18-4b for help in visualizing this step.

5. **Imagine you're a cow, and make the sound of a cow: mooo, mooo.**

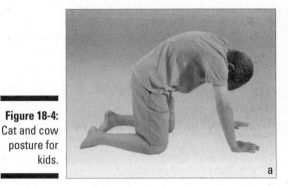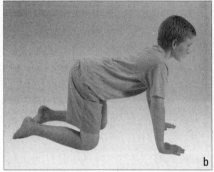

**Figure 18-4:**
Cat and cow posture for kids.

a

b

*Photograph by Adam Latham*

## Jumping frog

Use these instructions to lead your tot through jumping frog.

1. **Stand with your feet wide apart, and squat low (see Figure 18-5).**

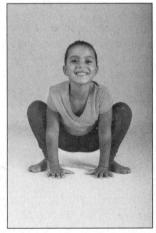

**Figure 18-5:**
Jumping frog for kids.

*Photograph by Adam Latham*

2. **Place your hands on the ground, and then jump and raise your arms.**

3. **Imagine you're a frog, and make the sound of a frog: ribbit, ribbit.**

## Tree posture

Work your child through tree posture by using the following instructions, and check out Figure 18-6 for an illustration. Flip to Chapter 7 for more information on the adult version.

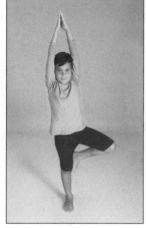

*Photograph by Adam Latham*

**Figure 18-6:**
Tree posture
for kids.

1. **Start in the mountain posture, standing tall and still.**

2. **Bend one of your legs, and place the bottom of that foot high on the inside of your other thigh.**

3. **Bring your hands together high above your head, and imagine that you're a tree as you make the sound of the wind blowing through your leaves: shhhhhhh.**

4. **Now try the same movements on the other side.**

### Cobra II

Chapter 11 gives you more information on the adult version of cobra II; the following instructions and Figure 18-7 help you lead your child through this version.

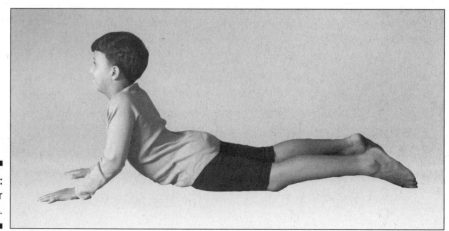

**Figure 18-7:**
Cobra II for
kids.

*Photograph by Adam Latham*

1. Lie flat on your belly, and place your hands on the floor near your armpits, with your fingers going forward.

2. Raise your head, shoulders, and back as you press down on your hands, keeping your hips on the ground.

3. Imagine that you're a cobra, and make the cobra's sound: ssssss.

### Lion posture

With the help of these instructions and Figure 18-8, your youngster can take pride in the lion posture. Chapter 6 provides additional information on the adult version.

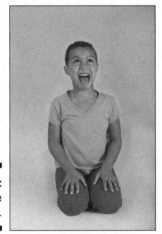

Photograph by Adam Latham

**Figure 18-8:**
Lion posture
for kids.

1. Sit on your heels, and place your hands on your knees.

2. Open your mouth wide, stick your tongue way out, and roll your eyes upward as though you're trying to see something high above you.

3. Imagine you're a mighty lion, and roar: ahhaahh!

### Downward-facing dog

We discuss the adult version of this posture in Chapter 7, but the following steps and Figure 18-9 lay out a child-friendly variety.

1. Start on your hands and knees.

2. Press through your arms, pushing down on your hands; straighten your legs and look down.

3. Imagine that you're a dog, and bark: woof, woof.

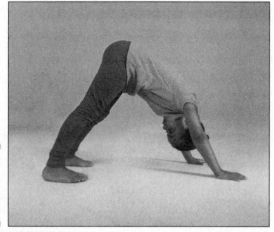

**Figure 18-9:**
Downward-
facing dog
for kids.

*Photograph by Adam Latham*

### Child's posture

This pose (one of the yummy poses) even has *child* in the name! Use the following instructions and Figure 18-10 to guide your tyke through the child's posture.

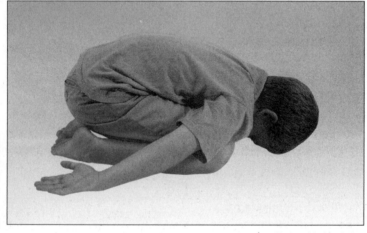

**Figure 18-10:**
Child's
posture for
kids.

*Photograph by Adam Latham*

1. **Kneel on the ground and fold up like a ball.**

2. **Place your hands at your sides, with your palms up.**

3. **Relax and think good thoughts.**

### The bridge

Figure 18-11 illustrates this easy posture. Give your child the following instructions to help him through the pose, and check out Chapter 14 for the adult bridge.

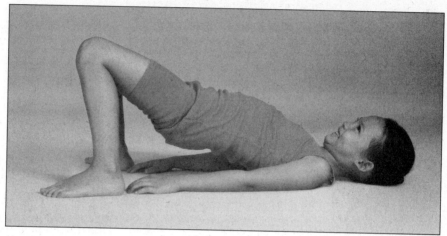

**Figure 18-11:**
Bridge for
kids.

*Photograph by Adam Latham*

1. **Lie on your back, bending your knees and letting your feet be firm on the ground.**

2. **Place your arms at your sides, with your palms down.**

3. **Raise your hips and become a bridge.**

4. **Imagine that you're a bridge, and make the sound of the cars traveling over you: chuga chuga chuga.**

### The wheel

The following directions and Figure 18-12 help your child get rolling with the wheel posture.

This advanced posture requires a fair amount of strength and flexibility. If your child isn't ready for it, come back to it when he's stronger and more flexible.

1. **Lie on your back with your knees bent and your feet on the ground.**

2. **Place your arms over your head, and turn your hands so that they're flat and your fingers are facing back toward the top of your shoulders.**

3. **Press up into the wheel.**

4. **Smile from the inside out.**

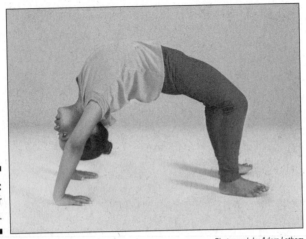

**Figure 18-12:**
Wheel for
kids.

*Photograph by Adam Latham*

### Knee-hugger

Knee-hugger is another of the yummy poses. These steps and Figure 18-13 show you how to help your child do it. You can find the adult version in Chapter 14 (there it's called knees-to-chest).

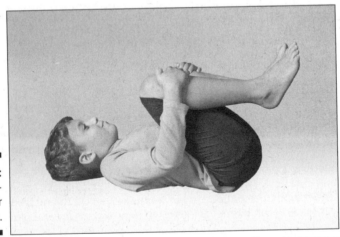

**Figure 18-13:**
Knee-
hugger for
kids.

*Photograph by Adam Latham*

For an added benefit, have your child rock his knees from side to side while he's hugging them — it gently massages the back.

1. **Lie on your back, and then bend and hug your knees.**

2. **Just relax and think good thoughts.**

### Easy posture

These instructions help you walk (sit?) your young yogini through the easy posture; check out Figure 18-14 for the proper sitting posture. (We cover the adult version in Chapter 6.)

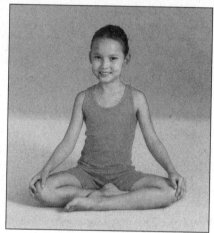

**Figure 18-14:**
Easy posture for kids.

*Photograph by Adam Latham*

Your child may be more comfortable with a blanket under his hips.

1. **Sit on the floor and cross your legs comfortably.**

2. **Keep your back and head tall, without straining.**

3. **Imagine a big balloon in your belly: When you breathe in, fill the balloon, and when you breathe out, let the air out of the balloon.**

## Ah, shavasana, the yummy part

No matter how short your child's Yoga session, be sure to include a period of final relaxation, or *shavasana*. Shavasana allows a child to relax her body without forcing it. It can be as simple as counting 5 breaths. This rest is especially helpful for children who are never ready for bedtime, for fear they may miss something — sound like a little one you know? Flip to Chapter 4 for more on shavasana.

### The big yummy posture: Shavasana

Use the following instructions to help your child relax at the end of the session. Figure 18-15 illustrates the pose, and you can read more about the adult version in Chapter 4.

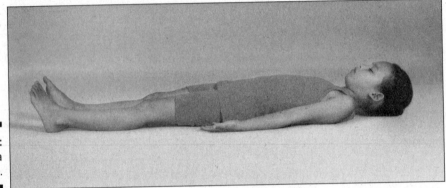

**Figure 18-15:**
Shavasana
for kids.

*Photograph by Adam Latham*

1. **Lie flat on your back, turning your palms up and letting your feet flop out.**

2. **Close your eyes gently, or keep them open and soft — whichever feels best.**

3. **Relax and think good thoughts.**

# Easing the Transition into Adulthood: Yoga for Teens

Yoga practice in the teenage years is so much more than an exercise program. Yes, it provides an energy outlet and a way to build muscle and flexibility — both important in their own right. But Yoga practice also provides an entry point for a healthful and balanced perspective on life and self that can remain for a lifetime. The following sections describe some benefits Yoga can offer teens.

## Calling all teens: The antidote to stress in an overscheduled life

Maybe you're vying for a place on the team or a high class ranking, juggling a part-time job, or caring for younger siblings while being a full-time student. More likely than not, your time and energy are stretched to the max.

## Integrating Yoga into the classroom

The lessons of Yoga aren't confined to the Yoga mat or the body. The skills and understanding acquired through Yoga practice help children of all ages, including teens, approach life in a more grounded, centered, and emotionally intelligent way. When presented as an exploration, traditional Yoga themes such as the practice of *ahimsa,* or nonharming (see Chapter 20), can translate into simple, practical distinctions, such as the difference between force and finesse. Consider the simple exercise of untying a knot: By using finesse rather than force, a child learns through his own experience which is the better way. This awareness applied to Yoga poses and balance allows a child to recognize which feels best in her own body; applied to personal relationships, it illustrates the better way to get along with the people in her life.

You don't need to be a Yoga teacher to bring this often-neglected aspect of learning into the classroom. Classroom teachers can learn to lead children through basic poses and routines to enhance their ability to learn throughout the day — for instance, morning sun salutations (see Chapter 14) to energize and focus their energy, balancing poses (see Chapter 9) after recess to regroup for academics, alternate nostril breathing (see Chapter 5) in a comfortable seated pose (see Chapter 7), or a simple forward bend (see Chapter 12) to help calm the mind as a prelude to creative writing. The list goes on. To date, more than 1,000 schools have integrated Yoga techniques into their curricula through the training and materials available through Yoga Playgrounds and Yoga Ed, both developed by Leah Kalish.

And your shifting hormonal levels may leave you feeling like a different person from day to day, hour to hour, and even minute to minute.

Yoga can be an oasis in a vast desert of stress. Yoga, a union of mind and body, can make weathering the demands of daily life easier. With regular practice, you may find that you have a greater ability to think for yourself and trust yourself — important at a time of life when peer pressure can feel overwhelming and poor judgment and bad decisions can impact your health, your well-being, and your future.

 Headstands, shoulder stands, and the lotus position may look like the popular idea of Yoga, but in fact, they can be dangerous. Young people are still growing and generally don't yet have the necessary musculature and stability to tackle these postures safely, so stay away from them for now.

## *Fit for life, and so much more*

Perhaps the most important benefit Yoga can offer you during your teen years is the opportunity to develop a lifelong friendship with your body. When you develop a Yoga practice, first under the guidance of a skilled and nurturing teacher and then later on your own, you tune in to your body, pay attention to what's happening, and respond appropriately — not unlike the good energy you put into your friendships with your best buddies. A regular Yoga practice can help you develop the focus, concentration, and discipline you need to study well and pursue your dreams. And when you're barefoot on your mat in the practice studio, you're free from the pecking order of your school campus. Yoga helps you become self-confident and courageous, without competing. How good is that?

Of course, Yoga is also a great way to become and stay fit. Both the USDA and Health Canada rank having an adequate level of physical activity as a high health priority. At ChooseMyPlate.gov, the United States Department of Agriculture (USDA) puts physical activity on par with eating a balanced diet, for a healthful life. As a form of physical fitness, Yoga is an attractive package:

- ✔ It's economical. You already have this book, so you can begin practicing right away, without anything else.

- ✔ You don't need a gym or a playing field. You just need enough floor space to practice safely. If you practice at home, try to find a private space. If your space is at a premium, consider following the lead of a highly respected Yoga teacher who's been known to practice "bathroom Yoga" when no other private space was available. Building codes require even the smallest bathrooms to have a certain amount of floor space. Check it out: Yours may just be long enough for a mat.

## Can Yoga help you maintain a healthy weight?

According to Robert M. Sapolsky's *Why Zebras Don't Get Ulcers* (Henry Holt and Company), modern garden-variety stressors can lead to overeating — in particular, choosing the wrong kinds of food to overeat. Stress floods your body with hormones that affect your appetite. If the stress is intense but short-lived, most people usually experience a loss of appetite — the way you feel when you're too nervous to eat. But when you experience frequent on-and-off stress throughout the course of the day, day in and day out, the hormonal levels in the body increase appetite — and not for the healthy stuff. What helps? Engaging in regular exercise that you look forward to doing, meditating, and cultivating a self-accepting, nonperfectionist approach to life are a few practices that have been shown to help. How handy to be able to find all that in Yoga!

# Developing Yoga Routines for the Young and Restless

The routines in this section have been specifically designed for teens. When done carefully, they also work for men and women well into their 30s, but we don't recommend them for the typical middle-aged person over 40. A lot of what group Yoga classes across America (especially in health clubs) offer today was originally designed for lightweight teenage boys in India whose lifestyles involved a lot of squatting. Middle-aged beginners often jump into that kind of Yoga in a competitive way and end up with injuries to show for it because it's just not built for them (or they for it).

Most professional athletes are usually at their highest physical prowess from their teens to early 30s. Then the body starts to change, and so should the training program, to prevent injuries. I (Larry) call the first stage "Yoga for the Young and Restless." Many of the popular styles of Yoga, such as Ashtanga Yoga, some components of Iyengar Yoga, and modern flow Yoga, were inspired by the teachings of the late Sri T. Krishnamacharya of Southern India earlier in his life and were originally intended for younger practitioners. The unpublished routines in this section were passed down to me (Larry) by Sri T. Krishnamacharya's son (and my teacher), T.K.V. Desikachar.

These routines are meant to be challenging. However, always keep in mind Yoga's fundamental principle: "Do no harm." Trust your inner teacher. If your body says it's time to rest, rest (even if others are still in their poses). Trusting yourself in this way is an important step toward becoming a balanced adult.

## Standing routine

As you get ready to begin your routine, remember that Yoga is a body, breath, and mind discipline. With the exception of the jumps, move slowly and stay in the moment.

Before you begin, here are some general tips and instructions to keep in mind:

- ✔ Choose either focus or chest-to-belly breathing from Chapter 5.
- ✔ Stay and breathe in each posture for 8 to 10 breaths.
- ✔ Do the whole routine twice on both sides.

✔ Refer to Chapter 7 for detailed instruction on all the postures in this routine (although note that some postures here are variations on Chapter 7's postures).

✔ This routine takes about 15 to 20 minutes.

When you're ready, follow these steps to complete the standing routine:

1. **Start in the mountain posture (see Figure 18-16a).**

   Initiate the Yoga breathing style of your choice from the list earlier in this section.

2. **As you exhale, jump or step out into a wide stance with your arms in a *T* parallel to the floor, as in Figure 18-16b.**

3. **As you inhale, raise your arms from the sides and overhead as you rotate your feet and torso to the right (see Figure 18-16c).**

4. **As you exhale, sink into warrior I position, with your right knee bent in a 90-degree angle (as in Figure 18-16d).**

5. **As you inhale, rotate your shoulders to the left and drop your arms into a *T*, with your palms down, for the warrior II position; open your back (left) hip to the left as far as it can go, and tuck your tail under comfortably.**

   Figure 18-16e gives you a visual.

6. **As you exhale, rotate your shoulders to the right, and reach forward with your left arm and back with your right arm so they're parallel to the floor (as in Figure 18-16f), for the reverse triangle variation I.**

7. **Inhale and then, as you exhale, drop your left hand to the floor and bring your right arm straight up for the reverse triangle variation II; keep your right leg bent and rotate your head up to the right (see Figure 18-16g).**

   If your neck gets tired, turn your head down.

8. **As you exhale, roll down with your arms, trunk, and head; turn your feet forward and parallel, and then hang down the middle, holding your elbows for the standing spread-legged forward bend (see Figure 18-16h).**

9. **Roll your body up, and then jump or step back into the mountain posture in Step 1.**

10. **Repeat Steps 1 through 9 on the left side.**

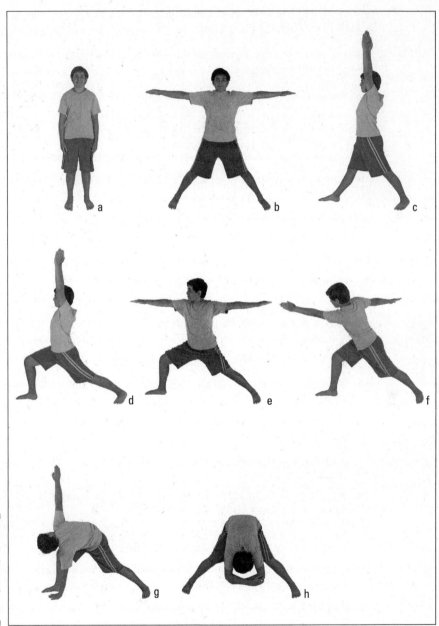

*Photograph by Adam Latham*

**Figure 18-16:**
Sequence
of poses for
the standing
routine for
teens.

## *Floor routine*

Some people call this routine the Lifetime Sequence because getting into wide-legged seated forward bend postures takes a lifetime if you aren't naturally flexible in the hips. And if you happen to believe in reincarnation, you have the luxury of another lifetime to work on it.

Before you begin, here are some tips to keep in mind:

- ✔ Choose focus or chest-to-belly breathing from Chapter 5.
- ✔ Stay in each posture (including each time you raise your arms) for 6 to 8 breaths.
- ✔ Do the whole sequence twice.
- ✔ This routine takes 20 to 25 minutes.
- ✔ Feel free to soften your knees in all the forward bends.
- ✔ Challenge yourself, but don't strain yourself.

This routine isn't recommended for people with lower back problems aggravated by rounding.

When you're ready, follow these steps to complete the floor routine:

1. **Start with your arms in the air and with a straight back, as in Figure 18-17a.**

2. **As you exhale, bend forward and down to the seated forward bend pose in Figure 18-17b.**

3. **As you inhale, raise your trunk and arms to a straight back, and separate your legs wide, as in Figure 18-17c.**

4. **As you exhale, bend forward and down to a spread-legged forward bend, as Figure 18-17d illustrates.**

5. **As you inhale, raise your trunk and arms up to a straight back position, as you did in Step 3 (see Figure 18-17c).**

6. **As you exhale, rotate to the right, as in Figure 18-17e, and bend forward and down, as in Figure 18-17f.**

7. **As you inhale, raise your trunk and arms to a straight back position, as you did in Step 5 (see Figure 18-17c).**

8. **As you exhale, rotate to the left as in Figure 18-17g, and bend forward and down (see Figure 18-17h).**

9. **As you inhale, raise your trunk and arms to a straight back position and bend your legs halfway, with your toes up (see Figure 18-17i).**

10. **As you exhale, bend forward and down, and try to move your toes down, as in Figure 18-17j.**

11. As you inhale, raise your trunk and arms to a straight back position, drop your knees to the sides, and join the soles of your feet together, as Figure 18-17k illustrates.

12. As you exhale, bend forward and down, and hold your feet (see Figure 18-17l).

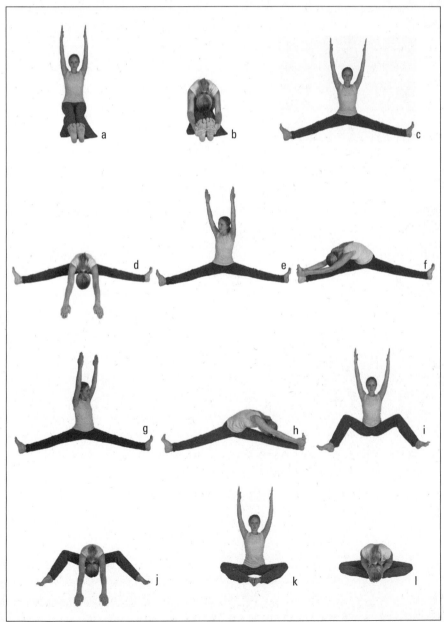

**Figure 18-17:** Sequence of poses for the floor routine for teens.

*Photograph by Adam Latham*

If you have back problems lifting up from the forward bends in this routine, try the roll-up: Keep your chin on your chest and roll up, stacking your vertebrae one at a time, with your arms hanging at your sides. When you're fully upright, bring your arms up and overhead from the front, and look forward.

# Chapter 19

# It's Never Too Late: Yoga for Midlifers and Older Adults

*I*f you're on the senior side of the life curve and you're considering taking up Yoga, you're not alone. A 2012 *Yoga Journal* study reported that approximately a third of the 20.4 million adults in America who practice Yoga are older than age 45.

Yoga can help practitioners of every age improve their health and well-being. The Yoga toolbox includes innumerable postures that, depending on how you modify them, can offer the appropriate level of challenge to each and every yogi and yogini, regardless of age or ability. Remember, the process and the practice are important, not the final form of the postures. One advantage more mature practitioners of Yoga have over more youthful adherents is greater patience to be still for breathing exercises and meditation, both of which become more important relative to the postures as you age.

This chapter presents safe Yoga routines for people in their middle-aged and senior years. The Prime of Life Yoga discussion addresses folks who fall within the vast expanse of the middle years — generally between 40-something and 70-something.

The "Cherishing the Chair" section addresses the needs of folks who are generally older than 70; however, people of any age can follow these routines. Yoga is a union of body, breath, and mind, and the best variations of Yoga postures for any individual are ones that meet physical, emotional, and lifestyle needs, regardless of age.

# Reaping the Benefits of Yoga through Midlife and Beyond

*Midlife*, as the word suggests, refers to the middle of life. It's not, as some people think, "The End," but rather a new beginning. The following sections show you how Yoga helps you navigate the physical and emotional changes associated with midlife and allows you to age gracefully, healthfully, and actively.

## Working through menopause

Menopause signals a major biochemical change in a woman, marked most obviously by the disappearance of her monthly flow. Her body's sexual glands go into relative retirement, and she can no longer bear children. The hormonal shifts that lead up to actual menopause can take up to a decade. *Perimenopause*, the term given to the longer process, can bring with it a host of undesirable side effects: hot flashes, palpitations, dizzy spells, insomnia, vaginal dryness, urinary problems, and irritability. This time of life can make women prone to depression, but with an attitude of acceptance for the change and the possibilities yet to come, it can actually be a satisfying time of life. Yoga comes into play here.

Regular Yoga practice can help alleviate the physiological side effects of menopause, especially if you start a few years before its onset, and help you cultivate a forgiving, accepting, and positive attitude important for your emotional well-being. Inversions (see Chapter 10), which have a profound effect on the glands and inner organs and (both literally and figuratively) allow you to view things from a new perspective, are especially helpful. For soothing rest and whole-person recovery, we particularly recommend that you cultivate the corpse posture we describe in Chapter 15. Just give your body a chance to rebalance its chemistry.

## Not just a "woman thing": Navigating andropause

Men experience something similar to menopause, called *andropause*. Although changes in their sexual glands may lessen their sex drives, men can continue to sire children into old age. But when they see their vitality and hairline recede a little, men are often thrown into an existential crisis.

Midlife offers a great opportunity to discover life's possibilities beyond sexual reproduction and raising children. Regular Yoga practice can buffer the unpleasant physiological side effects of andropause and stabilize the emotions triggered when you realize you're no longer quite so dashing — unless, of course, you have practiced Yoga all along.

## Developing bones of steel

With regular exercise, you can prevent the bone loss *(osteoporosis)* associated with midlife and old age. Regular weight-bearing exercises strengthen your bones, but stress causes acidity, which leaches the calcium from your bones. Many people don't realize that osteoporosis actually starts in your mid- to late 20s. Therefore, you can't begin Yoga too early — and it's never too late to take it up! Buns of steel ain't bad, but bones of steel are the better deal.

# Approaching Prime of Life Yoga with the Right Mindset

As you age, mobility is the new flexibility. So although you may have been able to do the most acrobatic postures in your youth, the important goal now is to maintain the mobility to remain fit and active. In the Prime of Life approach to Yoga postures, spinal freedom and movement take precedence over form. Adjustments to the posture, such as bending the knees *a lot*, if necessary, encourage movement of the spine.

The attitude you bring to your practice is critical. The right attitude on the mat allows you to practice postures safely and spills over to your life off the mat. Here are a few Yoga principles for a safe and fulfilling practice.

- ✔ Challenge yourself, but don't strain yourself.
- ✔ Yoga is a dialogue, not a monologue; keep body, breath, and mind linked.
- ✔ Think of your Yoga practice as a meditation in motion.
- ✔ You get no gain with *negative pain* (pain that does harm).
- ✔ You're the chairperson of the board; you decide when to come out of the posture.
- ✔ Let the posture fit you instead of trying to fit yourself into the posture.

# Developing User-Friendly Routines for Midlifers

In this section, we present routines for two different skill levels, both of which are equally ideal for men and women. (For true beginners with a few aches or pains, we recommend starting with the lower back routine in Chapter 22.)

You can find recommendations for DVDs on Yoga for this age group in the appendix.

## Prime of Life Yoga routine: Level 1

The routine in this section is a nice general-conditioning routine for midlifers and even younger folks who want to ease back into physical activity. This user-friendly sequence strings together a series of safe postures that work each side of the body separately, helping to achieve greater balance.

You can find detailed instructions for each of these various poses or their variations in Chapters 4, 7, 8, and 15. Choose a breathing technique from Chapter 5. Hold each posture and its variation for 6 to 8 breaths, with the exception of warrior I (Steps 2 and 3) and revolved triangle variation (Steps 9 and 10). For each of these postures, move into and out of the postures three times, and then hold for 6 to 8 breaths. This routine takes about 30 to 35 minutes.

1. **Start in the mountain posture (see Figure 19-1a); initiate the Yoga breathing style of your choice for 6 to 8 breaths (see Chapter 5).**

2. **As you exhale, step forward with the right foot about 3 to 3½ feet (or the length of one leg). Your left foot turns out naturally; turn it out more to increase stability. Place your hands on the tops of your hips, and square the front of your pelvis; release your hands and hang your arms (see Figure 19-1b).**

3. **As you inhale, raise your arms from the front up and overhead, and bend your right leg into a right angle for warrior I, as Figure 19-1c illustrates.**

4. **Repeat Steps 2 and 3 three times, and then stay in warrior I for 6 to 8 breaths.**

5. **As you exhale, bend both arms downward and draw your elbows back, as you turn your palms up and lift your chest (see Figure 19-1d); hold this proud warrior posture for 6 to 8 breaths.**

6. **As you inhale, keep your right leg bent, and join your palms together in front of you and bring them up and overhead as you look up and back (see Figure 19-1e); stay in the exalted warrior posture for 6 to 8 breaths.**

7. **As you exhale, come down over your bent right leg and place your hands on the floor for the standing asymmetrical forward bend (see Figure 19-1f); stay in the posture for 6 to 8 breaths.**

   Work on straightening your right leg based on your flexibility in the moment. A soft or bent leg is okay.

   If you want to feel the stretch more, square your hips by pulling your right hip back and putting your left hip forward. A more challenging option is to rotate the back foot inward, called *paralleling the feet.*

8. **As you inhale, roll your body up vertebra by vertebra, and then step your feet together back into the mountain posture from Step 1.**

9. **Repeat Steps 1 through 8 on the left side.**

10. **From the mountain posture, step out with your right foot about 3 to 3½ feet (or the length of one leg); as you exhale, bend forward from the hips, hang down, and place the palms of both hands on the floor directly below your shoulders, as in Figure 19-1g.**

11. **As you inhale, raise your right arm toward the ceiling and look up at your right hand for the reverse triangle variation, as Figure 19-1h illustrates.**

12. **Repeat Steps 10 and 11 three times, and then remain with your right arm up for 6 to 8 breaths; repeat on your left side.**

    Soften your knees and arms. Turn your head down if your neck gets sore.

13. **As you exhale, hang your torso, head, and arms down, holding your bent elbows with opposite-side hands for the standing spread-legged forward bend (see Figure 19-1i); stay for 6 to 8 breaths.**

14. **Transition to your hands and knees, and slide your right hand forward and your left leg back as you exhale, keeping your hand and your toes on the floor; as you inhale, raise your right arm and left leg to a comfortable height for the balancing cat posture (see Figure 19-1j).**

    Stay up for 4 to 8 breaths, and then repeat with opposite pairs, lifting your left hand and your right leg.

    If you want a bigger challenge in this posture, raise your bottom foot just off the floor.

15. **As you exhale, come back to all fours and fold down into the child's posture variation (with your arms in front of you), as in Figure 19-1k; hold for 6 to 8 breaths.**

16. Lie flat on your back, with your arms along the sides of your torso, your palms up, and your eyes closed for the corpse posture, as in Figure 19-1l.

17. To finish, use belly breathing from Chapter 5 or a relaxation technique from Chapter 4 for 3 to 5 minutes.

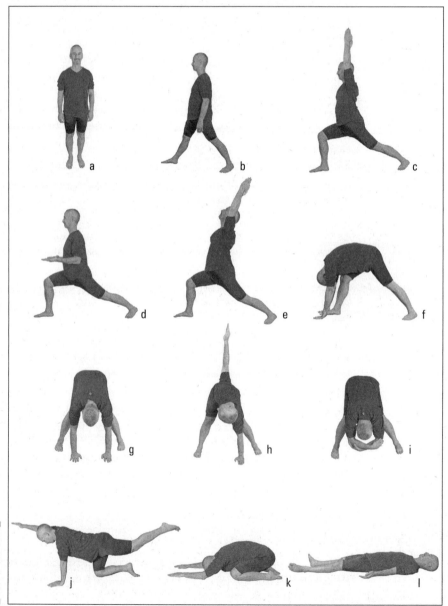

**Figure 19-1:**
Prime of Life Yoga routine: Level I.

*Photograph by Adam Latham*

# Prime of Life Yoga routine: Level II

After you master the level I sequence in the preceding section, enjoy the challenge of this section's level II sequence. It's a little longer and more physically demanding. Like the other routine, it brings balance by working each side of the body separately.

Plan to spend approximately 45 minutes to complete this sequence, which has two parts: standing postures and postures on the floor.

For detailed information on the various postures in this section or their variations, head to Chapters 4, 7, 8, 11, 12, and 15. Select a breathing technique from Chapter 5. Hold each posture and variation for 6 to 8 breaths, with the exception of the warrior II posture (Steps 3 and 4) and the seated forward bend posture (Steps 12 and 13) — in both of those postures, you move into and out of them three times before holding for 6 to 8 breaths.

1. **Start in the mountain posture (see Figure 19-2a).**

    Initiate the Yoga breathing style of your choice from Chapter 5 for 6 to 8 breaths.

2. **As you exhale, step out to your right with your right foot about 3 to 3½ feet (or the length of one leg); turn your right foot out 90 degrees, and turn your left foot slightly inward, or keep it straight if a slight inward turn isn't available to you.**

3. **As you inhale, raise your arms out to your sides in a *T* parallel to the line of your shoulders and the floor, for the warrior II ready posture (see Figure 19-2b).**

4. **As you exhale, bend your right knee to a right angle with the floor, and turn your head to the right, as in Figure 19-2c; repeat Steps 3 and 4 three times, and then remain in the warrior II posture for 6 to 8 breaths.**

5. **As you inhale, raise your right arm and turn your right palm up; as you exhale, reach back with your left hand (palm down) and hold the outside of your left leg, looking up at your right hand for the reverse warrior posture (see Figure 19-2d). Stay for 6 to 8 breaths.**

6. **As you inhale, move back briefly to the warrior II position, and then bend your right arm, lay your right forearm across the top of your right thigh, and extend your left arm over your head in alignment with your left ear, as in Figure 19-2e; stay in this extended right angle posture for 6 to 8 breaths.**

7. **Repeat Steps 1 through 6 on the left side.**

8. **From your wide stance, roll your body up, turn both feet forward (to the right), and hang your arms at your sides; as you exhale, bend forward from the hips and hang your torso, head, and arms down, holding your bent elbows with opposite-side hands in the standing wide-legged forward bend (see Figure 19-2f). Hold for 6 to 8 breaths.**

9. **Return to mountain posture (refer to Figure 19-2a.)**

10. **As you inhale, raise your arms from the front up and overhead; as you exhale, bend forward from the hips, and raise your left leg back and up until your arms, torso, and left leg are all parallel to the floor and you're balancing on your right leg in the warrior III posture (see Figure 19-2g). Hold for 6 to 8 breaths.**

11. **Repeat Steps 9 and 10, balancing on the other side with your left leg.**

12. **Lie on your back, with your knees bent and feet flat on the floor at hip width, and place your hands at your sides palms down; as you inhale, raise your hips and your arms overhead to touch the floor behind you in the bridge variation with arm raise posture (see Figure 19-3a). Hold for 6 to 8 breaths.**

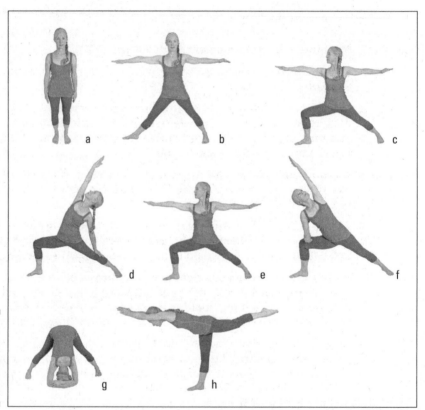

**Figure 19-2:**
Prime of Life
Yoga rou-
tine: Level II,
part 1.

*Photograph by Adam Latham*

13. **Lie on your abdomen with your left arm forward (palm down) and your right arm back at your right side (palm up), and then bend your right knee and hold your right foot with your right hand; lift your chest, left arm, and right foot to a comfortable level as you inhale into the half bow posture (see Figure 19-3b). Stay up for 6 to 8 breaths, and then repeat with opposite pairs, holding your left foot with your left hand and extending your right arm forward.**

14. **Move to your hands and knees, with both at hip width; as you exhale, sit back on your heels and fold your head and hips down into a comfortable position for the child's posture variation (see Figure 19-3c). Stay folded for 6 to 8 breaths.**

15. **Transition to a seated position, with your legs stretched out in front of you, and bring your back up nice and tall, moving your arms forward and up alongside your ears as you inhale (see Figure 19-3d).**

16. **As you exhale, bend forward from your hips, bringing your hands, chest, and head toward the floor, as in Figure 19-3e; repeat Steps 15 and 16 three times, and then stay down and folded for 6 to 8 breaths.**

    Soften your legs and arms as needed.

    Take extra caution or avoid seated straight-legged forward bends if you have back problems that rounding the back may exacerbate.

17. **Lie flat on your back, with your legs stretched out and your arms extended into a *T*, with your palms up; as you exhale, bring your right leg up and across your torso to the opposite side, slide your left arm overhead, and turn your head to the right until you're in the Swiss army knife (see Figure 19-3f). Stay in the posture for 6 to 8 breaths, and then repeat with opposite pairs.**

    Soften your limbs as needed.

18. **Stay on your back, and hug both knees to your chest with your hands as you exhale for the knees-to-chest posture (see Figure 19-3g); hold for 6 to 8 breaths.**

    Hold under your thighs if you have knee problems. As an alternative, rock gently from side to side.

19. **Lie flat on your back in the corpse posture (refer to Figure 19-2h), with your arms along the sides of your torso, your palms up, and your eyes closed to finish; use belly breathing from Chapter 5 or a relaxation technique from Chapter 4 for 3 to 5 minutes.**

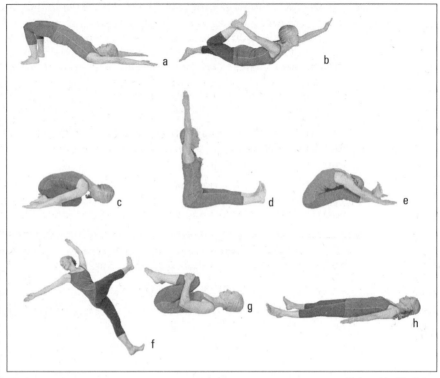

*Photograph by Adam Latham*

**Figure 19-3:**
Prime of Life
Yoga rou-
tine: Level II,
part 2.

# *Staying Active: Yoga for Older Adults*

According to the National Institute on Aging (www.nia.nih.gov), "'Too old' and 'too frail' are not, in and of themselves, reasons to prohibit physical activity. In fact, not very many health reasons can truly keep older adults from becoming more active." Many chronic conditions are actually a result of *not* exercising. As a form of exercise, Yoga has many benefits specific to seniors. Improved balance and flexibility reduce the risk for (and fear of) injury and increase mobility. Yoga also improves circulation and your ability to sleep, and adding even light weights to the postures increases bone density and lowers the risk of fracture. Plus, group practice promotes social interaction and a sense of connectedness.

Seniors interested in Yoga first need to check with their physician. After getting the green light, seek out a class that focuses on your age group, both for the social benefits and to be guided by a teacher who can adapt postures to your needs and abilities. Head to Chapter 2 for more on picking a teacher and a class. Be sure to mention any physical conditions or concerns (such as high blood pressure, hip replacement, osteoporosis, and so on), and check that your prospective teacher can modify the routines to ensure your safety. In a group setting, a skilled teacher offers a range of options so that each student can practice at a level appropriate for her abilities and limitations.

## How old is too old for Yoga?

Shelly Kinney, a Las Vegas–based Yoga therapist, recounts her experience with Ms. L, a 96-year-old student who was glued to her walker. After several months of Yoga practice, Ms. L was able to enter and leave the class without it. How did this happen? She executed warrior and side angle postures from a chair, added light weights over time, and worked with balance postures with a ballet bar on one side, a chair at the other, and Shelley there for support. Slowly but surely, Ms. L built up strength, flexibility, and confidence. She's proof that you're never too old to take up Yoga and enjoy its benefits.

# Cherishing the Chair: Safe Routines for Older Adults

You don't have to practice Yoga on the floor. If getting down to the floor or getting up and down is difficult, chair Yoga offers spinal freedom while allowing you to remain in your comfort zone. You can improve your flexibility, mobility, and balance even while seated. The following routines show you how.

You're in charge of whether you do a particular posture. If it doesn't feel right for you, don't do it. The National Institute of Aging provides a wealth of information to help guide you on what may be safe for you and what you may want to avoid. We also list books addressing the needs of older practitioners in the appendix, and your Yoga teacher may suggest other books or articles. Educate yourself, and enjoy the benefits of breath and movement.

## Cherish the chair routine: Level I

The postures in this seated Yoga routine give you the same main benefits of a regular Yoga class, including stress reduction, improved circulation, better concentration, and an overall sense of well-being. This routine takes about 15 to 20 minutes. Choose one of the Yoga breathing techniques in Chapter 5, and use it for this entire routine. Follow the instructions for breath and movement, and have fun!

Place blankets or a block under your feet if they don't sit flat on the floor in any of the chair postures.

### Seated mountain posture

Check out Figure 19-4 and the following steps for a visual of this posture.

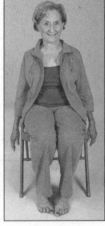

**Figure 19-4:**
Seated
mountain
posture.

Photograph by Adam Latham

1. **Sit comfortably in a chair, with your back extended and your eyes either open or closed.**

2. **Hang your arms at your sides, and visualize a vertical line down the middle of your ears, shoulders, hips, and backs of your hands; stay for 8 to 10 breaths.**

### Seated mountain arm variation

You can see how to do this posture in Figure 19-5. Just follow these steps.

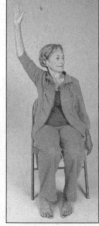

**Figure 19-5:**
Seated
mountain
posture
variation.

Photograph by Adam Latham

1. **Start in the seated mountain posture from the preceding section; raise your right arm and turn your head to the left as you inhale.**

2. **As you exhale, return to the seated mountain posture.**

3. **Repeat Steps 1 and 2 with your left arm and a right head turn, alternating right and left sides slowly for a total of 4 to 6 repetitions on each side.**

### Seated karate kid variation

Figure 19-6 illustrates this posture. Executing it is easy.

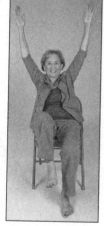

**Figure 19-6:** Seated karate kid variation.

*Photograph by Adam Latham*

1. **Start in the seated mountain posture, and raise your arms forward and up alongside your ears as you inhale.**

2. **As you exhale, bend your right knee and raise it toward your chest to a comfortable level.**

3. **Take another breath and then, as you exhale, lower your right knee and your arms back to the seated mountain posture.**

4. **Repeat Steps 1 through 3 with both arms and your left knee, alternating both your knees slowly as you raise your arms, for a total of 4 to 6 repetitions on each side.**

Be careful with this posture if you've have a hip replacement. If you aren't sure whether your hips can handle it, check with your doctor first.

### Seated wing-and-prayer

Figure 19-7 shows you this posture. Here's how you do it.

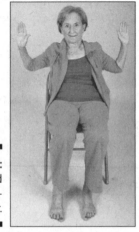

**Figure 19-7:**
Seated
wing-
and-prayer.

*Photograph by Adam Latham*

1. **Start in the seated mountain posture, with your hands together in prayer position and your thumbs at your breastbone.**

2. **As you inhale, open your hands outward and lift your chest like wings.**

3. **As you exhale, bring your hands and arms back together into the prayer position.**

4. **Repeat Steps 1 through 3 slowly for 4 to 6 repetitions.**

### Seated butterfly posture

Check out the seated butterfly in Figure 19-8, and then follow these steps to try it on your own.

1. **Start in the seated mountain posture, with your arms extended fully to the sides and parallel to the floor, and your palms facing forward.**

2. **Inhale and then, as you exhale, bring your right hand toward the inside of your left arm in a twisting motion.**

3. **Repeat Steps 1 and 2 slowly for 4 to 6 repetitions, and then do the same with your left hand and right arm.**

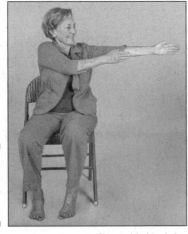

**Figure 19-8:**
Seated
butterfly
posture.

*Photograph by Adam Latham*

## Standing warrior I chair variation

Use Figure 19-9 and the following steps to guide you through this posture.

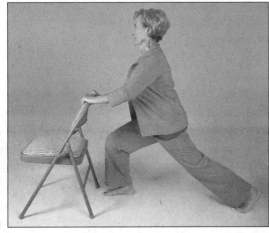

**Figure 19-9:**
Standing
warrior
I chair
variation.

*Photograph by Adam Latham*

1. **Stand in the mountain posture (see Figure 19-2a earlier in the chapter), facing the back of your chair from about 3 to 3½ feet away.**

2. **As you exhale, step forward with your right leg, place your hands on the back of the chair, and bend your forward leg into approximately a right angle.**

   You can keep your back foot flat or pivot on the ball of your back foot. Don't be tempted to force the angle.

3. **Stay in Step 2 for 4 to 6 breaths, and then repeat with your left leg forward for 4 to 6 breaths.**

### Seated sage twist

Check out Figure 19-10 and the following steps for the seated sage twist.

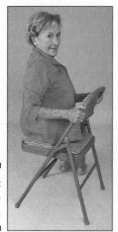

**Figure 19-10:**
Seated sage
twist.

*Photograph by Adam Latham*

1. **Sit in your chair sideways, with the back of the chair to your right and your feet flat on the floor.**

2. **As you exhale, turn to your right and grasp the sides of the chair back with your hands.**

3. **As you inhale, bring your back and head up nice and tall; as you exhale, twist deeper.**

4. **Continue this sequence three times, or until you reach your comfortable maximum, and then stay for 4 to 6 breaths; repeat Steps 1 through 4 on the left side.**

### Seated forward bend

These steps help you achieve this bend; see Figure 19-11 for an illustration.

1. **Start in the seated mountain posture.**

2. **As you exhale, bend forward from your hips and slide your hands forward and down your legs.**

3. **Let your head and arms hang down, and relax in the folded position for 4 to 6 breaths.**

4. **For a nice ending, use the seated mountain posture; close your eyes and choose focus breathing (Chapter 5) or a relaxation technique (Chapter 4) for 2 to 5 minutes.**

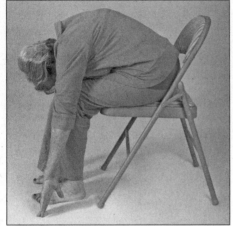

**Figure 19-11:**
Seated forward bend.

*Photograph by Adam Latham*

## Cherish the chair routine: Level II

This routine is more challenging than level I (see the preceding section) and takes about 15 to 20 minutes. (But don't let the word *challenging* scare you — our model Tony is well into his 80s!) Pick one of Chapter 5's Yoga breathing techniques and use it for the entire routine. The instructions and photos here show you how it's done.

This routine also works in an office environment for any age group.

### Seated mountain posture

Figure 19-12 illustrates this posture. Here's how it works.

1. **Sit comfortably in a chair, with your back extended and your eyes either open or closed.**

2. **Hang your arms at your sides, and visualize a vertical line down the middle of your ears, shoulders, hips, and backs of your hands; stay for 8 to 10 breaths.**

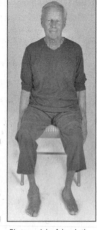

**Figure 19-12:**
Seated
mountain
posture.

*Photograph by Adam Latham*

### Seated mountain double arm variation I

For help with this posture, check out Figure 19-13 and the following steps.

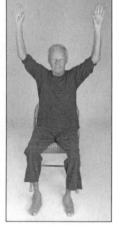

**Figure 19-13:**
Seated
mountain
double arm
variation I.

*Photograph by Adam Latham*

1. **Start in the seated mountain posture (see the preceding section).**

2. **As you inhale, raise your arms from the front up and overhead.**

   Try to bring your arms alongside your ears, with your palms forward (see Figure 19-13), but don't force it.

3. **As you exhale, lower your arms back to your sides.**

4. **Repeat Steps 1 through 3 four to six times.**

### Seated mountain double arm variation II

Figure 19-14 and the following steps show you how to achieve this pose.

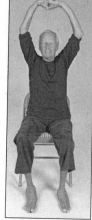

**Figure 19-14:**
Seated
mountain
double arm
variation II.

*Photograph by Adam Latham*

1. **Start in the seated mountain posture.**

2. **As you inhale, raise your arms from the front, up and overhead.**

3. **Interlace your fingers and reverse your palms toward the ceiling.**

4. **Keeping your arms soft, hold your arms alongside your ears for 4 to 6 breaths.**

### Seated triangle posture

Refer to Figure 19-15 for a visual of this posture, and then follow these steps.

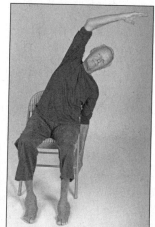

**Figure 19-15:**
Seated
triangle
posture.

*Photograph by Adam Latham*

1. **Start in the seated mountain posture and, as you inhale, raise your right arm out and up from the right side, with your palm rotated inward toward your head.**

2. **As you exhale, lean your right arm, head, and torso to the left as you drop your left arm.**

   Keep your bottom on the seat of the chair.

3. **Hold Step 2 for 4 to 6 breaths, and then repeat Steps 1 through 3 on the opposite side (with the left arm).**

### Seated pigeon posture

Figure 19-16 demonstrates this posture; here's how you do it.

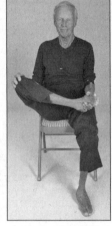

**Figure 19-16:** Seated pigeon posture.

Photograph by Adam Latham

Don't try this posture if you've had a hip replacement.

1. **Start in the seated mountain posture.**

2. **As you exhale, bring your bent right knee directly up, and then hold the outside of that knee with your right hand and the outside of your right heel with your left hand.**

3. **Place the outside of your right ankle on top of your left thigh just above your left knee; drop your right knee toward the floor to a comfortable level.**

4. **Stay for 4 to 6 breaths, and then repeat on the other side.**

You can slowly and gently move your top knee up and down a few times to limber your hip joint before you relax and breathe.

### Seated warrior I chair variation

Check out Figure 19-17 for the proper positioning on this posture, and then follow these steps to complete it yourself:

1. **Straddle your chair sideways, with the back of the chair on your right.**

2. **Keep your right knee bent in a right angle, and try to straighten your back (left) leg, with your toes or foot on the floor.**

3. **As you inhale, raise both arms forward and up until they're alongside your ears.**

4. **Stay in this position for 4 to 6 breaths, and then repeat Steps 1 through 3 on the other (left) side, holding Step 3 for 4 to 6 breaths.**

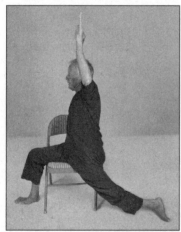

**Figure 19-17:** Seated warrior I chair variation.

*Photograph by Adam Latham*

### Seated camel posture

The following steps and Figure 19-18 show you how to execute this posture:

1. **Start in the seated mountain posture.**

2. **Move to the front edge of your chair; reach back with your hands and hold the back of your seat or the sides of your chair back.**

3. **As you inhale, lengthen your head and neck and then slowly look up at the ceiling; hold this position for 4 to 6 breaths.**

If you have neck problems, begin by just looking forward; then try looking up gradually over a period of time. If this head movement causes any pain or dizziness, leave it out.

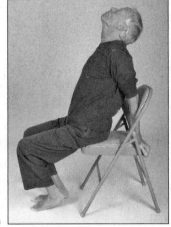

**Figure 19-18:**
Seated
camel
posture.

*Photograph by Adam Latham*

### Seated forward bend

Figure 19-19 and the following steps help you achieve this bend.

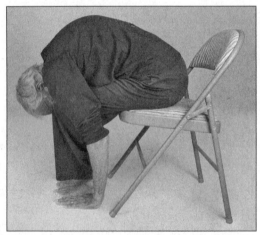

**Figure 19-19:**
Seated for-
ward bend.

*Photograph by Adam Latham*

1. **Start in the seated mountain posture.**

2. **As you exhale, bend forward from your hips and slide your hands forward and down your legs.**

3. **Let your head and arms hang down, and relax in the folded position for 4 to 6 breaths.**

4. **Finish the sequence in the seated mountain posture; close your eyes and use focus breathing (check out Chapter 5) or a relaxation technique (flip to Chapter 4) for 2 to 5 minutes.**

# Chapter 20

# Prop Art: The Why and How of Simple Props

· · · · · · · · · · · · · · · · · · · · · · · · · · · · · · · · · · · · · · · · · ·

## In This Chapter

▶ Weighing the pros and cons of using props

▶ Relying on props you probably already own

▶ Investing in store-bought props for Yoga practice

· · · · · · · · · · · · · · · · · · · · · · · · · · · · · · · · · · · · · · · · · ·

*T*he mainstay for any Yoga practice is, of course, the body-mind itself. However, props — physical means of support — may enhance your Yoga experience, especially if you're a beginner.

Traditionally, yogis and yoginis have relied on just a few basic props for their postural, breathing, and meditation practice — a bundle of grass or a tiger skin to sit on; a T-shaped arm rest (called *hamsa danda*) for prolonged meditation; and a *neti pot,* which looks like an undersize pitcher, for cleansing the nasal cavities with lukewarm (often salted) water before practicing breath control. Unfortunately, most Westerners' lifestyles and diets produce neither a naturally balanced mind nor a well-trained body, so a lot of these folks (especially beginners) often need to incorporate props into their Yoga to encourage proper alignment.

Even so, your own body is often all the prop you need. For example, the principle of *Forgiving Limbs* (which we cover in Chapter 3), in which you bend your knees and elbows, allows you to enjoy the function and benefits of a given posture even if your body isn't flexible enough to assume the posture's classic (traditionally taught) form. Many people may benefit from the use of simple aids in addition to their bent limbs, so we discuss some of these external props in this chapter. When you use them intelligently, props can help you practice with pleasure in spite of tight hamstrings, stiff hips, and an inflexible back.

Of course, using props has both pros and cons, but this chapter gives you enough information to make your own decisions about what you want to include in your Yoga practice; throughout the book, we point out where you may benefit from using a prop in a posture and show you how to use it.

# Examining the Pros and Cons of Props

As with anything in life, doing Yoga with props has its upsides and downsides. The following sections list some of the benefits and disadvantages of using props, but you have to determine on your own how props can help support your Yoga practice.

## Exploring the advantages of props

One of the great parts about using props in your Yoga practice is that you can use them as extensively as you want or not at all. A folded blanket under your hips can make all the difference when you want to sit cross-legged for more than a couple minutes, and a wall can be a welcome support for your legs or back while you're doing particular postures. Here are a few more prop plusses:

- Props give you the added advantage of leverage in many postures.
- They improve your alignment, balance, and stability.
- Props like the Body Slant (which we discuss later in the chapter) provide the benefits of a classic inversion such as a headstand without compressing your neck.
- They allow you to participate more fully in a group class. With safe tools, you can perform some postures that would otherwise be inaccessible to you instead of hanging out in easier or resting postures until the group comes back to your level.
- For the most part, props are relatively inexpensive and usually last for a long time.

## Looking at props' drawbacks

Although Yoga props have their benefits, they do have some downsides as well. Keep the following in mind as you evaluate whether a prop is right for you:

- Given the advantage of a prop, some people go too far in a posture and injure themselves. Don't try to look like a model on a magazine cover or a Yoga calendar; listen to your own body's needs.
- You can become too dependent on props, which inhibits your progress.
- If you are accustomed to practicing with props, you may have to carry them if you are practicing somewhere other than in a studio that supplies them or at your home, if you own them.
- Some props take time to set up and take down, which can break the flow of a class.
- Some props are expensive.

# Going Prop Hunting at Home

The human species prides itself on its use of tools, and Yoga's growing popularity in the Western world has spawned an industry of Yoga-related props — gear that can be complicated and costly. But useful props can be as simple as items lying around your house. Usually, a couple blankets, a strap, a chair, and a wall for support is all you need.

Yoga has always favored an experimental approach, and we recommend that you proceed in the same way. Find out for yourself what works for you and what doesn't. Instead of giving up on a challenging posture, experiment with recommended props. For instance, if you can't sit comfortably with your legs folded in the tailor's seat *(sukhasana)*, try placing a folded blanket or firm pillow under your hips. The following sections explain how common household finds can prop up your Yoga session.

## Working with a wall

Walls are a great prop — they're everywhere, they're free, and, best of all, they're versatile. You can use a wall in a great variety of postures: to support your buttocks and improve the angle of your forward bend, to brace your back heel in the standing postures, or to support the backs of your legs in the reclining raised-legs relaxation position. Walls also can support you in the more advanced inverted postures, such as the half shoulder stand (see Chapter 10), and they work as a frame of reference by which you can check your posture and alignment.

Check out Chapter 21 for the specifics of incorporating walls into your Yoga routine.

## Using a blanket for more than bedding

Besides the obvious use of keeping you warm during relaxation, blankets can prop your hips in sitting postures, your head and neck in lying postures, and your waist in prone back bends like the locust posture. You also can use blankets as protective padding under your knees when kneeling.

The firmness of the blanket is important. You want something under your knees or neck that doesn't sink or collapse, as does a padded blanket or comforter. Always use a firm, flat blanket, and be sure to fold it thickly (or use more than one) when you need to raise your hips (or head or shoulders).

---

# Prop proliferation

Yoga props and accessories from around the world are now big business in the United States. More than any other teacher, Yoga Master B.K.S. Iyengar of Pune (pronounced *poon-ah*) has influenced the development of props for Hatha Yoga in modern times. Americans, however, have made some of their own breakthroughs in the area of Yoga-inspired props.

Yoga teacher Larry Jacobs of Newport Beach, California, invented the Body Slant (which we describe later in "Turning to inversion props") and offers an entire line of safe and practical inversion furniture through mainstream national mail-order catalogs. Renowned sports medicine physician Leroy R. Perry, Jr., DC, in Los Angeles, California, has developed specialized inversion products known as Dr. Perry's spinal decompressor devices that Yoga teachers and Yoga enthusiasts use internationally.

---

Most blankets nowadays are made out of synthetic materials (or a synthetic/wool blend) — a relief for people with wool allergies.

## Choosing a chair for comfort

A folding metal chair or a sturdy wooden chair without arms can have multiple uses as a Yoga prop. Many (if not most) beginners have a hard time sitting on the floor for prolonged periods during meditation or breathing exercises, and sitting on a chair is a great alternative to sitting on the floor. Make sure, though, that your feet aren't dangling; if they don't easily touch the floor, place them on a phone book. Students with back problems often use a chair during the relaxation phase at the end of a Yoga class. Lying on your back and placing your lower legs up on a chair, combined with guided relaxation techniques from the instructor, can really help release back tension or pain. (Chapter 25 has more on using chair poses to alleviate chronic pain.)

You can find numerous books and magazine articles about doing your entire Yoga practice in a chair, with suggestions for ways to take Yoga chair breaks around the house or in your office for a quick pick-me-up.

## Stretching with a strap

You most frequently use a strap with postures that involve stretching the hamstrings, most commonly from a supine reclining (lying on your back) or sitting position. An old karate belt or necktie works great, but so does a rolled-up towel or a bathrobe belt. You also can order an "official" Yoga strap from one of the mail-order companies we recommend in the resources list online at www.dummies.com/extras/yoga.

# Seeking Out Props You May Want to Purchase

As you gain comfort and confidence in your Yoga practice, you're sure to become curious about the array of props you either see being used in class or hear about from your association with fellow Yoga practitioners. Whether you plan to spend freely as you experiment with the best props for your personal situation, or you expect to approach buying a bit more conservatively, keep in mind that you're likely to find a sweeping range of merchandise and price tags out there in consumer land. By investing wisely — combining product research with an understanding of your own needs — you can gain greater rewards from your Yoga experience.

Figure 20-1 shows you walls, straps, bolsters, blocks, and chairs — all common Yoga props. The following sections give you more information on buying them; check out the preceding section for ways you can mimic some props with household items. Be sure to consult our online resource guide as well at www.dummies.com/extras/yoga for reputable places to look for props.

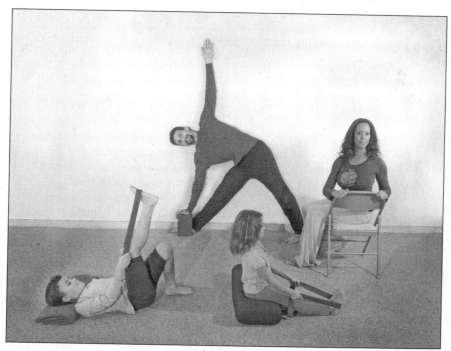

**Figure 20-1:**
Common
Yoga props.

*Photograph by Adam Latham*

## Supporting alignment with the help of blocks

Some styles of Yoga incorporate blocks for improving or facilitating certain postures. You may find a block helpful in standing twists when your bottom hand can't make it to the floor, or in standing forward bends to support your hands. Two blocks are ideal, but you can get by with one. If you use a block, it needs to be firm. Some students prefer the more substantial feel and heft of a wooden block, or they may like the lightness of foam or other light materials (especially if they drop the block on a floor or foot). Think of the block as a raised floor to support you. Depending on how you lay it on the floor beside or in front of you, you can "raise the floor" to various heights to aid you in your practice. Try not to clutch the block with your hands — just use it to aid your balance.

Commercially, blocks are available in a variety of materials, including wood, recycled and new foam, bamboo, and cork. The price varies with the size and material and ranges from $8 to $30; foam tends to be less expensive than wood, and cork falls somewhere in between.

If you decide to make your own block, a good standard is 9 inches high, 6 inches wide, and 4 inches deep. Be sure that the block is well sanded and varnished, to eliminate the possibility of splinters. You can also tightly wrap up an old hard-back book or two in some masking tape and use that for support.

## Bolstering support with pillows

*Bolsters* are large, firm, usually rectangular or cylindrical pillows. You use them to support your knees in reclining postures, to help release your lower back and raise your buttocks in forward bends, and to help soften tight hips and hamstrings. You can also place bolsters under your upper back to open your chest when you lie over them. During the stress of pregnancy, bolsters are a great support for the side-lying posture (see Chapter 16). A good standard size for bolsters is 6 x 12 x 25 inches for rectangular bolsters, and 9 x 27 inches for the cylindrical shape.

Bolsters are usually made of thick cotton batting with a removable canvas covering that you can wash, and they come in a range of sizes, materials, and prices. Expect to pay $35 to $70, depending on your taste and needs. You can also buy a pranayama bolster (see Chapter 5) that's long and thin (about 8 x 30 inches). One bolster is usually plenty for your personal use.

You can create your own bolsters by using thickly rolled blankets. In a pinch, sofa or bed pillows work, too — if they're not too soft.

## Eyeing the many uses of eye pillows

*Eye pillows* are small bags filled with light materials (usually plastic pellets) that yogis and yoginis use for various relaxation techniques. Although an eye pillow may seem self-explanatory, there's actually more to eye pillows than meets the, well, eye. Naturally, they block light and other visual stimuli, which helps quiet the brain; they also put gentle pressure on your eyes, which slows your heart rate. You can just cover your eyes with a towel, but the effect isn't quite the same.

Eye pillows are available in many shapes and sizes. Some eye pillows are packed with herbal essences, which adds the incentive (in-scent-ive?) of aroma therapy, but be sure the perfume isn't so strong it becomes bothersome. Eye pillows are usually about 4 x 8 inches and cost from $10 to $20, depending on which type you choose; some more expensive models tie down like a mask, which is usually unnecessary. (Check out the resource guide at www.dummies.com/extras/yoga for more on locating props.) You usually place one eye pillow across the top of both eyes while you're in a lying position on your back.

If you decide to make your own eye pillow, use materials such as cotton stuffed with rice, or silk stuffed with flaxseed. Even stuffing an old sock does the job. Be sure to do a good job on the seams — you don't want flaxseed in your eyes!

## Turning to inversion props

We purposely omitted the headstand and the full shoulder stand from this book because we feel that these postures require the guidance of a competent Yoga teacher. Because Western-world necks have become so weak and vulnerable, many physicians and a large number of chiropractors, orthopedists, and osteopaths aren't in favor of inverted Yoga postures such as the headstand, the full shoulder stand, and the plow because they can compress the neck. Because the benefits of inversion and reversing the pull of gravity are so great (as we cover in Chapter 10), many entrepreneurs have attempted to create safe and effective inversion devices.

You can now find quite a selection of inversion apparatuses to suit various bodies and budgets. One that we like for its effectiveness, safety, and convenience is the Body Slant, created by yogi Larry Jacobs (see Figure 20-2). It's the high-tech version of what used to be called Grandma's Slant Board. These three pieces of firm foam that fold and unfold easily make inversion safe and simple. Just lie back for 10 minutes to receive the rejuvenating effects of inversion.

Ask your physician before using any new exercise device to be sure the prop is right for your personal situation.

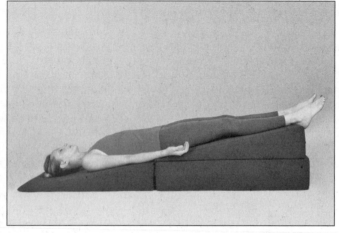

**Figure 20-2:**
The Body
Slant is
safe and
effective.

Avoid using the Body Slant or any other inversion prop if you have the following conditions: glaucoma or *retinopathy* (disease of the retina), hiatal hernia, high blood pressure, heart disease, or a past stroke.

# Chapter 21

# Yoga Against the Wall

. . . . . . . . . . . . . . . . . . . . . . . . . . . . . . . . . . . . . . . . . . . . . . . .

## *In This Chapter*

▶ Using the wall as a prop to build confidence, balance, and physical awareness

▶ Taking your Yoga to go

▶ Promoting world peace through wall Yoga

▶ Practicing standing, bending, and balancing postures at the wall

. . . . . . . . . . . . . . . . . . . . . . . . . . . . . . . . . . . . . . . . . . . . . . . .

Consider the wall your friend, one you can always turn to when you need a little extra support or a confidence boost — and one that doesn't shy away from giving you some honest and direct feedback.

The wall can give you some welcome benefits:

✔ Provides safety and stability

✔ Supports your balance

✔ Gives you feedback on your alignment

✔ Allows you to be curious and try something new

✔ Adds variety to reinvigorate your practice

If the walls in your home are flush with furniture and framed artwork, you can always use a door.

In this chapter, we discuss the ways in which using the wall as a prop can support your Yoga practice and give you new pose possibilities. We also illustrate a variety of safe postures you can easily do at the wall.

## The World Is Your Yoga Studio

When you embrace the wall as a prop, you open up a world of possibilities for practice. For starters, a wall allows you to practice when you're not dressed for Yoga. Some postures you can easily do in business dress in an office setting. Perhaps you've got high-powered business meetings, or you're someone who delivers important presentations, or you're waiting for a job interview. Imagine the benefits of taking a few minutes to stretch and breathe beforehand. Envision how a few moments of movement, breath, and focus can improve the parts of your day that follow.

Wall Yoga is a great option when the floor surface isn't inviting. Attention all backpacker travelers — how great does a few minutes of wall Yoga sound when you're staying in a super-budget hotel that has seen better days?

Yoga doesn't need to be solely an indoor practice, either. A tree or the side of a building can stand in for a wall. Hikers, runners, golfers, and tennis players alike can enjoy and benefit from a few minutes of Yoga as preparation for their main activity.

You can do many categories of postures, and the wall helps in each instance.

- **Standing postures:** The wall provides feedback on your alignment and orientation in space.

- **Safe inversions:** The wall provides safety and allows you to experience the benefits of inversions (refer to Chapter 10) without doing traditional inversions that can be risky for many people.

- **Forward bends and hamstring stretches in hanging postures:** The wall provides safety, precision, and guidance for your alignment.

## Wall Yoga is glamorous and exotic!

Here's a bit of fun historical trivia. Indra Devi was the first foreign woman the late Professor Sri T. Krishnamacharya, the father of modern Yoga, accepted as a student in the 1930s in India. After she received his blessing to teach, life events took her to Shanghai, where she taught Yoga to Madame Chiang Kai-Skek, among others. In the 1940s, she moved to Hollywood and opened a studio, where she offered Yoga adapted to the needs of Westerners. One posture she used was the headstand in the corner, to give the practitioner the support of two walls. Among her students were Gloria Swanson and Marilyn Monroe.

Wall Yoga has now traveled to the far north of the globe. In 1997, I (Larry) was the resident Yoga teacher aboard a trip to the North Pole on an icebreaker with members of the World Presidents Organization. To accommodate the compact surroundings, I developed a High Seas Brace Wall Yoga Program.

# A Wall-Supported Yoga Workout

You can do these postures in sequence for a full and varied Yoga session, sprinkle them into your floor-based practice, or use them as desired.

Most people spend way too much time leaning forward. Maybe you spend hours in front of a computer entering data, writing, or simply gaming or surfing. Or perhaps you're a health professional who leans in toward patients a good part of the day. Chances are, your posture is suffering because of it and you're feeling those effects. The first two Yoga postures we illustrate in this chapter are a perfect way to check your posture and remind yourself which way is up.

## Wall mountain pose

Doing the mountain pose against the wall gives you feedback on your body's alignment, improves posture and balance, and facilitates Yoga breathing. You can see it illustrated in Figure 21-1.

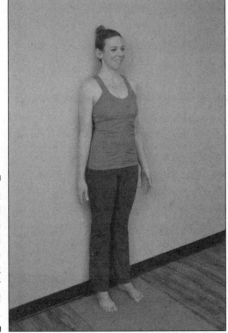

**Figure 21-1:**
In wall mountain posture, you get valuable feedback on your posture and alignment.

© John Wiley & Sons, Inc.

1. **Stand tall but relaxed, with your feet hip distance apart, and hang your arms at your sides, with your palms turned toward your legs.**

2. **Touch the wall with your hips and shoulders; visualize a string lifting the tip of your head and keeping your feet reaching down to the earth.**

3. **Choose a Yoga breathing technique to use throughout the routine (consult Chapter 5 to make your selection).**

4. **Stay in this posture for 6 to 8 breaths.**

## Mountain posture flow

This posture is great for everyone with a desk job. Try it two or three times a day, and you'll notice a dramatic improvement in your posture.

In addition to aligning the body and improving posture, mountain posture flow relieves stress and tension in the neck and shoulders. You can see it illustrated in Figure 21-2.

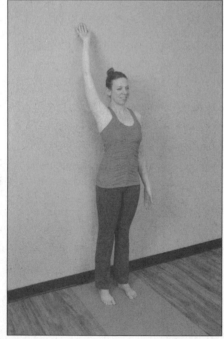

**Figure 21-2:**
Mountain posture flow helps relieve tension in the neck and shoulders.

© John Wiley & Sons, Inc.

1. **Stand in the mountain pose, with your feet and body about 6 inches away from the wall.**

2. **As you inhale, raise your right arm and touch the wall behind you with the back of your hand.**

   Adjust your distance from the wall as needed so that you can touch the wall with your extended hand.

3. **As you exhale, bring your hand back down to your side; repeat with your left arm, and then raise both arms and touch the wall.**

4. **Repeat the sequence of one arm, then the other arm, and then both arms two or three times.**

Try turning your head away from your arm as you raise your right arm and then your left to add in a nice neck stretch.

## Wall warrior flow

Wall warrior flow is a simple series of movements that warm you up before athletic activities, indoors or out, as well as within your longer Yoga session. It strengthens and stretches the legs, back, shoulders, and arms; it also improves flexibility in the hamstrings, calves, and Achilles heel. You can see it illustrated in Figure 21-3.

1. **Stand facing a wall about 3 feet away; place the toes of your right foot close to the wall, and place the palms of both hands on the wall, with your arms parallel at shoulder height.**

2. **Step back with your left foot 3 to 5 feet, and turn out your foot about 45 degrees (see Figure 21-3a).**

3. **Start with both legs straight, and look straight ahead. Take a deep breath and, as you exhale, bend your front leg to a 90-degree angle while keeping the outside edge of your back foot down (see Figure 21-3b); repeat three times, and then stay in the warrior posture, looking straight ahead, for 6 to 8 breaths.**

4. **Slowly straighten your right leg and raise the front half of your right foot off the floor as you bend your back leg and drop your left hip (see Figure 21-3c).**

5. **Stay in this posture for 6 to 8 breaths, and then repeat Steps 1 through 5 on the left side.**

Try this sequence on a wall or a tree outside to prepare for golf, tennis, or a hike.

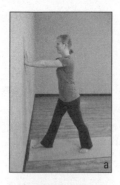
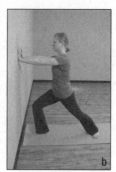
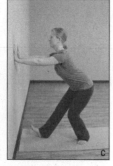

**Figure 21-3:** This multibenefit flow is a great way to warm up.

## Standing side bend at the wall

The standing side bend at the wall, also called the willow pose, stretches and tones the muscles along the sides of the abdomen, ribcage, and spine. It facilitates breathing and helps give you a supple spine. See Figure 21-4 for an illustration.

1. **Stand tall sideways next to a wall, with your feet hip distance apart and your inside arm extended until you touch the wall with your hand.**

   Keep your palm and fingers pointing up at shoulder height.

2. **As you inhale, bring your outside arm up toward the ceiling and, as you exhale, bring it toward the wall in alignment with your ear.**

   If you need to, you can bend your inside arm at the wall and your legs.

3. **Repeat step 2 three times, and then stay with your top arm toward the wall for 6 to 8 breaths.**

4. **Turn in the opposite direction and repeat Steps 1 through 3.**

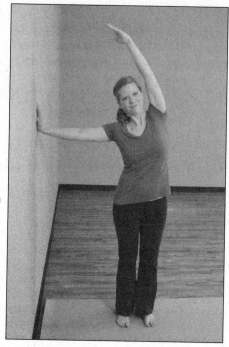

**Figure 21-4:**
The standing side bend at the wall tones you on the inside.

© John Wiley & Sons, Inc.

As you get more limber, straighten your inside arm at the wall more while holding the posture.

Avoid this posture if it causes back pain.

## Half chair at the wall

The half chair at the wall helps improve your overall stamina and strengthens your back, legs, shoulders, and arms. See Figure 21-5 for an illustration.

1. **Start with your back to the wall and your feet hip distance apart.**

2. **As you inhale, extend both arms forward and parallel to the floor. As you exhale, slide down the wall to a half squat position. If you can't see your toes when you're at 90 degrees, move your feet farther from the wall.**

   This posture also is great to use when you need to clean the walls.

3. **Repeat steps 1 and 2 three times, and then stay in the half squat position for 6 to 8 breaths.**

Avoid this posture if it causes knee or hip pain.

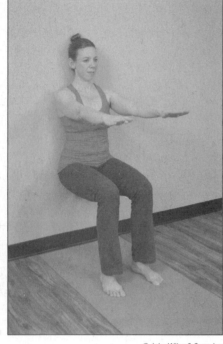

**Figure 21-5:**
The half chair at the wall posture builds stamina.

## Wall warrior III

Wall warrior III is a perfect illustration of how the wall can prepare you to eventually practice a highly beneficial posture away from the wall, without the extra support. With or without the wall, it's a good posture for overall stability and balance, and it strengthens the legs and arms. You can see it illustrated in Figure 21-6.

1. **Stand in the mountain posture (see Figure 21-1) and face the wall, about 3 to 4 feet away.**

2. **As you exhale, bend forward from your hips and extend your arms forward until your palms are flat against the wall. Alternatively, you may be comfortable with only your fingertips touching the wall for support.**

   Your folded upper torso makes a 90-degree angle with your legs and hips.

3. **As you inhale, raise your right leg back until it's parallel to the floor, as in Figure 21-6.**

4. **Stay in Step 3 for 6 to 8 breaths, and then repeat Steps 1 through 4 with the opposite leg.**

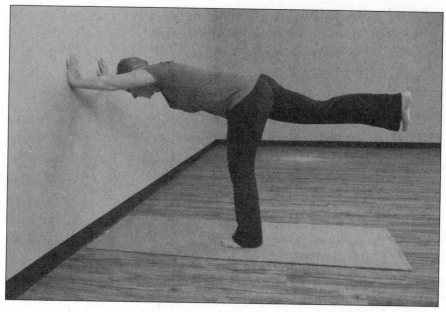

**Figure 21-6:**
Wall warrior III is a go-to posture for improving stability and balance.

© John Wiley & Sons, Inc.

# Wall hang

The wall hang lengthens the entire spine and stretches the hamstrings, shoulders, neck, and arms. Because the head is below the heart in this pose, it also offers the benefits of inversion (refer to Chapter 10 for more on inversion). You can see the wall hang illustrated in Figure 21-7.

1. **Stand with your back to the wall about 3 feet away, with your feet hip distance apart or slightly wider.**

2. **Keep your feet planted, and move your hips backward until they rest on the wall.**

3. **Bend forward from the hips, bend your arms, and hold your opposite elbows as you hang.**

4. **Soften your knees and breathe slowly. Stay for 8 to 10 breaths.**

For a shorter, simpler stretch, just hang your chest, head, and arms downward and stay a few breaths.

Avoid this posture if it causes back pain.

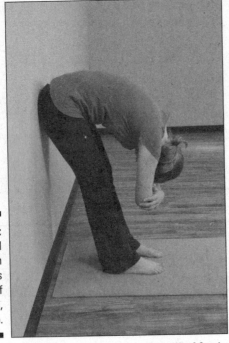

**Figure 21-7:**
This total
body stretch
offers
benefits of
inversion,
too.

© John Wiley & Sons, Inc.

# Yogi wall sit-ups

The Yogi wall sit-ups strengthen the abdomen (especially the upper abdomen) and the neck and shoulders. Check out Figure 21-8 for an illustration.

1. **Lie on your back about 3 feet away from the wall; place your feet on the wall, and adjust your floor position so you can bend your knees at a 90-degree angle.**

2. **Interlace your hands behind your head lightly. Inhale deeply and, as you exhale, sit up slowly, keeping your elbows wide so you don't throw your head forward; draw in your belly as you sit up.**

3. **Repeat 6 to 10 times.**

To make this posture more challenging, stay folded at the top for an extra breath, and then return to the floor on the next exhalation.

To strengthen the oblique muscles of the abdomen, try twisting with one elbow as you come up.

Avoid this posture if it hurts your back.

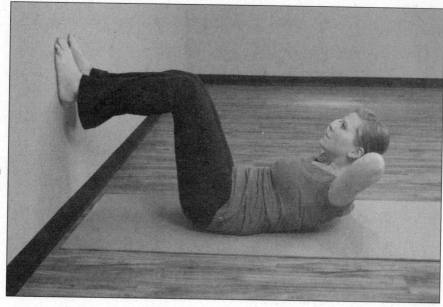

**Figure 21-8:**
The stability
of the wall
enhances
this
variation of
the sit-up.

© John Wiley & Sons, Inc.

# Wall splits

This simple supported posture does a body much good! Wall splits stretch the hips, hamstrings, claves, and inner thighs (called adductors). You can see it illustrated in Figure 21-9.

1. **Sit sideways, close to the wall, with your legs straight; when you're ready, swing both legs up on the wall, turn your upper body away from the wall, and lie flat on your back, with your palms down.**

2. **Scoot your hips as close to the wall as you comfortably can; as you inhale slowly, open your legs into a split until you reach your comfortable maximum.**

3. **Upon exhalation, slowly bring your legs straight up again.**

4. **Repeat Steps 2 and 3 three times, and then stay in the open position for 6 to 8 breaths.**

Don't force this posture. Take it nice and easy, allowing for gradual movement when you're opening your legs.

If your hamstrings are tight, you can move farther away from the wall and soften your knees in the splits.

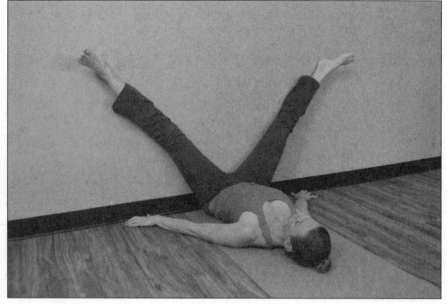

Figure 21-9: With the support of the wall, the benefits of the splits are widely accessible.

# Inverted hamstring pose at the wall

This wall inversion enables you to stretch your hamstrings, hips, calves, and ankles. See Figure 21-10.

1. **Lie flat on your back, with your hips about 3 feet away from the wall.**

2. **Place the soles of your feet up on the wall, with your knees bent at a right angle and your thighs parallel to one another.**

3. **As you exhale, straighten your right leg, bring it back toward you, and reach with both arms to hold your leg evenly.**

   Be sure to keep your hips on the ground and your shoulders dropped as you hold your right leg.

4. **Stay for 6 to 8 breaths, and repeat Steps 1 and 2 with the other leg.**

If you have difficulty reaching your extended leg, try using a strap behind the heel of your foot. (Check out Chapter 20 for more on props in Yoga.)

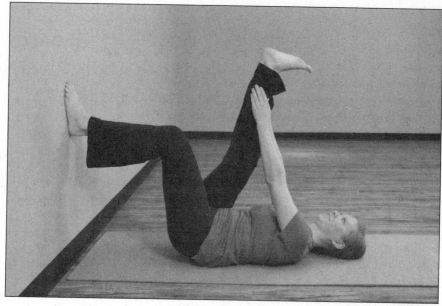

**Figure 21-10:**
The inverted hamstring pose does just what the name implies — and more.

© *John Wiley & Sons, Inc.*

# Legs up against the wall

The legs up against the wall posture calms the nervous system and improves circulation to the legs, hips, and lower back. Imagine the possibilities if everyone, especially world leaders, spent 5 minutes each day with their feet up the wall and breathing — the world would be a more peaceful place. Figure 21-11 illustrates this posture.

1. **Sit sideways as close as possible to the wall, with both legs extended forward; swing both legs up on the wall, and lie flat on your back.**

2. **Turn your palms up, soften your knees as necessary, and close your eyes.**

3. **Stay in this posture for 2 to 10 minutes.**

Try adding an eye pillow while you're relaxing in the pose. Not only do eye pillows block out the light, but the gentle pressure they provide promotes relaxation.

Avoid this pose if you have high blood pressure; have problems with your eyes, such as retinopathy or other conditions sensitive to pressure; or are more than 3 months pregnant.

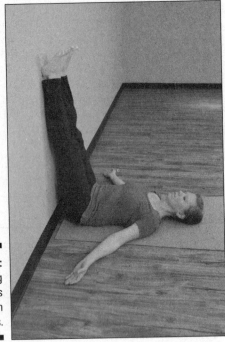

**Figure 21-11:**
This relaxing
pose has
circulation
benefits.

© John Wiley & Sons, Inc.

# Part IV
# Living Life the Yoga Way

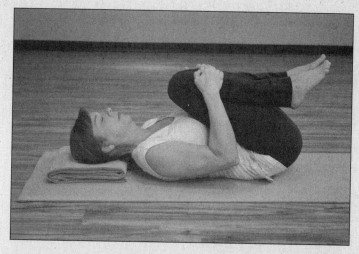

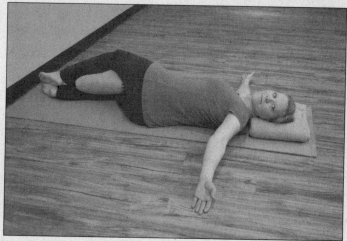

Greater clarity and awareness of the moment are two of the benefits dedicated yogis enjoy. Maintaining consciousness while dreaming is also possible. Check out www.dummies.com/extras/yoga for more info on these topics.

# In this part . . .

✔ Go beyond the physical postures, to understand the basic precepts of Yoga philosophy

✔ Find inner peace and happiness by adopting Yoga as a spiritual lifestyle based on moral integrity

✔ Find out about having a healthy back through our five-step plan to prevent your back's aches and pains from becoming chronic

✔ Explore how particular Yoga movements and postures serve therapeutic purposes, and see how to find a Yoga therapist if you need one

✔ Understand the mind-body connection in chronic pain, and get a primer on using Yoga techniques to address common pains that may ail you, including lower back pain, headaches, and overall body pain

# Chapter 22

# Yoga throughout the Day

The postures and breathing exercises of Hatha Yoga — some of which we cover in preceding chapters — are just some of the tools from Yoga's well-stocked storehouse. When you practice them correctly, they're extremely useful and potent in helping you regain or maintain your physical and mental health. Practicing postures and breathing can stabilize and boost your body's vitality, and even harmonize your emotions and strengthen your mind.

But even more fundamental to the postures and breathing (Steps 3 and 4 in the eightfold path of Raja Yoga — see Chapter 1 for more about Raja Yoga and the eightfold path) are Steps 1 and 2; they provide guidance for relating to the world around you. When you approach Yoga as a lifestyle or spiritual path, you unlock the real power of Yoga. Yoga is a conscious way of life; it gives you the means to tap into your full potential as a human being.

In this chapter, we show you how you can connect with your deeper potential and live your entire day the Yoga way. This approach includes paying proper attention to moral values, which are an important aspect of all branches and schools of Yoga but often get overlooked by Western practitioners.

## Making Yoga a Habit

The classic definition of Yoga is that it's the stilling of the fluctuations of the mind. Achieving Yoga in this respect involves more than an occasional workout on the mat; it encompasses how you live off the mat as well. When you pursue Yoga as a lifestyle or spiritual discipline, your new habits create and strengthen new pathways in your brain; the improvements in how you live your life and how you relate to others and yourself become second nature.

## Turning your face toward a Yoga morning

For thousands of years, Yoga practitioners have begun the day at sunrise, a time considered favorable and especially potent for meditating, praying, and tapping into your highest potential. Quiet and peaceful, sunrise is also a time charged with symbolic significance in Yoga. Traditionally, the sun is celebrated as the first teacher, or *guru,* who brought the teachings of Yoga to humanity. The sun is seen as a symbol for the spirit, which shines with undiminished brightness forever. Through the sun salutation sequence, an exercise we describe in Chapter 13, yogis acknowledge their reverence for the inner sun.

Philosophical and historical significance aside, with today's busy lifestyles, research says you're more likely to complete your Yoga practice if you do it in the morning. However, if you can't practice then, make sure you leave room in your schedule for Hatha Yoga or meditation at some other time during the day or in the evening. Even a few minutes of postures and breathing exercises can refresh you and help you refocus for whatever else you have on your plate that day — and motivate you to do the same tomorrow.

## Practicing Yoga throughout the day

When you view Yoga as approaching your life mindfully, you find that daily life offers many opportunities to practice. Consider a few examples of when a little Yoga can improve your approach to and experience of various situations.

- ✔ Encountering heavy traffic during your daily commute to and from work
- ✔ Dealing with customers, a demanding boss, or fellow employees
- ✔ Enjoying your meals
- ✔ Experiencing pregnancy and childbirth
- ✔ Responding when your child's behavior leaves much to be desired
- ✔ Living through a health crisis
- ✔ Enjoying life's pleasures, such as vacations and holidays
- ✔ Doing the daily shopping and other chores
- ✔ Grieving the death of a loved one

You can bring awareness, which is the foundation for all other positive attitudes and practices, to all these situations. You can also bring understanding, patience, calmness, forgiveness, kindness, compassion, love, good humor, and a host of other virtues. By practicing various Yoga techniques, you also calm your mind and raise your energy level or bring energy to others.

Don't think of the world as "out there" and your Yoga practice as "in here." Because Yoga connects inside and outside, such a distinction is artificial. Allow your practice to flow into all situations. You're never so busy that you can't transform a few seconds of free time into meaningful time through Yoga: Exhale deeply, center yourself, silently recite a *mantra,* or bless someone.

# Seeking Your Higher Self

However they may conceive the ultimate goal, all schools of Yoga seek to open a door to your true nature, which we call the *spirit* or *higher Self.* You can find as many approaches to self-realization (or enlightenment) as you can human beings. Everyone's spiritual journey is unique, yet everyone's inner evolution follows certain universal principles. That fundamental process is marked by progressive *self-observation, self-understanding, self-discipline,* and *self-transcendence,* which are all interconnected practices. The most significant principle is that, to discover your essential nature, you must overcome the gravitational pull of your ordinary habits and patterns.

## Observing yourself

In Yoga, you simply begin to observe yourself. Staying in tune with yourself is different from being neurotically self-involved. *Self-observation* means being consciously aware of how you think and behave, without judging yourself.

Self-observation includes noticing — in a nonjudgmental way — how you react to people and situations. For instance, you may discover that, in many ways, you're often overly critical or too gullible and accommodating. Or you may determine that you tend to be rather inward and afraid of engaging life, or that you never think before you leap. The natural calmness that you create through Yoga's physical exercises can help you start uncovering your tendencies — without collapsing into self-recrimination or exploding into anger with others.

## Understanding yourself

Based on self-observation, self-understanding involves grasping the deeper reasons for your habit patterns. Ultimately, *self-understanding* is the realization that all your thoughts and behaviors revolve around the ego, an artificial psychological pole. Your ego allows you to identify yourself in a very specific way. For example:

I'm Frank, a 35-year-old Caucasian male and a United States citizen. I'm 5 feet 11 inches tall, have an athletic build, weigh 165 pounds, and have blue eyes and brown hair. I'm married, have two children, and am an investment advisor and a cyclist. I'm ambitious and not very religious.

These ego identifications are useful in your daily life — as long as they don't cause you to feel separated from your spiritual core or create barriers to other people.

Yoga sees the ego as nothing more than a way of quickly identifying yourself both verbally and psychologically. It's not your true nature, the spirit or Self. It's not an actual entity in its own right, but merely something you habitually do. The ego is based on the process of self-contraction *(atma-samkoca,* pronounced *aht-mah sahm-koh-chah).* The symbol for the ego is a clenched fist. Yoga shows you how to release that fist and engage life from the viewpoint of the spirit or Self, which is in harmonious relationship with everyone and everything.

## Practicing self-discipline

When a seed sprouts, it must push through the soil before it can benefit from the sunlight. Similarly, before you can experience the higher levels of Yoga, you must overcome the built-in lethargy of your ego-driven personality, which doesn't want to change. Self-observation and self-understanding become increasingly effective through the practice of *self-discipline* — the steady cultivation of spiritual practices.

By exercising voluntary self-control over your thoughts, behaviors, and energies, you can gradually transform your body-mind into a finely tuned instrument for higher spiritual realizations and harmonious living. You can't practice self-discipline without frustrating the ego a little because the ego always tends to move along the path of least resistance. Yogic practice creates the necessary resistance to spark further growth in you.

## Transcending yourself

*Self-transcendence* is at the heart of the spiritual process. This impulse and practice of going beyond the ego-contraction in every moment — through self-observation, self-understanding, and self-discipline — comes to full blossom in the great event of enlightenment, when your entire being is transformed by the spirit, or Self (see Chapter 23).

# Making Inroads into the Eightfold Path with Moral Discipline

The eightfold path of Yoga, as we outline it in Chapter 1, is a useful model for the stages of the yogic process. In the following sections, we explain the first limb of the eightfold path in more detail because, along with the second limb, it gives you the essential moral foundation for practicing Yoga success-fully. We start with the five practices of moral discipline *(yama)*, which Yoga insists you practice under all circumstances. They're the same moral virtues you find in all the world's great religious traditions:

- ✔ Nonharming, or *ahimsa* (pronounced *ah-heem-sah*)
- ✔ Truthfulness, or *satya* (pronounced *saht-yah*)
- ✔ Nonstealing, or *asteya* (pronounced *ahs-the-yah*)
- ✔ Chastity, or *brahmacarya* (pronounced *brah-mah-chahr-yah*)
- ✔ Greedlessness, or *aparigraha* (pronounced *ah-pah-ree-grah-hah*)

These five disciplines are meant to harmonize your interpersonal life and are especially important in today's enormously complex world. Yoga reminds you that you can't attain self-fulfillment in isolation from others. You can't hope to realize your higher nature without fostering what's good and beautiful in your day-to-day life in interactions with others and the environment. Thus, universally recognized moral virtues are the rich soil in which you plant all your other efforts on the path of inner growth and ultimate self-realization.

Yoga understands these virtues to be all-comprehensive, extending not only to your actions, but also to your language and even your thoughts. In other words, you're called to abstain from doing wrong to others, speaking wrong of them, and poisoning them with your thoughts.

## Vowing to do no harm

Opportunities to practice nonharming come into play hundreds of times a day. The more sensitive you become to the effect you have on others, the more you're called to live with moral mindfulness. How do you practice the virtue of nonharming in your life? You may think of yourself as a fairly harm-less individual because you don't physically or verbally abuse anyone, but have you ever started or listened to gossip? And what about a reflexive nega-tive reaction toward an annoying client or an inconsiderate driver?

Nonharming is not only abstaining from harmful actions, speech, and thoughts, but also actively doing what's appropriate in a given moment to avoid unnecessary pain to others. For example, even withholding a smile or kind word from someone when you sense that the gesture may benefit that person is a form of harming.

To live, humans involuntarily harm and even kill other beings — just think of the billions of microorganisms in your food and even in your own body that give up their lives so that you can stay alive and be healthy. The ideal of nonharming is just that: an ideal to which you may aspire. The concept calls for abstaining from deliberately harming other beings. As a useful exercise, ask yourself these questions:

- How many times today have I spoken harshly?
- Do I kill harmless spiders instead of leaving them alone or relocating them?
- Are my thoughts about things and people predominantly pessimistic, overly optimistic, or simply realistic?
- When I have to correct someone's behavior, do I do so constructively, with encouragement, or do I merely criticize?

Yoga expects you to control your anger and murderous thoughts — not to be confused with merely suppressing your feelings (which never works anyway). Yoga also encourages you to cultivate, step by step, better habits and mental dispositions. As you become more peaceful and content, you don't react as strongly and irrationally to life's pressures. Instead, you're better able to go with the flow — with awareness, a smile, and a helping hand.

If you become aware of the various ways in which you harm others through your thoughts, words, and actions, don't succumb to feeling overwhelmed with guilt. That negative response is just another way of perpetuating violence. The practice of nonharming includes applying the approach to your dealings with yourself. Simply acknowledge the situation, feel remorse, resolve to behave differently, and then actively change your mental, verbal, and physical behavior.

## Telling the truth all the time

Yoga sees that facts and perspectives are many, but that both truth is always one and truthfulness (satya) is a supreme moral virtue. Truth is the cement that holds together good relationships and entire societies.

Consider the following questions. Have you ever . . .

- Told a little white lie, not to protect someone's feelings, but because it was more convenient than telling truth?
- Omitted certain facts from your résumé to appeal to a prospective employer?
- Failed to declare taxable income, even small amounts?
- Lied about your age?
- Failed to keep your promises?

Unless you're lying to yourself, you probably had a few "yes" responses. Admittedly, lies appear to vary by degree of severity. You may consider these examples fairly insignificant, and from a conventional point of view, they are. However, Yogic practice values simplicity and clarity, whereas lying usually ends up being more complicated and confusing. Yoga is also concerned about the pathways you build in your brain. If you become accustomed to not telling the truth in little matters, sooner or later, you may not be able to distinguish truth from falsehood in big matters as well.

Truthfulness is a marvelous tool for keeping your energy pure and your will undiluted. Of course, in your attempts to be truthful, you must bear the principal moral virtue of nonharming in mind. Life isn't black and white; many gray areas exist. If speaking the truth may bring more harm than good to another, you're wise to remain silent. Your intention is the key.

## Seeing how stealing means more than material theft

Nonstealing (*asteya*), the third moral discipline, is trickier than it looks at a casual glance. You need not be a pickpocket, shoplifter, bank robber, or embezzler to violate this virtue. From the perspective of Yoga, depriving someone of his due reward or good name is also theft. Appropriating someone's ideas without due acknowledgment, stealing someone's boyfriend or girlfriend, and denying your child proper parental guidance are all examples of theft as well.

To ponder the ideal of nonstealing, consider the following questions:

✔ What percentage of your income do you allocate for charitable causes?

✔ Are any of your computer programs bootlegged copies?

✔ Did you ever withhold love from a family member or friend as punishment?

Traditionally, people who are well established in the virtue of nonstealing are described as always being sustained by life; they never lack anything for their further growth. The greatest antidote to the vice of stealing is generosity. A fulfilling life is a life that elegantly balances giving and taking.

Highly competitive Western society is designed to promote self-centeredness to the point that people constantly infringe on the virtues of nonharming, truthfulness, and nonstealing. The kind of aggressive competitiveness rampant in the business world is all about elbowing your way to the top, beating the other guy, using any means necessary to outsmart your opponent, and winning the game at all costs.

## Observing chastity in thought and deed

Chastity (*brahmacarya*, pronounced *brah-mah-chahr-yah*) means abstention from inappropriate sexual behavior. According to Yoga, only adults who are in a committed marriage or partnership should be sexually active; all others should practice sexual abstinence. For many Westerners, this standard is difficult.

Yogically speaking, you must extend the ideal of chastity to action, speech, and even thought. We leave it up to you to determine where, in your own case, you can change your behavior to bring it more in line with Yoga's moral orientation. Bear in mind that Yoga isn't asking you to go against human nature, which includes sexuality. Instead, Yoga invites you to consider your higher spiritual potential. The Yoga masters recommend chastity not for prudish reasons, but because it's an effective way of harnessing your body's vital energy. The practitioner who's firmly grounded in chastity supposedly obtains vigor or vitality.

If you engage Yoga as a lifestyle or spiritual discipline, periodically taking stock of your virtues and vices can help you build toward achieving your higher Self. Considering your sexuality, ask yourself these questions:

- ✔ Do I tend to use sexually suggestive or explicit language?

- ✔ Do I use sex for emotional security or for personal power?

- ✔ Am I flirtatious and, if so, why?

- ✔ Do I know the distinction between sex and love?

- ✔ Am I capable of true intimacy, or do I treat my partner as a sex object?

## Acquiring more by living with less

Greed is a vice that underlies much of modern consumerism. From a yogic point of view, greed is a failed search for happiness because whatever possessions you may acquire can't fulfill you. On the contrary, the more you're surrounded by "stuff," the more likely you are to experience a gaping hole in your soul. Intrinsically, money and possessions aren't "wrong," but few people ever master the art of relating to them properly. Instead of owning things, most people are owned (controlled) by them.

Yoga holds high the ideal of voluntary simplicity — the choice to live simply. How do you measure up to it? Try to answer these questions honestly:

- ✔ Have you ever been called a miser?

- ✔ Do you have too much "stuff"?

- ✔ Do you expect to be pampered?

- ✔ Do you tend to overeat?

- ✔ Do you accumulate money and possessions for the sake of having more?

- ✔ Do you crave being the center of attention?

- ✔ Are you envious of your neighbors?

Yoga encourages you to cultivate the virtue of greedlessness in all matters. The Sanskrit word for this value is *aparigraha* (pronounced *ah-pah-ree-grah-ha*), which means "not grasping all around." The Yoga practitioner who is well trained in the art of greedlessness is said to understand the deeper reason for life. Behind this traditional wisdom lies a profound experience: As you loosen your grip on material possessions, you also let go of the ego, which is doing the gripping or grasping. As the ego-contraction relaxes, you increasingly become in touch with the abiding happiness of your true Self. Then you realize how little you need to be happy. You live fully in the present, and you aren't afraid to give freely to others and also share with them your inner abundance.

## Adding other moral practices

In addition to the five moral virtues Yoga master Patanjali lists in his Yoga-Sutra, other Yoga texts mention the following as belonging to the first limb of the eightfold path:

- Sympathy, or *daya* (pronounced *dah-yah*)

- Compassion, or *karuna* (pronounced *kah-roo-nah*)

- Integrity, or *arjava* (pronounced *ahr-jah-vah*)

- Patience, or *kshama* (pronounced *kshah-mah*)

- Steadfastness, or *dhriti* (pronounced *dhree-tee*)

- Nonattachment, or *vairagya* (pronounced *vie-rah-gyah*)

- Modesty, or *hri* (pronounced *hree* — the initial letter *h* is sounded out loud)

- Humility, or *amanitva* (pronounced *ah-mah-neet-vah*)

As you can see, Yoga has high expectations for a serious practitioner. But becoming a saint isn't the goal. Yoga is about freedom and happiness. The moral virtues are natural side effects of a life dedicated to spiritual enlightenment.

# Exercising Yogic Self-Discipline

The second category or limb of the eightfold path is known as restraint *(niyama)*, also translated as "self-restraint." We explain the second limb here because it's an integral part of the moral orientation of Yoga, which Western practitioners frequently give short shrift. According to Patanjali, restraint comprises five practices:

- Purity, or *shauca* (pronounced *shau-chah* — the *au* sounds similar to *ow* in *cow*)

- Contentment, or *samtosha* (pronounced *sahm-toh-shah*)

✔ Austerity, or *tapas* (pronounced *tah-pahs*)

✔ Study, or *svadhyaya* (pronounced *svahd-hyah-yah*)

✔ Dedication to a higher principle, or *ishvara-pranidhana* (pronounced *eesh-vah-rah prah-need-hah-nah*)

## Purifying mind and body

An old saying from the Puritan tradition suggests, "Cleanliness is next to godliness." Yoga goes further, stating that perfect purity and divinity are one and the same. All of Yoga is a process of self-purification. It begins with mental purification (through the practice of the moral disciplines described earlier in this chapter), proceeds to bodily cleansing (through various purification techniques, including postures and breath control), follows with more profound mental purification (through sensory inhibition, concentration, meditation, and the ecstatic state), and ends with realizing the perfect purity of the spirit itself.

The Sanskrit word for purity is *shauca*, which has the root meaning of "being radiant." The ultimate reality, or spirit, is pure radiance. As you clean the windows of your body-mind, you invite in more of the spirit's light. Accomplished Yoga masters have a radiance about them.

## Calming the quest through contentment

Contentment *(samtosha)* is traditionally defined as being satisfied with what life presents to you. When you're content, you have joy in your heart. You can face life with great calm. You can still strive to improve your situation, perhaps by earning a degree or getting a better job. But your quest for improvement doesn't come from a place of neediness or gnawing dissatisfaction.

## Focusing with austerity

Austerity *(tapas)* entails all kinds of practices designed to test your willpower and awaken the energy locked away in your body. Traditionally, these tests have included strict dieting or prolonged fasting, staying awake for several days, or sitting completely still in meditation directly under the hot Indian sun. Few of these practices are possible for modern Westerners, but the basic principle behind *tapas* (literally meaning "heat") is as valid now as it was thousands of years ago: Whenever you want to make progress on the path of Yoga, you must avoid wasting your energy on activities that are irrelevant to your inner development. By carefully regulating your mental and physical behavior, you generate more energy for yogic practice.

But progress calls for overcoming all kinds of inner resistances. *Tapas* makes a demand on you, which creates a certain amount of inner heat. Change is never easy, and for many people, self-discipline is a big stumbling block. They tend to give up too soon. Yet self-discipline — through the strength of your will — is within reach. Just persist and observe how your goals move closer. For instance, your effort to overcome laziness and practice Yoga regularly is a form of *tapas*, which gradually strengthens your willpower.

A good way to practice *tapas* is by periodically going on a retreat, where you have nothing to distract you from your inner work. Retreats provide an opportunity to see all your tendencies clearly and start turning them around by creating better patterns of thought and behavior. Austerity isn't about self-chastisement; it's an intelligent way of testing and strengthening your willpower. Remember, Yoga seeks not to increase pain and suffering, but to remove it. Always be kind to yourself, and as your commitment to inner growth increases, don't hesitate to challenge yourself firmly.

## *Partnering research with self-study*

Self-study *(svadhyaya)*, which Western practitioners often neglect, is an important part of traditional Yoga. *Self-study* means both studying for yourself and studying yourself. Traditionally, this commitment has involved poring over sacred scriptures, reciting them, and meditating on their meanings. In this way, practitioners have stayed in touch with tradition and also gained self-understanding because study of the scriptures always confronts you with yourself. For basic study, we recommend the following Yoga texts, which are all available in good English translations; flip to Chapter 1 for more on the specific branches of Yoga:

- ✔ *Yoga-Sutra* of Patanjali, the standard text on Raja Yoga

- ✔ *Bhagavad-Gita*, the earliest available Sanskrit text on Jnana Yoga, Karma Yoga, and Bhakti Yoga

- ✔ *Hatha-Yoga-Pradipika*, one of the classical manuals of Hatha Yoga

- ✔ *Yoga-Vasishtha*, a marvelous work on Jnana Yoga, filled with traditional stories and beautiful poetic imagery

- ✔ *Bhakti-Sutra* of Narada, a classical work on Bhakti Yoga

You can find full or partial translations of numerous Yoga texts in my (Georg's) *The Yoga Tradition* (Hohm Press).

Why study the Yoga scriptures? They're the distillations of several thousand years of experimentation and experience. If you're serious about Yoga, why not benefit from the wisdom of the accomplished adepts of this tradition?

Today you can usefully extend your study to include not only important Yoga scriptures, but also contemporary philosophy and historical analysis. Yoga practitioners who recognize the great ideas and forces that are shaping modern civilization are better equipped to study themselves. To understand yourself, you must also understand the world you live in. Studying the various components of human nature is wonderful mental training, and it can help you thoroughly comprehend the wisdom of Yoga.

## Relating to a higher principle

The third element of self-restraint (*niyama*) is devotion to a higher principle. The Sanskrit term is *ishvara-pranidhana*, where the word *ishvara* means "lord," referring to the divine. We translate it as "higher principle," to emphasize that you don't need to believe in a personal God to perform this practice. Devotion to a higher principle essentially means keeping your sight fixed on realizing your highest spiritual potential. If you happen to believe in a personal deity, you can use the traditional practice of repeating whatever name you have for the divine until your mind becomes absorbed in the state of contemplation. Or you can employ prayers and invocations to feel near to God or Goddess. But always remember that, according to Yoga, the divine isn't a separate being, but the essence of everything.

# Chapter 23

# Meditation and the Higher Reaches of Yoga

. . . . . . . . . . . . . . . . . . . . . . . . . . . . . . . . . . . . . . . . . . . . .

## In This Chapter

▶ Concentrating on finding your focus

▶ Making the most of your meditation practice

▶ Exploring states of ecstasy and enlightenment

. . . . . . . . . . . . . . . . . . . . . . . . . . . . . . . . . . . . . . . . . . . . .

*Y*ou've probably heard the saying, "You give as good as you get." The same goes for Yoga. Doing a few postures now and then certainly gives you some benefits; however, to reap Yoga's full rewards, you need to live a yogic lifestyle — a lifestyle that encompasses the physical, mental, and spiritual.

Yoga postures are a great place to start. Yoga postures can have a huge positive effect on your physical and emotional well-being. Remember, though, Yoga alone isn't enough. A nutritious diet, adequate sleep, meaningful work, and a reasonably happy family life are other important pieces of the puzzle of good physical and mental health.

Beyond the basic benefits of a healthy body, the physical practice of Yoga can help you continue to explore your deeper mental and spiritual potential. In fact, a vital, healthy body is the best foundation for meditation (yogic concentration) and the higher reaches of Yoga. Try meditating when your nose is blocked from a cold, when you're running a fever, or when your back is killing you. Pain and discomfort may make you philosophical ("Why me?"), but they don't contribute to a basically relaxed mind. And that's exactly why you need to meditate.

Many chapters in this book deal specifically with Yoga postures designed to relax your body and thus prepare your mind for the higher stages of Yoga. This chapter explains how to integrate meditation into your routine so that you can reach the top rung of the Yoga ladder.

# Understanding Concentration

How busy is your mind? Can you concentrate easily? The following little exercise gauges your CQ (Concentration Quotient):

Think of a beautiful white swan. It looks neither left nor right, but just slowly and majestically glides across the surface of a pond. It barely causes ripples in the water. Keep thinking of that swan. Try to form a clear image, and then hold it as steadily as possible in your mind while slowly counting down from 100.

How far did you manage to count before your mental image of the swan faded into thin air or another thought intruded? Was it 97 or 96? Perhaps you lost your concentration with the count of 99. You may have been able to continue your counting for several more numbers, but reaching much beyond 96 is unusual for most beginners. If you did, your power of concentration is good — only a yogi or yogini can count all the way to 0 and think of the swan.

If you think you didn't do well with this exercise because visualizing isn't your strong suit, try this one for good measure:

Sit quietly. Take a few deep breaths, and then let your mind go totally blank. No thoughts, no images, no counting — no ripples in your mental pond at all. Just sit. Just be.

How did you do? Don't feel bad if your concentration exercise went something like this:

Okay, I'm not thinking. Heck, that's a thought, isn't it? Let me try again. . . . That's much better. See? Having no images isn't that difficult. And what was that about counting? I didn't do too well with the counting test, but I hate tests. Oh darn, I'm thinking again. Okay, back to no thoughts. . . .

## The inner limbs of Yoga

According to Raja Yoga in the Yoga-Sutra of Patanjali, the yogic path comprises eight limbs *(anga)*. The first five limbs — moral discipline, self-restraint, posture, breath control, and sensory inhibition — are called *outer limbs*. These practices belong to the entrance hall of Yoga's vast mansion. In the interior of the estate, you find concentration, meditation, and ecstasy, known as the *inner limbs*. You can successfully practice these inner limbs only after you achieve a certain degree of mastery in the other five practices.

Don't be discouraged if your mind is a veritable speed train and your concentration is too poor to slow it down. Your mind's forward charge merely means that you have room for improvement, and you *will* improve with practice. Distraction isn't negative in itself. Instead, you can look at your lack of clear concentration as an opportunity to gently refocus your attention. As you refocus repeatedly, your mind can become more obedient. Think of your mind as a spirited foal that exuberantly gallops around the meadow. With a little training, that frisky colt can become an excellent racehorse. The following sections delve into how concentration works and what it can do for you.

## Unleashing your essence

The ability to concentrate is a boon to everything you do. Without it, you'd constantly hammer your finger rather than a nail, you'd miscalculate your taxes, and you'd be unable to follow the razor-sharp logic of Sherlock Holmes.

Yogic concentration is far more demanding than the kind of concentration you use in daily life — but it's also much more rewarding. Yoga can help you unlock the hidden chambers of your own mind. When you're able to focus your attention on your inner world like a laser, you can discover the most subtle aspects of your mind. Above all, yogic concentration ultimately enables you to discover your spiritual essence.

Concentration leads to meditation (which we discuss later in the chapter) and brings you clarity and peace of mind — two qualities that stand you in good stead in any situation. They enable you to live your life more fully, more meaningfully, and more competently. Whether you're a busy mother and homemaker or a top executive, the mental tranquility you produce through regular concentration and meditation exercises can transform your entire day.

## Gaining focus

When you gain skill with concentration and meditation on the Yoga mat or meditation cushion, you gradually become able to apply this mindfulness to every aspect of your life. The Sanskrit word for concentration is *dharana*, which means "holding." You hold your attention by focusing on a specific bodily process (such as breathing), a thought, an image, or a sound (as we discuss in "Practicing Meditation," later in the chapter). Through *concentration*, you seek to become *concentric*, or properly centered and harmonious with yourself. When you're out of center (*eccentric*), or out of touch with your spiritual core, all your thoughts and actions are out of sync; they don't flow from your innermost core and thus make you feel alienated, uneasy, and unhappy.

You can determine whether you're currently *concentric* or *eccentric* by checking in with your body. How do you feel? How does a decision you're about to make feel? How does a relationship feel? What does your body tell you about your present activity or your job? How do you feel about your life as a whole? This kind of mindfulness is called *focusing*, which means paying careful attention to how your mind is registering in your body. Body and mind go together, so keeping mentally in touch with your body regularly is vital and even fundamental to a good meditation practice.

Through focusing, you also become aware of your own baggage — old resentments, disappointments, fears, and expectations. People tend to store negative experiences in their bodies, which makes them predisposed to sickness. Sooner or later, all people need to work through these stored memories for their own good health and to share their liberated selves with the world around them.

One way to begin replaying and diffusing negative experiences recorded in your body is to ask yourself, "Is anything preventing me from feeling good and happy right now? What, if anything, is keeping me from experiencing bliss?" Your body contains the answer(s): a sensation of tightness in the chest, a hollow feeling around the heart, a contraction in the pit of your stomach, fearful pounding in the head — you get the idea. All these reactions are physical expressions of corresponding emotional states.

When doing this kind of focusing work, don't settle for the first answer that comes to mind. Instead, ask yourself, "What else is there to prevent me from feeling good and happy?" If you encounter too much inner pain, you may want to consider doing this work in the company of a trusted friend or under the guidance of a competent counselor or therapist.

# Practicing Meditation

*Meditation* is a mental process involving focused attention (also known as calm awareness or mindfulness). Many people confuse meditation with stopping all thoughts, but that type of meditation is only one (rather advanced) kind. In the beginning, meditation is simply noticing the endless stream of thoughts flickering on your mental screen; consider your observations an important part of your overall effort to be *mindful*, or attentive.

Many forms or styles of meditation exist, but two basic approaches stand out: meditation with a specific focus and objectless meditation. The latter is pure mindfulness without narrowing attention to any particular sensation, idea, or other phenomenon. Most beginners find this kind of meditation difficult, although some are drawn to it. We recommend that you start with meditation on a specific focus. The following categories of objects are suitable for this exercise:

- A bodily sensation, such as breathing, which makes an excellent focus

- A bodily location, such as one of the seven cakras, or energy centers, (we discuss the cakras in the next section)

✔ A process or action, such as eating, walking, or washing dishes

✔ An external physical object, such as the flame of a candle

✔ A *mantra* (a single sound, a phrase, or a chant)

✔ A thought, such as the idea of peace, joy, love, or compassion

✔ A visualization of light, emptiness, a saint, or one of the many deities of Hindu or Buddhist Yoga

Experiment with all these various focal points for meditation until you find what appeals to you the most. Then stick with it. For instance, if you choose to visualize a particular saint or deity, you benefit by always using the same figure in your daily visualization practice.

The following sections give you more information on mastering meditation.

## Getting a handle on cakras: Your wheels of fortune

If you choose to focus your meditation on a cakra (one of the options in the earlier list), you first need to understand the concept of cakras. According to Yoga, the physical body has a more subtle energetic counterpart that consists of a network of energy channels called *nadis* (pronounced *nah-dees*) through which the life force *(prana)* circulates. The most important channel, called the *sushumna-nadi* (pronounced *su-shum-na*), or "gracious channel," runs along the axis of the body from the base of the spine to the crown of the head. In the ordinary individual, this central conduit of subtle energy is said to be mostly inactive. The purpose of many Hatha Yoga exercises is to clear this channel of any obstructions so that the life energy can flow freely in it, leading to better health and also higher states of consciousness.

When the central channel is thus activated, it also sets the seven psychoenergetic centers of the body in motion. These centers are the *cakras*, which are aligned along the central channel. The word *cakra* simply means "wheel" and refers to the fact that these areas are whirlpools of energy that keep the physical body in balance and functioning properly. In ascending order, the seven cakras are listed here:

✔ *Muladhara* ("root prop," **pronounced** *moo-lahd-hah-rah*): Located at the base of the spine between the rectum and genitals, this center is the resting place of the dormant "serpent power," the great psychospiritual energy that Hatha Yoga seeks to awaken. This center is connected with elimination as well as fear.

✔ *Svadhishthana* ("own place," **pronounced** *svahd-hisht-hah-nah*): Located at the genitals, this center is connected with the urogenital functions and also with desire.

- ✔ *Manipura* **("jewel city," pronounced** *mah-nee-poo-rah*): Located at the navel, this center distributes the life force to all parts of the body and is especially involved in the digestive process and willpower.

- ✔ *Anahata* **("unstruck," pronounced** *ah-nah-hah-tah*): Located in the middle of the chest, this center, which is also called the heart cakra, is the place where you can hear the "unstruck," or inner sound, in meditation. It's also linked with love.

- ✔ *Vishuddha* **("pure," pronounced** *vee-shood-hah*): Located at the throat, this center is associated with both speech and greed.

- ✔ *Ajna* **("command," pronounced** *ah-gyah*): Located in the middle of the head between the eyebrows, this center is the contact place for the guru's telepathic work with disciples. It's also associated with the experience of higher states of consciousness.

- ✔ *Sahasrara* **("thousand-spoked," pronounced** *sah-hahs-rah-rah*): Located at the crown of the head, this special cakra is associated with higher states of consciousness, notably the ecstatic state (which we cover in "Working toward Ecstasy," later in the chapter).

## Following a few guidelines for successful meditation

Think of your meditation as a tree that you must water every day — not too much and not too little. Trust that, one day, your nurturing will bring the tree to bear beautiful blossoms and delicious fruit.

Consider these vital tips to help you set the stage for a meditation routine:

- ✔ **Practice regularly.** Try to meditate every day. If daily meditation isn't possible, meditate at least several times a week.

- ✔ **Cultivate the correct motivation.** People meditate for all kinds of reasons: health, wholeness, peace of mind, clarity, spiritual growth, and so on. Be clear in your own mind why you're sitting down to meditate. The best motivation for meditation (and Yoga practice in general) is to live to your full potential *and* to benefit others by your personal achievements.

   In Buddhism, this motivation is known as the *bodhisattva* ideal. The bodhisattva ("enlightenment being") seeks to realize enlightenment (the ultimate spiritual state) for the benefit of all other beings. As an enlightened being, you can be far more efficient in helping others in their own struggle for wholeness and happiness.

- ✔ **Meditate at a regular time.** Take advantage of the fact that your body-mind is a creature of habit. After a few weeks of meditating at the same time during the day or night, you may find yourself looking forward to your next meditation session. Traditionally, Yoga practitioners prefer the hour of sunrise, but this time isn't always practical. (Head to Chapter 18 for more on morning meditation.)

Inevitably, you have moments when meditation is the last activity you want to do. In this case, resolve to sit quietly for at least 5 minutes. Often this break is enough to get you in the mood for full-fledged meditation. If not, don't beat yourself over the head; just go on to something else and try again later or the next day.

✔ **Meditate in the same place.** Choose the same place for the same reason you use the same time: Your body-mind enjoys what's familiar. Use this fact to your advantage by setting aside a room, or even a corner of a room, that your mind can associate with meditation.

✔ **Select an appropriate posture for meditation, and do it correctly.** Sit up straight, with your chest open and your neck free (see the following section for instructions about posture). To avoid falling asleep, don't recline while meditating, and don't meditate on your bed, even in a sitting position; your mind is likely to associate the experience with sleep. If you're not used to sitting on the floor, try sitting on a straight-backed chair or on a sofa with a cushion behind your back. If you can comfortably sit on the floor, you have a variety of yogic postures to choose from; several appear in Chapter 7.

✔ **Select a meditation technique, and stick with it.** In the beginning, you may want to try out various techniques to see which appeals to you the most. But when you find a good technique for your particular needs, don't abandon it until it bears fruit (in terms of increased peace of mind and happiness), a meditation teacher advises you to change to a different technique, or you feel really drawn to a different technique.

When you have your routine sorted out, keep the following suggestions in mind as you grow your meditation tree:

✔ **Begin with short sessions.** Meditate only 10 to 20 minutes at a time at first. If your meditation naturally lasts longer, simply rejoice in the fact. But never force yourself if the timing creates conflict or unhappiness in you. Also beware of overmeditating. Often what beginners regard as a nice long meditation is just self-indulgent daydreaming. Make sure your meditation contains an element of alertness. When you start drifting off into a comfortable space, you can be sure that you're no longer meditating. Like the practice of the Yoga postures, your meditation must have an edge (that is, you must push against the limitations of your mind, but without frustrating yourself).

✔ **Be alert, yet relaxed.** Inner alertness, or mindfulness, isn't the same as tension or stress. Cats are good examples of this alertness. Even when a cat is completely relaxed, its ears move around like radar dishes, catching every little sound in the environment. The more relaxed you are, the more alert your mind can be, so make sure your body is relaxed by regularly practicing some of the relaxation exercises we describe in Chapter 4.

✔ **Don't burden yourself with expectations.** Entering meditation with a desire to grow spiritually and to benefit from the experience is certainly acceptable. However, don't expect every meditation to be wonderful and pleasant.

✔ **Prepare properly for meditation.** As a beginner, don't expect to be able to jump from the fray of your daily activities straight into meditation. Allow your mind a little time to unwind before you sit for meditation. Have a relaxing bath or shower, or at least wash your face and hands.

✔ **At the end of your meditation, integrate the experience with the rest of your life.** Just as going straight from overdrive into a meditative gear isn't prudent, you need to refrain from jumping up from meditation to return to your other activities. Instead, make a conscious transition into and out of meditation. At the end of the session, briefly recall your reasons for meditating and your overall motivation. Be grateful for any energies or insights your meditation generates. Equally important, don't feel negative about a difficult meditation experience. Instead, be grateful for *any* experience. Sometimes important insights surface during meditation; then your challenge is to translate these messages into daily life. When you continually perform this kind of integration, your meditation deepens more quickly as well.

✔ **Be prepared to practice meditation for a lifetime.** You don't grow a tree overnight. On the yogic path, no effort is ever wasted. Therefore, don't give up if your meditation isn't what you think it should be after a month or two. Don't conclude too hastily that meditation isn't working or that the technique you're using isn't effective. Instead, correct your understanding about the nature of meditation and carry on. Your very effort to meditate counts.

## Roses come with thorns

If you're a beginner and your meditations are consistently comfortable, you have every reason to be suspicious. The purpose of meditation is to clear your mind, and doing so entails clearing away the debris (or what one teacher has called "the frogs deep down in the well").

In the beginning, meditation consists largely of discovering just how unruly your mind is. If your meditation practice is successful, you encounter your shadow side (all aspects of your character you prefer not to think about). As you go on, more profound insights into your character can and do occur, which then requires you to make the necessary changes in your attitudes and behaviors.

Few meditations are spectacular, which isn't at all what meditation is about. Even a seemingly bad meditation is a good meditation because you're applying mindfulness. Don't be surprised to find that your meditation is calm and uplifting one day and then turbulent and distracted the next, for no apparent reason. Until your mind reaches clarity and calmness, you can expect this fluctuation. Just keep a sense of humor and graciously accept whatever happens in your meditation.

Be wary of weekend workshops that promise immediate success, if not enlightenment itself. Meditation and enlightenment are lifelong processes.

# Maintaining proper bodily posture

Correct posture is important for meditation. This seven-point checklist can help you develop good sitting habits:

- ✔ **Back:** Your back position is the single most important physical feature of your meditation. Your back should be straight but relaxed, with your chest open and your neck free. Correct posture enables your bodily energies to flow more freely, which prevents sleepiness. (Flip to "Getting a handle on cakras: Your wheels of fortune," earlier in the chapter, for details on the bodily energies.) Most Westerners need a firm cushion under their *sits bones* (the bones directly under the flesh of the buttocks) to encourage good posture during meditation and to stop their legs from going to sleep. If you go that route, however, make sure your pelvis doesn't tilt forward too much. Alternatively, you can sit on a chair. Any posture is acceptable, as long as you can comfortably maintain it for the desired duration.

- ✔ **Head:** For the correct position of your head, picture an attached string pulling the back of your head upward so that your head is tilted slightly forward. Too much of a forward tilt invites drowsiness, but not enough of a tilt can cause mental wandering.

- ✔ **Tongue:** Allow the front part of your tongue to touch the palate just behind the upper teeth. This position reduces the flow of saliva and the number of times you have to swallow, which many beginners find disturbing.

- ✔ **Teeth:** Don't clench your teeth — keep your jaws relaxed. Be sure that your mouth doesn't hang open, either.

- ✔ **Legs:** If you can sit cross-legged for an extended period of time without experiencing discomfort, we especially recommend the perfect posture (*siddhasana*), which we describe in Chapter 6. The folded legs form a closed circuit, which aids your concentration. If sitting cross-legged is a problem for you, just meditate in a chair.

- ✔ **Arms:** Keep your hands cupped in your lap, with your palms up and your right hand on top of your left. Relax your arms and shoulders, leaving a few inches between your arms and your trunk, which allows the air to circulate and prevents drowsiness.

- ✔ **Eyes:** Most beginners like to close their eyes, which is fine. As you develop your power of concentration, however, you may want to experiment with keeping your eyes slightly open while gazing downward in front of you, to signal your brain that you aren't trying to go to sleep. Advanced practitioners are able to keep their eyes wide open without becoming distracted. In any event, make sure your eye muscles are relaxed.

## *Overcoming obstacles to meditation*

Whenever you deal with change, you also deal with resistance to change. Thus, the path of meditation is littered with various obstacles that can trip you up. Here are the most important potential hindrances: doubt (about the yogic path or yourself), negative thoughts (about yourself, others, life, and so on), haste, boredom, pretense, and the hunt for spiritual experiences. The ego lurks in many niches, especially when you travel on the yogic path.

## *Adding sounds to meditation*

Using a sound or phrase to focus the mind is a popular approach in many spiritual traditions, including Hinduism, Buddhism, Christianity, Judaism, and Islamic Sufism. In Sanskrit, these special sounds are called *mantras* and are thought to better focus attention. Mantra Yoga made its debut in the Western world in the late 1960s with the Transcendental Meditation (TM) movement, founded by Maharishi Mahesh Yogi, whose most famous disciples were The Beatles.

Here are some well-known *mantras:*

- The syllable *om* is composed of the letters *a, u,* and *m,* and stands for the waking state, dream state, and deep sleep, respectively. Hindus consider this syllable to be sacred and to symbolize the ultimate reality, or higher Self *(atman).* The sound begins from the belly and moves upward; the long-drawn, nasalized humming sound of *m* represents the ultimate reality.

- The mantra *so'ham* (pronounced *so-hum*) means "I am that" — that is, "I am the universal Self." You repeat it in sync with breathing: *so* on inhaling and *ham* on exhaling.

- Buddhist Yoga widely uses the mantric phrase *om mani padme hum* (pronounced *om mah-nee pahd-meh hoom*). It means *"Om. Jewel in the Lotus. Hum,"* which conveys that the searched-for higher reality is present here and now.

- The mantric utterance *om namah shivaya* (pronounced *om nah-mah shee-vah-yah*) is a favorite phrase among Hindu devotees of the Divine in the form of Shiva. It means "*Om.* Salutation to Shiva."

- Members of the Krishna Consciousness movement made the mantric utterance *hare krishna* (pronounced *hah-reh krish-nah*) famous in the West. It invokes the Divine in the form of Krishna, who is also called Hari.

According to the Yoga tradition, sounds are considered mantras only after a guru passes the sound to a worthy disciple. Thus, the syllable *om* on its own — without proper initiation — isn't a mantra. Many Western Yoga teachers take a more relaxed approach and recommend both traditional and contemporary words for mantra practice.

### Reciting your mantra

Whether you choose your own *mantra* or are given one, you must repeat it over and over again, either mentally or vocally (whispered or aloud), to make it effective.

This practice of recitation is called *japa* (pronounced *jah-pah*), meaning "muttering." So what happens after you recite a *mantra* a thousand, ten thousand, or a hundred thousand times? As you repeat the sound, your attention becomes more focused and your consciousness becomes absorbed into the sound. The *mantra* begins to recite itself, serving as an anchor for your mind whenever you don't need to engage your thoughts in specific tasks. This shift simplifies your inner life and gives you a sense of peace. Ultimately, your *mantra* can guide you to enlightenment. Of course, to achieve enlightenment, you must fulfill the other requirements of Yoga as well, notably honoring the moral disciplines, which we cover in detail in Chapter 22. We also discuss the road to enlightenment further in "Reaching toward Enlightenment," later in this chapter.

We recommend that beginners recite their mantra aloud, at a slow, steady pace. When you have some experience with this form of meditation, you can begin to whisper your mantra so that only you can hear it. Traditionally, the most powerful form of mantric recitation is silent or mental recitation. However, this exercise calls for a certain degree of skill in maintaining your concentration, so start with a vocal mantra.

### Using a rosary

Yoga practitioners often tell rosary beads while reciting their mantras — a practice that helps focus the mind. The typical rosary *(mala)* consists of 108 beads plus an extra-large bead that represents the cosmic mountain Meru. You tell the beads by using the thumb and middle finger. Your fingers must not cross the master or Meru bead. After 108 recitations (or beads), you simply turn the rosary around and start counting again.

## Breathing mindfully

Mindful observation of the breath is a meditation exercise, taught particularly in Buddhist circles, that any beginner can try. As we note in Chapter 5, the breath is the link between body and mind. Since ancient times, the Yoga masters have made good use of this connection. Mindful breathing, or breathing meditation, is a simple and effective way of exploring the calming effect of conscious breathing. Here's how it works:

1. **Sit up straight and relaxed.**

2. **Remind yourself of your purpose for meditation, and resolve to sit in meditation for a given period of time.**

   We recommend at least 5 minutes for this exercise. Gradually extend the duration.

3. **Close your eyes or keep them half open while looking down in front of you.**

4. **Breathing normally and gently, focus your attention on the sensation created by the breath flowing in and out of your nostrils.**

   Carefully observe the entire process of inhalation and exhalation as it occurs at the opening of your nostrils.

5. **To prevent your mind from wandering, you can count in inhalation/exhalation breath cycles from 1 to 10.**

*Note:* Don't be concerned if you notice that your attention has wandered. Especially don't be judgmental about any thoughts that may pop into your head. Instead, rededicate yourself to the process of observing your breath.

## Walking meditation

Mindfulness is possible in any circumstance. You can eat, drive, wash dishes, have a conversation, watch television, or make love mindfully. For beginners, mindfulness while walking is an excellent form of meditation. Just follow these steps to get started:

1. **Remind yourself of your purpose for meditation and resolve to meditate for a given period of time.**

   For a first try, we recommend at least 5 minutes for this exercise.

2. **Keep your eyes open but unfocused, looking down and a few steps ahead of you.**

   Don't lower your head, but keep your neck relaxed.

3. **Stand completely still, and feel your entire body.**

4. **Focus your attention on your right foot, especially the toes and sole.**

5. **Slowly raise your right foot and take the first step.**

   Feel the sensation of the pressure lifting from your right foot and leg and shifting over to your left leg.

6. **As you slowly place your right foot back on the ground, become aware of the contact between the sole and the ground.**

   Also notice the rest of your body: your swinging arms that keep you balanced, your neck and head, and your pelvis.

7. **Acknowledge any thoughts that arise, without being judgmental; return your attention to your whole body, not merely one limb or movement.**

8. **At the end of your walking meditation, stand completely still for a few seconds, observing the clarity and calmness within you.**

## Associating prayer with meditation

A close relationship exists between meditation and prayer. Prayer practices mindfulness in relation to a being — a *guru*, a great master (dead or alive), a deity, or the ultimate spiritual reality itself — deemed "higher" than the participant. Prayer, like meditation, involves a feeling of reverence.

# Working toward Ecstasy

When you start meditating, you're well aware that "you" — the subject — are quite different from the object of meditation. You experience the white or blue light or the visualized deity as distinct from yourself. But as meditation deepens, the boundary between subject and object — consciousness and its contents — becomes increasingly blurred. Then at one point, the two merge completely. You *are* the light or deity. This point is the celebrated state of ecstasy called *samadhi* in Sanskrit (pronounced *sah-mahd-hee*).

Yoga distinguishes two fundamental levels of ecstasy. At the lower level, the ecstatic state is associated with a certain form or mental content. The higher type of ecstasy is a state of formless consciousness.

Many Yoga practitioners never experience the ecstatic state, but some definitely encounter it in the course of their lives. What matters isn't how often or how long you enter into *samadhi*, but whether and how much you embody spiritual principles in your daily life. Are you compassionate and kind? Do you see others not as total strangers, but as fellow beings going through their own struggle of self-realization? Can you love unconditionally? Are you forgiving and encouraging toward others?

*Samadhi* isn't identical with enlightenment, which is the real goal of Yoga. You can attain enlightenment without ever experiencing *samadhi*. The following section enlightens you about the state of enlightenment.

## Wherever you go, there you are

Sri Ramana Maharshi was one of the great Yoga masters of the 20th century. As he was on his deathbed, his disciples expressed their sorrow at losing him. He calmly said, "They say that I am dying, but I am not going away. Where could I go? I am here." He had realized the eternal Self, which is everywhere. To this day, his spiritual presence can be felt in the hermitage that disciples built for him long ago.

# Reaching toward Enlightenment

People usually associate the word *enlightenment* with profound intellectual understanding. However, in Yoga, *enlightenment* refers to the permanent realization of your true nature, which is the ultimate or transcendental Self (*atman*). The Sanskrit word for enlightenment is *bodha* (pronounced *bohd-ha*), which means "illumination." The same realization also is referred to as *liberation* because it liberates you from the misunderstanding that you're a separate self, referred to as *I* in a unique body and gifted with a mind that's disconnected from everything else.

This chapter has taken you on a journey through some of the philosophy and terminology of yogic meditation. Here's the bottom line: If you remember nothing else, remember that it's the doing, not the knowing, that's most important; the regular day-to-day practice is what counts.

# Chapter 24

# Yoga Therapy: Customizing Your Back and Body Treatments

*Y*oga therapy applies the principles of Yoga to people with physical, psychological, or spiritual needs that a group class can't normally address. A Yoga therapist is a Yoga teacher with advanced training who can adapt Yoga to the client's unique needs. The regular and mindful practice of carefully adapted Yoga postures can bring relief from pain, increase mobility and strength, and confer a sense of well-being.

This chapter introduces you to the field of Yoga therapy, helps you make informed decisions about whether Yoga therapy may be right for you, and shows you what to look for in a Yoga therapist. If your back is calling for more TLC (but not crying out for a doctor — if you're in acute pain, see your medical professional), the suggestions and postures in this chapter can help you become more aware of your needs and make peace with your back.

## What You Need to Know about Yoga Therapy

If you've ever suffered from a back problem, you aren't alone. More than 80 percent of Americans seek professional help for back pain at some point in their lives, and back pain is second only to the common cold for illness-related absences from work. Back-health experts recommend that people learn how to prevent pain and self-treat when they can safely do so.

## Everything old is new again: The evolution of Yoga as therapy

The therapeutic use of Yoga dates back thousands of years as a component of ayurveda. *Ayurveda* (*ayus* meaning "life" and *veda* meaning "related to knowledge or science") is an Indian system of medicine with ancient roots that's becoming well known in the West as well. It has a strong focus on disease prevention and takes a whole-person approach. Yoga therapy came into its own in India in the early part of the 20th century. Sri T. Krishnamacacharya, teacher to T.K.V. Desikachar, B.K.S. Iyengar, and Pattabhi Jois, used his own blend of Yoga and ayurveda. The Kaivalyadhama Yoga Hospital in Lonovola (www.kdham.com) and the Yoga Institute of Santacruz, Mumbai (www.theyogainstitute.org), both started almost a century ago and still operate today.

Yoga therapy has continued to develop in the United States, sometimes combined with ayurveda, but increasingly utilized as a complement to Western-style integrative medicine. Early pioneers in the field include Nischala Devi; Gary Kraftsow, MA; Judith Lasater, PT; Michael Lee; Richard Miller, PhD; Dean Ornish, MD; your humble coauthor, Larry Payne, PhD; and Makunda Stiles. Founded in 1989 by Richard Miller and me (Larry), the International Association of Yoga Therapists (www.iayt.org) supports research and education in Yoga and serves as a professional organization for more than 3,600 Yoga therapists and teachers in 50 countries worldwide.

Yoga therapy helps people in the chronic or rehabilitation stage of their pain (after the acute stage has passed) and is generally an adjunct to medical and/or chiropractic care. Acute pain is the body's distress signal and mustn't be ignored. What may feel like a musculoskeletal pain may, in fact, be a serious medical problem involving an organ, or a pinched nerve requiring spinal adjustment. People with acute pain need to seek help from a medical, chiropractic, or osteopathic physician or physical therapist.

In addition to its most common use with back problems, Yoga therapy is helpful with knee and hip problems, arthritis, and carpal tunnel syndrome. It can also benefit people who suffer from a host of other conditions, including anxiety, chronic pain, depression, diabetes, digestive problems, heart disease, hypertension, insomnia, painful menstrual periods and hot flashes, multiple sclerosis, Parkinson's disease, and more. Though not a cure, Yoga therapy can help improve the quality of life for people with serious chronic and progressive conditions.

If you think you may be a candidate for Yoga therapy, the next step is to find a qualified Yoga therapist who can meet your needs. The following sections help you with that search and also clue you in on what you can expect from Yoga therapy.

# How to find a good Yoga therapist

Finding a good Yoga therapist who fits your needs takes a bit of research. Following are some tips to help you in your search:

- ✔ **Visit the website of The International Association of Yoga Therapists.** You can browse a directory of 3,600 members worldwide and view their Yoga qualifications.

- ✔ **Find out where the Yoga therapist has received training.** Look for someone who has successfully completed a respected training program. The Yoga Therapy Rx training program at Loyola Marymount University in Los Angeles is the first of what is sure to become many university-based programs to prepare Yoga teachers to apply the tools of Yoga to bring relief and improvement.

- ✔ **Ask a trusted source.** Yoga therapists work with a range of healthcare practitioners. Ask your practitioner for a referral.

- ✔ **Visit the website of a respected training program.** Many training programs publish the names and contact information of therapists they've trained. While at the site, you can explore the training course descriptions and evaluate their appropriateness for your needs.

# What to expect if you see a Yoga therapist

Visiting any new practitioner can make a person uneasy. In this section, we guide you on ways to be an informed patient in discussing the Yoga therapy approach to healing and in exploring treatment length and cost.

## A whole-person approach

Yoga therapy takes the whole person into account. Although your chief complaint may be your achin' lower back, during the course of the assessment, your Yoga therapist may observe, ask about, and consider related factors beyond your tense muscles: how and how much you move and sit during the course of your typical day, your general level of stress (without becoming your psychotherapist), how you breathe, your typical diet and sleep patterns, and so on. In addition to an individualized program of coordinated movement and breath, your Yoga therapist may suggest journaling to help you learn more about your lifestyle and pain triggers, as well as modifying your daily routine to help you meet your goal.

## An initial series of sessions and beyond

About six sessions are generally helpful when working with a Yoga therapist. This duration allows time for you to get a handle on your personalized program and for your Yoga therapist to observe and adjust your movements and breath so that you have a program that works for you.

The goal is to develop a personal practice that you can continue on your own for further improvement in mobility, strength, and well-being. Your goal is to eventually participate in group classes, if you want to. Periodic tune-ups are a good idea, especially if you aren't participating in a group class where a skilled Yoga teacher can help you modify postures as necessary.

### Cost

As you may expect, private sessions with someone who has advanced training cost more than what you may pay for a group Yoga class. Individual sessions in large metropolitan areas range from about $75 to $200 each, depending on the experience of the therapist.

# A Five-Step Plan for a Healthy Back

The best way to prevent back problems or to keep them from becoming chronic is to use Yoga as part of a five-step plan, which we outline here.

- ✔ **Re-educate yourself on biomechanics.** How you sit, stand, walk, lift, sleep, and work can cause you pain or help you relieve pain.

- ✔ **Practice your Yoga or back exercise program regularly.** Be realistic about how much you can do each day, and *do it.*

- ✔ **Keep a back journal.** Journaling can help you discover more about how your lifestyle (such as sleeping, lifting, and sitting habits) affects your back.

- ✔ **Make healthful food choices.** Nutrition experts recommend a balanced diet rich in fruits and vegetables, whole grains, legumes, olive oil, low-fat dairy products, fish, and limited amounts of lean meat (if you eat meat).

- ✔ **Rest and relax consciously.** Be mindful about what you expose yourself to in the hours before bedtime. The last thing you see or listen to before bed affects your subconscious mind and can affect your sleep pattern.

# Yoga Rx for Lower Backs

We speculate that many readers can say that they've had a lower back problem at some point in their lives. Because lower back problems are the most common, we've focused this chapter on them. We address Yoga for the aches and pains in your upper back and neck online at www.dummies.com/extras/yoga.

Your "lower back" is actually the *lumbar vertebrae* section of the spinal cord. Spine movement brings much-needed circulation to the vertebral discs and helps keep them supple. The health of your hamstring and *psoas* (hip flexor) muscles, as well as the strength of your abdominal and core muscles, also affects your lower back. Helpful Yoga therapy postures allow you to stretch and strengthen key muscle groups, release tension, and bring your whole body back into harmony. The following sections give you some general guidelines on what kinds of Yoga movements work well for different lower back issues and offer a routine to help you segue into a regular group class.

## Lower back conditions that need more arching

If a forward bend or rounding is painful to your lower back, chances are, you may have strained your lower back muscles or you have a disc problem or sciatica. Be wise — if it hurts, don't do it! Consider some tips:

✔ **Avoid forward bends of any kind.** If you try a forward bend, keep your back flat, not rounded. Remember the concept of Forgiving Limbs (which we cover in Chapter 3), and bend your knees as necessary.

✔ **Try postures that allow you to arch, such as those in the cobra family (see Chapter 11), instead of bend forward.** Gentle extensions such as transitioning to warrior I from the mountain posture are also helpful. (Check out Chapter 7 for warrior I and the mountain posture.)

✔ **Use the "Lower back routine" later in this section.** You can also find DVD resources in the appendix.

## Lower back conditions that need more folding

Certain back conditions, including arthritis and *spondylolisthesis* (slipped vertebrae), can cause the vertebrae to jam, making arching painful. As we stress in the preceding section, if it hurts, don't do it. The following list gives you some pointers on Yoga for these conditions:

✔ Avoid postures that extend your back, such as ones in the cobra family, and athletic postures or sequences that involve jumping.

✔ Try postures that lengthen your back, such as gentle forward bends, downward-facing dog, and folding cat. (Flip to Chapter 7 for more suggestions.)

## What about scoliosis?

Scoliosis, a condition in which the spine curves from side to side, can be structural or functional. If you think you have scoliosis, consult your medical or chiropractic physician.

✔ *Structural scoliosis* is a hereditary disorder more common in girls than boys.

✔ *Functional scoliosis* may occur as a result of a problem elsewhere in the body, such as one leg that's shorter than the other, or

can even result from frequently holding a position that causes a twist in the spine. Postures that stretch one side of the spine at a time, such as *asymmetrical* (one-sided) forward bends, side bends, and twists, are generally helpful and may reduce or eliminate the curve in time. (Chapters 11 and 12 give you more info on postures that bend and twist.)

## *Lower back routine*

The following exercises aren't meant for acute back problems. If any part of this routine causes you back or neck pain, omit that part and check with your medical or chiropractic physician before you continue.

A session or two of Yoga or back exercise during your week doesn't help much if you misuse or abuse your back the rest of the time.

No single Yoga routine is appropriate for all back problems. When your doctor feels that you're ready for a regular group class, the following routine can help you make the transition. Keep in mind that the Yoga breathing we recommend for this routine (Chapter 5's focus breathing or belly breathing) is just as important as the Yoga postures. Inhale and exhale slowly through your nose, with a slight pause after both the inhalation and the exhalation. We give you various options for many of the postures so that you can find the right moves for you. And remember that executing the postures in the proper sequence is important.

### *Corpse posture with bent legs: Shavasana variation*

Relaxation and breathing are important ingredients for a healthy back. The corpse posture is a classic position to start the process.

If your back feels uncomfortable, place a pillow or blanket roll under your knees. If your head tilts back, place a folded blanket or small pillow under your head.

1. **Lie flat on your back, with your arms relaxed along the sides of your torso and your palms up.**

2. **Bend your knees, and place your feet on the floor at hip width.**

3. **Close your eyes and relax (see Figure 24-1).**

4. **Stay in the posture for 8 to 10 breaths.**

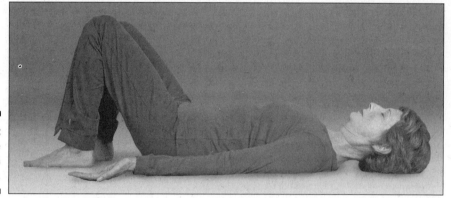

**Figure 24-1:**
Corpse
posture with
bent legs.

*Photograph by Adam Latham*

### Knee-to-chest posture: Ekapada apanasana

Keeping your back healthy is like tuning a piano. The knee-to-chest posture helps you adjust and relax your lower back. If you have knee problems, hold the back of your thigh instead of just below your knee. Remember, this pose isn't a biceps exercise. Just hold your knee, breathe, and relax.

1. **Lie on your back, with your knees bent, palms down, and feet flat on the floor.**

2. **As you exhale, bring your right knee toward your chest, holding your shin just below your knee (see Figure 24-2).**

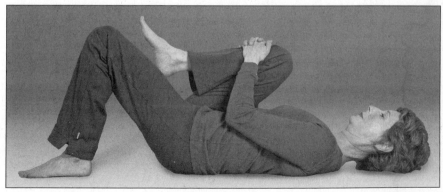

**Figure 24-2:**
Knee-
to-chest
posture.

*Photograph by Adam Latham*

3. Stay in the posture for 6 to 8 breaths.

4. Repeat Steps 1 through 3 with your left leg.

### Lying arm raise with bent leg: Shavasana variation

Many back sufferers have more problems on one side of the torso than the other. The lying arm raise is a safe, classic way to gently stretch and prepare each side of the back and neck for the rest of the routine.

1. **Lie in the corpse posture (see Chapter 14), with your arms relaxed at your sides and palms down; bend just your right knee, and put your right foot on the floor, as in Figure 24-3a.**

2. **As you inhale, slowly raise your arms overhead and touch the floor behind you, with your palms up (see Figure 24-3b); pause briefly.**

**Figure 24-3:**
Lying arm raise with bent leg.

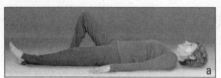 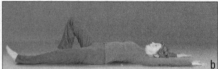

*Photograph by Adam Latham*

3. **As you exhale, bring your arms back to your sides, as in Step 1.**

4. **Repeat Steps 2 and 3 six to eight times, and then repeat Steps 1 through 3 with your left knee bent and your right leg straight.**

### Push-downs I: Urdhva prasrta padasana I

*Note:* We recommend that you start with this posture and replace it with push-downs II (in the following section) when you're ready to advance.

The abdomen is considered the front of your back (see Chapter 9). Keep this key area strong and toned if you want to prevent back problems. Push-downs are a great way to get that party started because they strengthen your abs without involving your neck and improve your core strength.

1. **Lying on your back with your knees bent and your feet on the floor at hip width, rest your arms near your sides, with your palms down.**

2. **As you exhale, push your lower back down to the floor for 3 to 5 seconds (see Figure 24-4); then inhale.**

As you inhale, your back releases from the push-down.

3. **Repeat Step 2 six to eight times.**

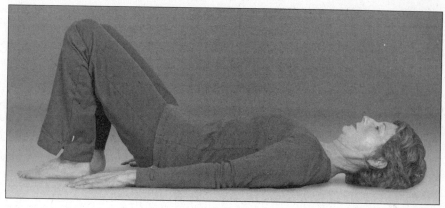

**Figure 24-4:**
Push-
downs I.

*Photograph by Adam Latham*

TIP

### Push-downs II: Urdhva prasrta padasana II

When you're ready for push-downs II (the advanced version of push-downs I in the preceding section), move your bent leg slowly. Resist the temptation to speed up.

1. **Lying on your back with your knees bent and your feet on the floor at hip width, rest your arms near your sides, with your palms down.**

2. **As you inhale, draw your right, bent knee in toward your chest, keeping your palms on the floor, as in Figure 24-5.**

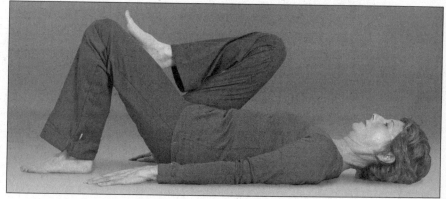

**Figure 24-5:**
Push-
downs II.

*Photograph by Adam Latham*

3. **As you exhale, push your lower back down to the floor, moving your bent right leg down until your right foot returns to touch the floor.**

   Repeat Steps 2 and 3 six to eight times, alternating slowly with the right and left legs.

To make push-downs II more challenging, draw both bent knees in toward your chest on the inhalation, and then push your lower back into the floor as you bring both your feet back to the floor on the exhalation. Be sure to keep both hands palms down on the floor the whole time.

### Dynamic bridge: Dvipada pitham

The gentle action of the bridge compensates the abs and relaxes the back for the hamstring stretch in the following section. (Head to Chapter 15 for more on sequencing and compensation.)

1. **Lie on your back with your knees bent and feet flat on the floor, at hip width.**

2. **Place your arms at your sides, with your palms down.**

3. **As you inhale, raise your hips to a comfortable height, as Figure 24-6 demonstrates.**

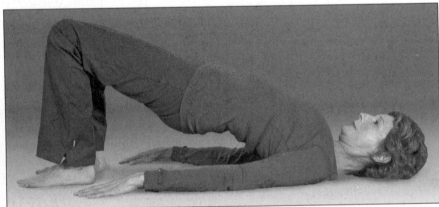

**Figure 24-6:**
Dynamic
bridge.

*Photograph by Adam Latham*

4. **As you exhale, return your hips to the floor.**

   Repeat Steps 3 and 4 six to eight times.

If the bridge causes you problems, try just tilting your pelvis toward your chin as you exhale; then try the bridge again later when you're ready.

### *Hamstring stretch: Supta padangustasana variation*

Tight hamstring muscles are a key factor in many cases of chronic back problems. A fine balance exists between stretching your hamstrings and not aggravating a chronic back condition. For this reason, we recommend keeping one leg bent, with the foot on the floor, to support your back.

1. **Lying on your back with your legs straight, place your arms along your sides, with your palms down.**

2. **Bend just your left knee, and put your left foot on the floor, as in Figure 24-7a.**

3. **As you exhale, raise your right leg until it's perpendicular to the floor (or as close as you can manage).**

4. **As you inhale, return your leg to the floor, keeping your head and the top of your hips on the floor.**

   Repeat Steps 1 through 4 three to four times, and then hold the back of your raised thigh in place just below your knee for 6 to 8 breaths, as in Figure 24-7b.

5. **Repeat Steps 1 through 4 on the other side, with your right knee bent and your left leg straight.**

   Make sure you feel the stretch in your hamstrings, not in your back.

If the back of your neck or your throat tenses when you raise or lower your leg, rest your head on a pillow or folded blanket.

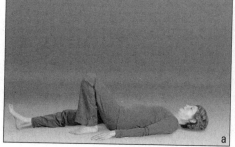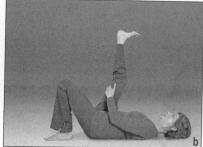

**Figure 24-7:** Hamstring stretch.

*Photograph by Adam Latham*

### *Balancing cat: Chakravakasana variation I*

This posture has been proven to strengthen core muscles throughout the spine, making it a great back exercise.

1. Starting on your hands and knees, position your knees about hip width and your hands just below your shoulders, with your fingers turned forward and your arms straightened; see Figure 24-8a for an illustration.

2. As you exhale, slide your right hand forward and your left leg back, keeping your hand and your toes on the floor.

3. As you inhale, raise your right arm and left leg to a comfortable height, as in Figure 24-8b.

4. Stay in Step 3 for 6 to 8 breaths, and then repeat Steps 1 through 3 with opposite pairs (left arm and right leg).

**Figure 24-8:**
Balancing
cat posture.

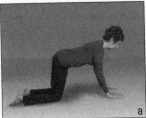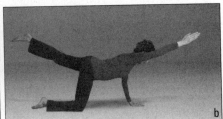

Photograph by Adam Latham

To make this posture easier, keep both hands on the ground as you extend each leg.

### Child's posture with arms in front: Balasana variation 1

If you listen for feedback from your body after doing a number of back bends, you hear a clear desire to fold as compensation (which we cover in Chapter 15). The child's posture is a smooth and easy way to fold when you're concluding hands and knees postures or front-lying back bends. The arms-in-front variation here distributes the stretch along the upper and lower back.

1. Starting on your hands and knees, place your knees about hip width, with your hands just below your shoulders and your elbows straight but not locked.

2. As you exhale, sit back on your heels, rest your torso on your thighs, and place your forehead on the floor.

3. Lay your arms on the floor, outstretched comfortably in front of you, with your palms down, as Figure 24-9 indicates.

Close your eyes and breathe easily. Stay for 6 to 8 breaths.

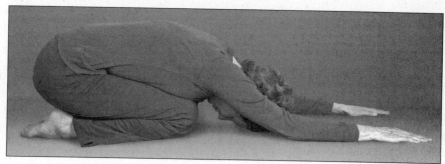

**Figure 24-9:**
Child's
posture
variation.

*Photograph by Adam Latham*

You can also try the regular child's posture with your arms back near your hips, with your palms up and hands on the floor. You may feel a little more stretch in your lower back, so choose the one that's most comfortable in the moment.

If you have knee or hip problems, lie on your back and do the knees-to-chest posture we cover later in this routine instead of the child's posture.

### Half warrior: Ardha virabhadrasana variation

This posture stretches your main hip flexors (the *iliopsoas*), one of the key muscle groups for maintaining a healthy lower back.

1. **Start by standing on your knees at hip width, and then take a big step forward with the right foot, keeping your left knee on the ground; square your hips forward, and place your hands on your right thigh, fingers forward just above your knee (see Figure 24-10a).**

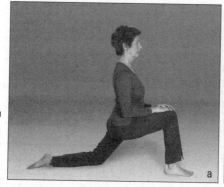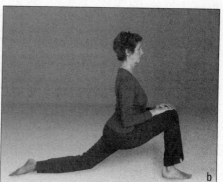

**Figure 24-10:**
Half warrior
variation.

*Photograph by Adam Latham*

2. **As you exhale, sink your hips forward and down, as Figure 24-10b demonstrates.**

   Be sure to keep approximately a 90-degree angle with your forward leg.

3. **As you inhale, return to the starting position in Step 1.**

4. **Repeat Steps 2 and 3 three to four times, and then stay in Step 2 for six to eight breaths.**

5. **Repeat Steps 1 through 4 in the same sequence on the left side.**

### Cobra II: Bhujangasana

*Note:* We recommend that you use either this posture or the cobra I posture in the following section, not both. Cobra I is less strenuous than cobra II, so go with cobra I if you aren't sure. Flip to Chapter 11 for further clarification.

As we explain in Chapter 11, most folks simply do too much forward bending. Finding a way to compensate with some form of back bend is important.

1. **Lie on your abdomen, with your legs at hip width and the tops of your feet on the floor.**

   You can also separate your legs further and roll your heels outward and your toes inward.

2. **Bend your elbows, and place your palms on the floor, with your thumbs near your armpits.**

   Rest your forehead on the floor and relax your shoulders (see Figure 24-11a).

3. **As you inhale, press your palms against the floor, and lift your chest and head forward and up (like a turtle coming out of its shell), keeping your buttocks loose.**

4. **Look straight ahead, as in Figure 24-11b.**

   Keep the top front of your pelvis on the floor and your shoulders relaxed. Unless you're very flexible, keep your elbows slightly bent and roll them inward toward your trunk.

5. **As you exhale, lower your torso and head slowly back to the floor.**

   Repeat Steps 3 through 5 six to eight times.

**Figure 24-11:**
Cobra II.

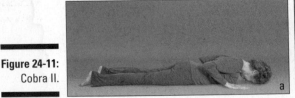 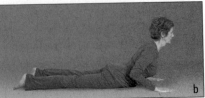

*Photograph by Adam Latham*

Move slowly and cautiously in all the cobralike postures. Avoid any of the postures that cause pain in your lower back, upper back, or neck. If cobra II is too strenuous, use cobra I, which appears in the following section, or repeat the lying arm raise, which we cover earlier in this chapter.

### Cobra I: Sphinx

*Note:* We recommend that you use either this posture or the cobra posture in the preceding section, not both. Cobra I is less strenuous than cobra II, so go with cobra I if you aren't sure.

If the cobra postures aggravate your lower back, separate your legs wider than your hips and turn your heels out with your toes inward. Also, if you move your hands farther forward, these postures are less difficult.

1. **Lie on your abdomen with your legs at hip width and the tops of the feet on the floor.**

2. **Rest your forehead on the floor and relax your shoulders.**

   Bend your elbows and place your forearms on the floor, with your palms turned down and positioned near the sides of your head.

3. **As you inhale, engage your back muscles, press your forearms against the floor, and raise your chest and head, as in Figure 24-12.**

   Look straight ahead, and keep your forearms and the front of your pelvis on the floor. Continue to relax your shoulders.

4. **As you exhale, lower your torso and head slowly back to the floor.**

5. **Repeat Steps 2 through 4 six to eight times.**

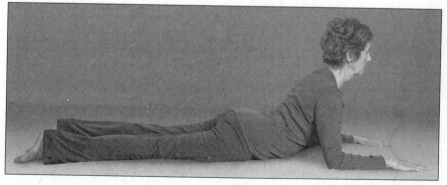

**Figure 24-12:**
Cobra I.

*Photograph by Adam Latham*

### Prone resting posture: Advasana variation

Resting at the right times is an important part of a Yoga sequence, and back bends may be the most strenuous part of your back routine. Remember, you don't ever want your Yoga routine to feel like you're in a hurry.

1. **Lie on your abdomen, with your legs at hip width and the tops of your feet on the floor.**

2. **Rest your forehead on the floor, or turn your head to one side and relax your shoulders.**

   Bend your elbows and place your forearms on the floor, with your palms turned down and positioned near the sides of your head, as in Figure 24-13. Stay for 6 to 8 breaths.

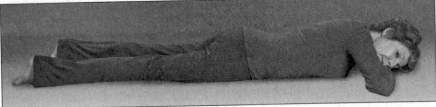

Figure 24-13:
Prone
resting
posture.

*Photograph by Adam Latham*

If this resting position is uncomfortable for you, use the bent knee corpse posture we describe earlier in the chapter.

### Locust I: Shalabhasana

The cobra postures in the preceding sections work primarily to stretch your back and restore its natural curves, but the locust posture works more on strengthening your back. Both postures are important to your back health.

1. **Lie on your abdomen, with your legs at hip width and the tops of your feet on the floor.**

   Rest your forehead on the floor.

2. **Extend your arms back along the sides of your torso, with your palms on the floor.**

3. **As you inhale, raise your chest, head, and right leg, as in Figure 24-14.**

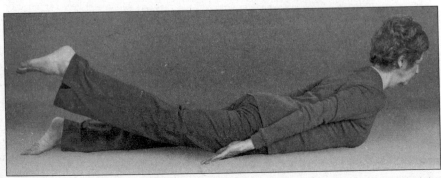

Figure 24-14:
The locust
posture
helps
strengthen
your back
and neck.

*Photograph by Adam Latham*

4. As you exhale, lower your torso and head slowly to the floor.

5. Repeat Steps 3 and 4 three times, and then stay in Step 3 (the last raised position) for 6 to 8 breaths.

6. Repeat Steps 1 through 5 with your left leg.

For a little extra challenge, and to open your shoulders and chest, try this pose with your palms facing down.

If this posture is too strenuous for you, try it without lifting your leg or by bending one leg at the knee, with both thighs still on the ground.

### Child's posture with arms back: Balasana variation II

Repeat the child's posture from earlier in the chapter, but keep your arms at your sides, pointing back to your feet (see Figure 24-15).

Close your eyes and breathe easily. Stay for 6 to 8 breaths.

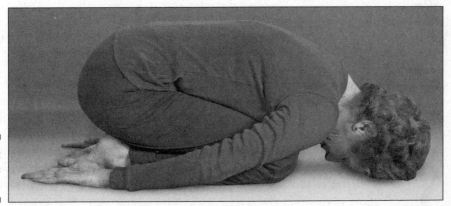

**Figure 24-15:**
Child's posture.

*Photograph by Adam Latham*

### The butterfly: Jathara parvritti variation I

Back pain sufferers often forget that the lower and upper back are very connected. Often an upper back twist like the butterfly has a safe ripple effect all the way down when a lower back twist isn't possible.

If you're having a disc-related problem, be very careful of twists for both the upper and lower back. If you have any negative symptoms, such as pain or numbness, leave out the twist and speak to your physician before adding it back into your program.

1. **Lie on your left side, with your knees bent and your arms extended parallel and not higher than your shoulders; join your palms together on the floor (see Figure 24-16a).**

   Place pillows or folded blankets under your head and between your knees for stability.

2. **As you inhale, raise your right hand up and over, turning your head to follow your hand until it touches the floor on the other side (see Figure 24-16b).**

   Don't force it! Move your hand and head only as far as you can comfortably go.

3. **As you exhale, return to the starting position in Step 1.**

4. **Repeat Steps 2 and 3 four to six times.**

5. **Repeat Steps 1 through 4 on the right side.**

Figure 24-16:
The
butterfly.

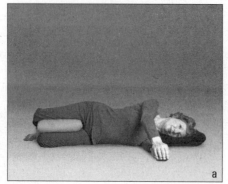 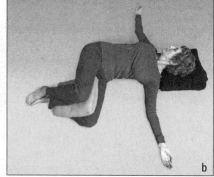

Photograph by Adam Latham

### Bent-leg supine twist variation: Jathara parvritti variation II

A good back routine often includes both an upper and a lower back twist. The bent-leg supine twist variation is appropriate here because it's easy to execute. We offer you a number of other effective twists in Chapter 12.

If you're having a disc-related problem, be careful of twists. If you have any negative symptoms, such as pain or numbness, leave out the twist and speak to your physician before adding it back to your program.

1. **Lie on your back, with your knees bent and feet on the floor at hip width; extend your arms out from your sides like a *T*, with your palms down and in line with the top of your shoulders.**

2. **As you exhale, cross your right leg over your left leg, slowly lower your bent legs to the left side, and then turn your head to the right, as in Figure 24-17.**

   Keep your head on the floor.

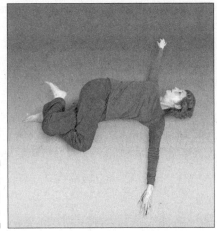

**Figure 24-17:**
Bent-leg
supine twist.

*Photograph by Adam Latham*

   3. **As you inhale, bring your bent knees back up to the middle; as you exhale, slowly lower them back down to the same side.**

   4. **Repeat Steps 1 through 3 three times, and then stay down on the left side for 4 to 6 breaths.**

   5. **Repeat Steps 1 through 4 with the left leg on top to the right side.**

If the cross-over twist variation is too difficult, try this same twist with your legs uncrossed and both feet on the ground.

### Knees-to-chest posture: Apanasana

One of the rules of sequencing (which we cover in Chapter 15) is to always follow a twist with some kind of forward bend. Knees-to-chest is a classic forward bend to use when the posture preceding it is a floor twist, as in this back routine.

   1. **Lie on your back and bend your knees in toward your chest.**

   2. **Hold your shins just below your knees (see Figure 24-18a).**

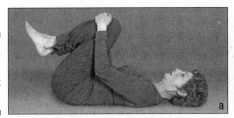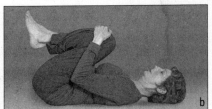

**Figure 24-18:**
Knees-
to-chest
posture.

*Photograph by Adam Latham*

3. **As you exhale, draw your knees inward, closer to your chest, as in Figure 24-18b.**

4. **Repeat Steps 2 and 3 three to four times, and then relax and breathe, holding your shins for 6 to 8 breaths.**

If you have any knee problems, hold the backs of your thighs instead.

### Corpse posture with bent legs, repeated

When you come to the end of our back routine, the corpse posture variation we discuss at the beginning of the routine gives you a stable position to focus on your breathing and deeply relax your back. You don't want to skip this part. Stay in this posture for 25 to 30 breaths, making your exhalation slightly longer than your inhalation.

Covering your eyes can give a deeper relaxation effect. Use an eye pillow or a scarf to cover your eyes to see whether you like it. (You can read more on eye pillows and other props in Chapter 20.) Placing your feet comfortably up on a chair or a bed also adds a calming effect and improves the circulation in your legs. It can even help improve your sleep.

# Chapter 25

# Using Restorative Postures to Relieve Stress and Chronic Pain

*P*ain serves a useful and critical purpose. Can you imagine lacking the ability to feel pain? The acute pain that comes from breaking a bone tells you to get to the emergency room ASAP, and an aching tooth propels you to the dentist's chair. Sometimes, however, pain persists or recurs and becomes an unwelcome part of daily life. This type of pain is referred to as chronic pain. Fortunately, relief is at hand: Yoga is just what the doctor ordered as part of the chronic pain relief toolkit.

But restorative Yoga isn't just for people in pain, although it's ideally suited for that purpose. Even people with intensely physical Yoga practices benefit from restorative Yoga. As the name suggests, it encourages a deep state of relaxation that's also suitable for releasing stress and unwinding at the end of a busy workweek.

In this chapter, we provide you with a number of postures that may look familiar, but in a specifically restorative form here. As restorative postures, they use props such as blankets, bolsters, blocks, and chairs to help you hold the poses longer and surrender into them rather than move through them.

## Your Yoga Toolkit for Relieving Chronic Pain

An estimated 50 million to 75 million Americans live with chronic pain. Most commonly reported issues are back pain, particularly in the lower back, and headaches. Joint pain stemming from arthritis, injury, and other traumas is also common.

Eastern wisdom teaches that pain is inevitable; suffering is optional. *Pain* is a physical sensation; *suffering* is how we choose to experience it. Westerners may be surprised at this distinction. In essence, what starts as a protective pain response to a real physical threat becomes entangled with our thoughts and emotions, and leads to suffering. Recognizing this interplay between the mind and body in how pain is experienced, Yoga approaches chronic pain relief with practices that address both the body and the mind:

✔ Physical postures, both active and restorative

✔ Breathing practices to elicit the relaxation response

✔ Meditation (see Chapter 23)

With chronic pain, the pain signals remain active in the nervous system long after the body has resolved the initial injury. The roots of present pain may lie in past trauma, stress, and illness.

Restorative Yoga can help get to the bottom of chronic pain, but you may need to try different techniques before you discover the right combination for you. When dealing with chronic pain, one size doesn't fit all, nor does the same technique necessarily suit you each day. Become familiar with a variety of techniques, and be willing to experiment to find the mixes that work for you.

## Relieving back and body pain with gentle movement

Back troubles plague most people at some point in their lives. Gentle movements coordinated with the breath stretch and strengthen muscles and also decrease stress. The stress relief component is critical. Remember, pain + stress = a heightened experience of pain.

The Five-Step Plan for a Healthy Back and the illustrated movements for a lower back routine in Chapter 24 provide sound guidelines and instructions for back care. You can find a safe routine for the upper back and neck in the online bonus content. If you're looking for relief from overall body pain, you can find a good beginner's routine in Chapter 14.

## Reducing the intensity and frequency of headaches

The good news is that about 95% of headaches are classified as primary headaches, meaning that they don't signify an underlying condition. Nonetheless, a headache can stop you cold until you can resolve the pain. Knowing what triggers your headaches can help you manage your life to avoid or minimize them. Stress often plays a key role.

What triggers your own headaches?

- ✔ Anxiety?
- ✔ Changes in the weather?
- ✔ Dehydration?
- ✔ Lack of sleep?
- ✔ Particular foods?
- ✔ Stress?

You may not be able to change the weather or reconfigure your life, but you can address your experience of stress. Breathing exercises that elongate the exhalation phase promote relaxation. You can experience an immediate stress reduction effect by simply inhaling slowly through the nostrils and then exhaling even more slowly through the nostrils. Chapters 4 and 5 lay out the basics of yogic breathing and present several breath-based relaxation techniques to choose from.

Vigorous routines with extreme postures that heat you up or make use of overheated rooms can trigger migraines in some people. If you suffer from headaches and are turning to Yoga for relief, seek out a class that's both gentle and breath based.

# Helpful Postures for Chronic Pain

The restorative postures that follow are a sampling of postures that are particularly helpful for various types of chronic pain. You can arrange the postures into a customized routine, use each one *a la carte* as needed, or incorporate them into your Yoga routine as additions or modifications.

Simple props can support your body and help you relax into restorative postures. Yoga studios often have bolsters handy, and the photographs in this chapter illustrate their use. However, if you don't have bolsters at home, folded blankets or pillows are just as good. Eye pillows are another handy prop when settling into a posture with closed eyes. Alternatively, a small towel can block out light and promote relaxation.

## For your aching lower back

All these postures help you release your lower-back tension, aided by support from either a prop or the floor. The magic is in the execution of these ancient postures to suit *your* body, as you simply breathe and allow yourself to surrender to the moment and release your stress.

### Knees-to-chest posture

The knees-to-chest posture in Figure 25-1 relieves tension in the lumbar spine and calms your nervous system.

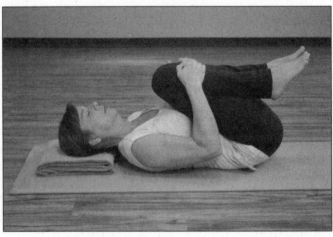

**Figure 25-1:**
The knees-to-chest posture is the go-to posture for the most common low back aches and pains.

© John Wiley & Sons, Inc.

1. **Lie on your back, and bend your knees in toward your chest.**

2. **Hold your shins just below your knees.**

3. **As you exhale, bring your knees toward your chest a comfortable distance.**

4. **Close your eyes, relax, and simply breathe through your nose; stay in the posture 1 to 3 minutes.**

   If you have any knee problems, hold the backs of your thighs instead. If your head tilts back, place a folded blanket or small pillow under your head.

5. **To come out of this posture (and any of the lying, or supine, postures), roll to one side like a log and push up from there; don't start the upward motion by lifting your neck forward.**

### Bent-leg feet-on-a-chair pose

In addition to addressing back pain, the bent-leg feet-on-a-chair pose relaxes the entire nervous system and improves circulation throughout your whole body. Check it out in Figure 25-2.

1. **Sit on the floor in a simple cross-legged position, facing a sturdy chair, and lean back on your forearms.**

2. **Slide your buttocks along the floor toward the chair until they're a comfortable distance from the front edge of the chair seat.**

3. **While exhaling, lift your feet off the floor and place your heels and calves on the chair seat.**

4. **Lie back on the floor, with your arms near your sides and your palms up.**

5. **Close your eyes, relax, and simply breathe through your nose; stay in the pose for 3 to 10 minutes.**

If your head tilts back, place a folded blanket or small pillow under your head.

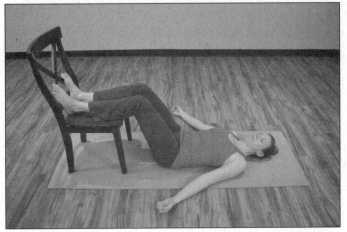

**Figure 25-2:** The bent-leg feet-on-a-chair pose is another classic therapeutic posture for the low back, for when you have more time.

© John Wiley & Sons, Inc.

## Supported corpse variation

In life, we all bend forward too much. This supported corpse variation, which Figure 25-3 illustrates, reverses that process and allows you to slowly and safely restore the natural curves in both the lower and upper back and the neck.

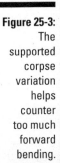

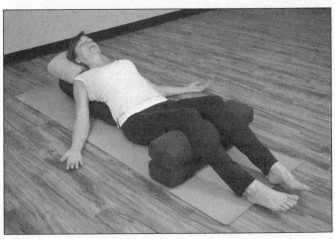

**Figure 25-3:** The supported corpse variation helps counter too much forward bending.

© John Wiley & Sons, Inc.

1. **Sit on the floor and place a bolster or two under your knees so that they're comfortably bent; your heels can lightly touch the floor or be suspended a few inches — it's all about how it feels in your lower back.**

   Refer to Chapter 20 for more on using props.

2. **Position another bolster vertically on the floor behind your hips, and place a rolled blanket on the bolster.**

3. **Lie back on top of the vertical bolster, and let your hips come down to the floor. Position the rolled blanket under your head, and move your arms out to a comfortable distance, with your palms up.**

4. **Close your eyes, relax, and simply breathe through your nose. Allow your chest to open and your neck to release; stay in the posture for 3 to 5 minutes.**

   If the vertical bolster creates an uncomfortable arch, replace it with two folded blankets.

Don't practice this pose if you experience pain in your lower or upper back, or if you've been diagnosed with disc disease.

### Supported cobra

If you feel pain when you round your back, the supported cobra, in Figure 25-4, can help you heal and take the pain away. It also helps restore the natural curve in your lower back, known as the lumbar curve.

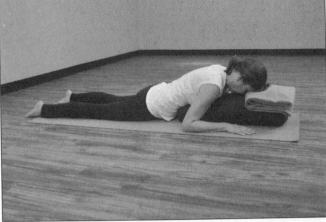

**Figure 25-4:** The supported cobra position helps if you feel pain on rounding.

© John Wiley & Sons, Inc.

1. **Place a bolster on the floor, and lie face down (prone) so that the bolster is positioned underneath you from the bottom of your chest to the top of your head.**

2. **Stretch your legs back, spread comfortably apart, with the tops of your feet on the floor.**

3. **Fold your arms comfortably underneath you, with your palms down, under the side of your head.**

4. **Relax, with your eyes closed; breathe through your nose and stay in the posture for 2 to 5 minutes.**

Don't practice this pose if you experience pain in your lower or upper back, or if you've been diagnosed with disc disease.

# For relief from headaches and from upper back and neck pain

Most headaches and upper back and neck pain result from muscle contraction or tension, often caused by extended periods of poor sitting or standing postures. These restorative postures, self-massage techniques, and supported inversions reduce tension and realign the natural curves of the spine in a safe, supportive manner.

## Supported crossed-legs forward bend

Use the supported crossed-legs forward bend (see Figure 25-5) as soon as you feel a headache coming on, either at home or at work. It has the added bonus of relieving tension in the lower abdomen and relaxing the digestive system.

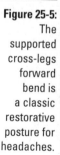

**Figure 25-5:** The supported cross-legs forward bend is a classic restorative posture for headaches.

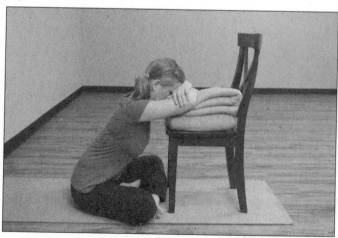

© John Wiley & Sons, Inc.

1. **Place two folded blankets on top of a sturdy chair, and then sit on the floor in front of it.**

2. **Cross your legs and scoot up to the chair as close as possible.**

3. **Cross your arms and hold them just above your opposite elbows.**

4. **Bend forward and place your arms on top of the blanket; place your head on top of your arms.**

5. **Close your eyes and breathe through your nose with long, smooth breaths; stay in the posture for 3 to 5 minutes.**

Placing two folded blankets under your hips can help you hold the posture longer.

### Self-massage

Not only does self-massage relieve tension in your neck, shoulders, and upper back, but it also helps prevent and reduce tension headaches by using the Yoga techniques of light touch (effleurage) and compression (ischemia). You can see this pose in Figure 25-6.

1. **Sit comfortably in a chair, with your back nice and tall and your feet either on the ground or supported by blankets.**

2. **Bring your left hand to the top of your right shoulder, and move your right hand in a slow, circular, massaging motion between your shoulder and your neck ten times.**

3. **As you massage yourself, be aware of any tight spots. When you find one, squeeze it firmly with your left hand and hold for 8 to 10 seconds.**

4. **When you release, repeat step 2.**

5. **Repeat with the left hand on your right side.**

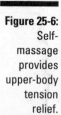

**Figure 25-6:**
Self-
massage
provides
upper-body
tension
relief.

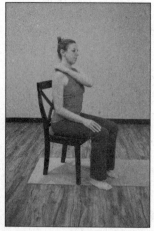

© John Wiley & Sons, Inc.

If it feels comfortable to do so, tilt your head sideways away from the massage while practicing on each side.

### Supported seated camel pose

If you sit too long at the computer or during a lecture, the supported seated camel pose (see Figure 25-7) can bring relief to your upper back and neck. It also restores the curve in your lower back (lumbar curve).

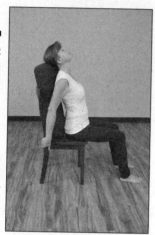

**Figure 25-7:** The supported seated camel pose brings relief from sitting too long when standing isn't appropriate.

© John Wiley & Sons, Inc.

1. **Find a sturdy chair, and place a bolster or firm pillows vertically at the back of the chair (see Chapter 20 for more on using props in your Yoga routine).**

2. **Sit on the front half of the chair, and reach back with your arms and hold the back of the chair at the level of the seat.**

3. **Lift your chest, squeeze your shoulder blades, and, if it feels comfortable, tilt your head back.**

4. **Breathe through your nose, with your eyes closed; stay for 1 to 3 minutes.**

### Supported fetal pose

The supported fetal pose, in Figure 25-8, is great for relieving pain in the upper and lower back, calming the nervous system, and relaxing the neck.

1. **Lie on your left side, with a folded blanket or a pillow between your knees and under the side of your head.**

2. **Add a bolster on its side, close to your chest and chin.**

   See Chapter 20 for more on using props in your Yoga routine.

3. **Snuggle up with the bolster, and place your hands and arms in a comfortable position on the top of the bolster.**

4. **Relax, close your eyes, and make your exhalation slightly longer than your inhalation; stay for 3 to 10 minutes.**

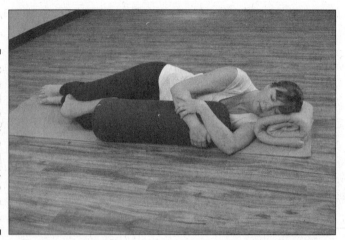

**Figure 25-8:**
The supported fetal pose relieves pain in the upper and lower back and also relaxes the neck.

© John Wiley & Sons, Inc.

### Supported reclined twist

The supported reclined twist, in Figure 25-9, works as an all-purpose pose. It promotes circulation to the lower and upper back, improves respiratory function, stimulates the kidneys, and creates an overall sense of well-being.

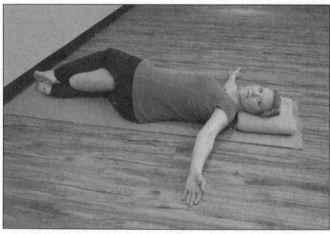

**Figure 25-9:**
The supported reclined twist creates an overall sense of well-being.

© John Wiley & Sons, Inc.

1. **Lie on your right side, with a folded blanket or a pillow between your knees and under the side of your head.**

2. **Open your left (top) arm up and over toward the floor on the left side, not higher than your shoulder; turn your head to the left well.**

3. **Repeat this movement three times, opening as you inhale and folding as you exhale; then stay in the open position and try to rest your left arm on the floor.**

Place as many folded blankets as you need under your left arm to rest comfortably.

**4. Stay in this position for 1 to 3 minutes; breathe slowly through your nose, and then reverse the process on the left side.**

### Supported half shoulder stand

The supported half shoulder stand, in Figure 25-10, calms the nervous system and relieves insomnia. It's also good for swollen legs and varicose veins.

**1. Sit sideways 6 to 8 inches away from a wall; have a bolster or a yoga block nearby.**

See Chapter 20 for more on using props in your Yoga routine.

**2. Swing your legs up onto the wall; lift your hips and place the bolster or block under the tops of your hips (your sacrum).**

**3. Rest your arms comfortably at your sides, with your palms up.**

**4. Breathe slowly through your nose; stay for 3 to 10 minutes.**

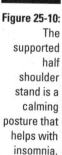

**Figure 25-10:**
The supported half shoulder stand is a calming posture that helps with insomnia.

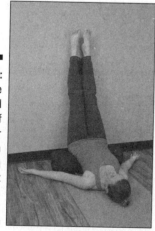

© John Wiley & Sons, Inc.

# For when it hurts all over: Joint and overall body pain

Some of the most common conditions in this category are fibromyalgia, chronic pain, and chronic fatigue. The American Medical Association tells us that stress plays a major role in these ailments. This group of restorative postures is especially good for stress reduction.

### *Supported corpse pose*

The supported corpse pose, in Figure 25-11, is the great relaxer. It also opens the upper back and chest, improves respiration, and reduces fatigue.

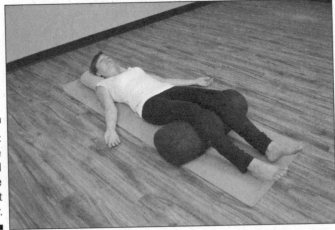

**Figure 25-11:**
The supported corpse pose is the great relaxer.

© John Wiley & Sons, Inc.

1. **Sit next to a bolster and a folded blanket.**

2. **Lie back, with the bolster under your knees and the blanket under your head.**

3. **Rest your arms comfortably at your sides, with your palms up.**

4. **Close your eyes and breath slowly through your nose; stay for 5 to 10 minutes.**

Don't practice this pose if you are more than 3 months pregnant.

### *Supported reclined bound angle posture*

The supported reclined bound angle posture, in Figure 25-12, is good for many ailments, including high blood pressure, insomnia, and digestive problems, because it reduces fatigue and has a positive effect on the liver and the stomach. It's also good for women during their menstrual cycle and during menopause.

1. **Place bolsters or a rolled blanket near both legs, place a bolster behind you vertically near your hips, and place a folded blanket on the vertical bolster; then sit comfortably.**

2. **Bend your legs and join the soles of your feet together; move the bolsters or rolled blankets to comfortable positions under the sides of your bent legs.**

3. **Lie back on the vertical bolster supporting and opening your upper back, and gently place the back of your head on the folded blanket.**

4. **Let your arms rest comfortably at your sides, palms up.**

5. **Close your eyes and breathe slowly and comfortably through your nose; stay for 3 to 5 minutes.**

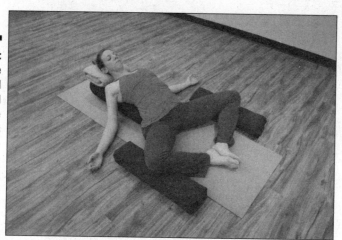

**Figure 25-12:**
The supported reclined bound angle posture is a multipurpose posture that's especially good for women.

© John Wiley & Sons, Inc.

Don't practice this posture if you experience pain in your lower back or if you're more than 3 months pregnant.

### Supported child's pose

The supported child's pose, in Figure 25-13, gently stretches the lower back, relieves tension in the upper back and neck, and calms the nervous system.

1. **Place a bolster vertically on your Yoga mat, with a folded blanket at the top.**

2. **Kneel at the back of the bolster.**

3. **Separate your bent knees slightly and scoot up until you can sit back, bend forward, and lie comfortably with your head and chest on the bolster in front of you.**

   Make sure everything is the right height for you to relax, and release your arms downward.

4. **Close your eyes and breathe slowly through your nose; stay for 3 to 5 minutes.**

Don't use this posture if it causes pain in your lower back, knees, or hips.

### Supported full bridge pose

The supported full bridge pose, in Figure 25-14, stretches the muscles of the neck and upper back and can be good for headaches. It also opens the chest and enhances breathing.

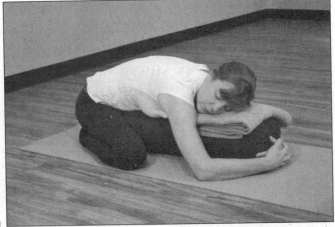

**Figure 25-13:** The supported child's pose is a popular posture for its tension relief and calming ability.

© John Wiley & Sons, Inc.

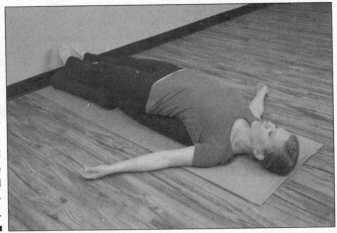

**Figure 25-14:** The stretch of the neck and upper back in the supported full bridge pose is good for headache relief.

© John Wiley & Sons, Inc.

1. **Place bolsters end to end vertically, 1 to 2 feet high and 5 to 6 feet long.**

2. **Sit on the middle of the stack, and lie back so that your shoulders and head are resting comfortably on the floor or a small folded blanket.**

3. **Close your eyes and breathe through your nose; stay for 3 to 5 minutes.**

Don't practice this posture if you experience pain in your lower back or if you're more than 3 months pregnant.

# Part V
# The Part of Tens

You can bring your yogic consciousness to the food you eat, for the betterment of your health and the well-being of the planet and our global neighbors. For a list of tips on eating like a yogi, check out www.dummies.com/extras/yoga.

# In this part . . .

✔ Understand the basic principles of safe Yoga practice

✔ Adopt both the mindset and the practical steps to ensure a great Yoga experience

# Chapter 26

# Ten Tips for a Safe Yoga Practice

### In This Chapter

▶ Focusing on being in the moment
▶ Listening to your body
▶ Modifying and adapting to make the posture fit you

*Y*oga offers a complete body and mind workout, with a complement of benefits you rarely find elsewhere. Yet as Yoga has become more popular, Yoga-related injuries have also become more common. With the proper intention and attitude, you can keep your Yoga practice safe and injury free.

Not everyone knows that some popular styles of Yoga originated from the training routines of athletic youths who preformed acrobatic Yoga shows around India. No wonder some forms of Yoga practice aren't suitable for everyone! Fortunately, the true benefits from Yoga derive from the practice itself — the process of being in the moment, not the outward expression of the posture.

The following tips help keep your Yoga practice safe for the duration of your routine.

## Avoid Seeing Yoga as a Competition — Even with Yourself

Yoga was never meant to be a competitive sport. Going beyond your limits makes you a prime candidate for an injury. Furthermore, one of the benefits of Yoga practice is the inward focus and sense of peace it brings; competition is a perfect antidote for inner peace. If you find yourself comparing yourself to the people around you during a Yoga class, bring your attention back to your own body and mind. You can generally always find someone who's more advanced than you and someone who's lagging behind. And the truth is, it doesn't matter how "good" or "bad" you are. Was your stretch deeper yesterday than today? Did you not hold poses today as long as you wanted to? It doesn't matter. Let it go.

## Listen to Your Body and Be in the Moment

Yoga is about the moment. It's a meditation in motion. Listen to what your body and breath are telling you, and learn to adjust your practice accordingly. Is your breath choppy? If so, scale back your physical practice until your breath becomes even again. Has the stretch crossed the line from being a sweet and focused exertion to pain? Then scale it back. You're not racing toward a finish line — and there's no prize for whoever has the most body aches afterward.

## Challenge Yourself, Don't Strain Yourself

Whichever style of Yoga you choose, remember that Yoga is a "work-in," not just a workout. While the more athletic forms of Yoga can be physically challenging as well as meditative, you need to find the line for *you* between challenge and strain — and then don't cross it. When you strain yourself in a pose, you're more apt to suffer an injury. Working at your edge can be quite enjoyable and rewarding, but stay within sensible limits. Honor the reality that what makes sense for you and your body can — and will — vary with the time of day and from day to day.

## Forget about What You Used to Do

Our bodies and physical abilities change over time. Generally, most people who are in their 40s, 50s, and older credit time with having had greater physical prowess. But time doesn't have to limit your practice and experience of Yoga. As we age and mature, we find wisdom in our lives and greater depth in our Yoga practice. In general, older practitioners tend to enjoy and benefit from practices with slower gentler movements and a greater emphasis on breath.

# Don't Buy into "No Pain, No Gain"

That feeling of physical exertion at just the right level, where you find the sweet spot of alertness and comfort, can be exquisite. So go ahead and find your edge, and feel the joy of your body at work. But if you reach the point of a wince, or if your breath becomes rapid, it's your direct message that you need to scale back a notch or two.

# Choose Function over Form

How your posture looks in a posture isn't important. Instead, you need to focus on how the posture benefits your body and mind. Try not to muscle yourself into the postures; relax into them. Don't twist yourself into a posture your body is unhappy with — it's a recipe for injury. Simple adaptations, such as bending your knees or elbows, enable you to reap the benefits of many postures without crossing the line into unsafe practice. When you focus on the function of a posture — for example, developing a more flexible spine or a stronger core to avoid an aching back — you can see that you don't need to achieve a perfect outward form to enjoy the benefits.

# Find the Intersection of Focus and Ease in Your Postures

The basic requirement for any Yoga posture is alertness or focus, and comfort or ease. If you keep this in mind, you can avoid injury. What's "ease-full" for you may be very different from what's "ease-full" for an adept practitioner. Knowing this, you can expect your postures to look different from the postures of someone with a long and advanced Yoga practice.

# Seek Out a Yoga Teacher Who Respects Your Limits

Learn to recognize the difference between a teacher who encourages you to give it your best and one who tries to push you beyond your healthful limits. If your instructor is of the second variety, exercise your right to decide what you will and won't do with your body in that class — and choose a different teacher next time.

Sometimes your own inner voice is the one pushing you beyond your limits. In those cases, refer back to this chapter's first tip: Yoga isn't a competition, even with yourself.

## Find Your Personal Comfort Zone

Your Yoga practice isn't a one-way street. Imagine that the teacher gives an instruction to take the pose to the next challenging level — you want to do it, you think you can do it, and you try to do it, but you find that it's too much for you. Well, you *can* change your mind. Work at the level that suits you best at that time, and give yourself a pat on the back for having been curious to explore just where that level is.

## Give Yourself the Benefit of Time and Allow Yoga to Unfold

Nowhere is it written that you must master certain Yoga postures to have a thriving and beneficial Yoga practice. If you hold on to an image of what a Yoga posture or practice should look like and push through regardless of warning signs that your breath and body are giving you, you're bound to hurt yourself.

We reap what we sow, and if you approach your practice with dedication and focus, as well as some loving-kindness for yourself, you can experience the benefits Yoga offers, regardless of which postures work for your body or how your posture looks when compared to the beautiful models on the covers of the popular Yoga magazines.

# Chapter 27

# Ten Ways to Get the Most out of Your Yoga Practice

*I*n this chapter, we give you ten tips for growing your Yoga practice into a sturdy, fruit-laden tree.

## Understand Yoga

Even if you seek only physical benefits from Yoga, try to take time to learn about its rich philosophical and spiritual foundations. Not only can it improve how you approach your Yoga practice, but it also can add insight to your life.

## Set Clear and Realistic Goals

Consider your personal situation carefully and then set your Yoga goals based on your abilities and needs. When you're realistic, you're less likely to experience disappointment or guilt when your schedule seems overwhelming, and you're better able to get back onto the mat when that happens.

## Commit Yourself to Growth

Allow your Yoga practice to transform not only your body, but also your mind. Don't put a ceiling on your own development or assume that you're incapable of ever achieving a certain Yoga posture or learning how to meditate. Let Yoga meet you where you are and gently expand you physically and mentally.

## Stay for the Long Haul

To derive the full benefits from Yoga, you have to apply yourself diligently, which also nicely strengthens your character. The longer you practice Yoga, the more enjoyable and beneficial it becomes.

## Start with Good Habits

Cultivate good Yoga habits from the outset. Seek out a qualified Yoga teacher, either in a group class or privately. Use this book as a guide to help you gain insight into what you're doing as you follow the step-by-step instructions.

## Vary Your Routine

You have hundreds of Yoga postures and variations to choose from. When you learn a core set of postures, you can create a different practice each day.

## Breathe to Increase Your Awareness

Conscious breathing during Yoga exercises *on* the mat greatly enhances the effects of your practice on your body and mind, equipping you with the vitality you need to meet the challenges of a busy life *off* the mat.

## Do Your Best, Don't Worry about the Rest

Be diligent but relaxed about your Yoga practice. Focus on practicing now, and leave the rest to the power of Yoga, providence, and your good karma.

## Allow Your Body to Speak Up

Your body is your best friend and counselor. If something doesn't feel right, it probably isn't. Trust your bodily instincts.

## Share Yoga

Plan to practice Yoga with others until you find your own momentum. Everyone needs a little encouragement from time to time.

# Index

# About the Authors

**Larry Payne, PhD,** is an internationally prominent Yoga teacher, author, workshop leader, and pioneer in the field of Yoga therapy since 1980. He discovered Yoga when he was challenged by his own serious back problems and injuries from numerous competitive sports he played in his youth.

Larry is the founding president of the International Association of Yoga Therapists and cofounder of the Yoga curriculum at the UCLA School of Medicine. He was the first Yoga teacher at the World Economic forum, was named "One of America's most respected Yoga teachers" by the *Los Angeles Times,* and was selected as a leading Yoga expert by Dr. Mehmet Oz, *Reader's Digest*, Web-MD, Rodale Press, and the *Yoga Journal.*

In Los Angeles, Larry is the founding director of the Yoga Therapy Rx and Prime of Life Yoga certification programs at Loyola Marymount University. He also has a thriving private practice in Yoga therapy as a back specialist. Larry is the coauthor of five books and is featured in the DVD series *Yoga Therapy Rx* and *Prime of Life Yoga.* His website is www.samata.com.

**Georg Feuerstein, PhD (1947–2012),** studied and practiced Yoga since his early teens and was a practitioner of Buddhist Yoga. Internationally respected for his contribution to Yoga research and the history of consciousness, he has been featured in many national magazines both in the United States and abroad. He has authored more than 40 books, including *The Yoga Tradition, The Shambhala Encyclopedia of Yoga*, and *Yoga Morality*, which have been translated into eight languages. Since his retirement in 2004, he has designed and tutored several distance-learning courses on Yoga philosophy for Traditional Yoga Studies, a Canadian company founded and directed by his wife, Brenda (see www.traditionalyogastudies.com).

# Dedication

**From Larry:** My contribution to this book is dedicated to the love of my life, Merry Aronson, and my beloved family, Dolly, Harry in heaven, Chris, Harold, Susan, Lisa, Natale, Maria, Sasi, and Alex, as well as to my students, who have been my greatest teachers.

# Acknowledgments

**From Larry:** Unless you are truly gifted like my coauthor, Georg, who, sadly, passed away in 2012, writing a book takes a village, and I have many people to thank in mine. Merry of MerryMedia first encouraged me to do this third revision. Sri T.K.V. Desikachar and his family have inspired my Yoga path since 1980. My editor, Deborah Myers, was simply grand. My council of advisers is always there for me: Professor Zhuo-Yi Qiu, OMD; David Allen, MD; Richard Usatine, MD; Rick Morris, DC; Richard Miller, PhD; Art Brownstein, MD; Christopher Chapple, PhD; Mike Sinel, MD; Fancy Fechser; Professor Sasi Velupillai; Sir Sidney Djanogly; Steve Ostrow, JD; Steve Paredes, DC; and my personal assistants, Darshana Thacker and Evelyn Floyd.

I would also like to thank Brenda Feuerstein, Georg's widow, who supported this project and continues his work at Traditional Yoga Studies, which they cofounded.

Tracy Boggier at Wiley initiated this revision project, and her patience and persistence made it happen. Thanks also go to our editorial team at Wiley, led by Alissa Schwipps, who is talented and compassionate.

I am very grateful to our photographer, Adam Latham, and our photo and video models, starring Jeffrey Aronson, Michael Aronson, Deborah Barry, Holly Beaty, Paul Blodgett, Anna Brown, Jamie Corydon, Lisa Daugherty, Chauncey Dennis, Lili Foster, Mia Foster, Terra Gold, Eden Goldman, Gilliam Hadlock, Anna Inferrera, Marvin Jordana, Chris Joseph, the Ketterhagen family (Kourtney, Luke, Mangala, and Prakash), Dolly Payne, Tony Ransdell, Heidi Rayden, Elizabeth Rea, Vivian Richman, and Connie Tellman.

---

## Publisher's Acknowledgments

**Senior Acquisitions Editor:** Tracy Boggier

**Senior Project Editor:** Alissa Schwipps

**Copy Editor:** Krista Hansing

**Technical Editor:** Lisa Daugherty

**Art Coordinator:** Alicia B. South

*Special Help*

Paige Newman, Paige Sandgren

**Project Coordinator:** Erin Zeltner

**Video Producer:** Paul Chen

**Photographer:** Adam Latham

**Cover Image:** ©iStockphoto.com/ Neustockimages